Pituitary Disorders

Editor

NIKI KARAVITAKI

ENDOCRINOLOGY AND METABOLISM CLINICS OF NORTH AMERICA

www.endo.theclinics.com

Consulting Editor
ADRIANA G. IOACHIMESCU

September 2020 • Volume 49 • Number 3

ELSEVIER

1600 John F. Kennedy Boulevard • Suite 1800 • Philadelphia, Pennsylvania, 19103-2899

http://www.theclinics.com

ENDOCRINOLOGY AND METABOLISM CLINICS OF NORTH AMERICA Volume 49, Number 3
September 2020 ISSN 0889-8529, ISBN 13: 978-0-323-75502-3

Editor: Katerina Heidhausen
Developmental Editor: Nicole Congleton

Endocrinology and Metabolism Clinics of North America (ISSN 0889-8529) is published quarterly by Elsevier Inc., 360 Park Avenue South, New York, NY 10010-1710. Months of issue are March, June, September, and December. Periodicals postage paid at New York, NY and additional mailing offices. Subscription prices are USD 375.00 per year for US individuals, USD 799.00 per year for US institutions, USD 100.00 per year for US students and residents, USD 454.00 per year for Canadian individuals, USD 988.00 per year for Canadian institutions, USD 497.00 per year for international individuals, USD 988.00 per year for international institutions, USD 100.00 per year for Canadian students/residents, and USD 245.00 per year for international students/residents. To receive student/resident rate, orders must be accompanied by name of affiliated institution, date of term, and the signature of program/residency coordinator on institution letterhead. Orders will be billed at individual rate until proof of status is received. Foreign air speed delivery is included in all *Clinics* subscription prices. All prices are subject to change without notice. **POSTMASTER:** Send address changes to *Endocrinology and Metabolism Clinics of North America*, Elsevier Health Sciences Division, Subscription Customer Service, 3251 Riverport Lane, Maryland Heights, MO 63043. **Customer Service: Telephone: 1-800-654-2452** (U.S. and Canada); **1-314-447-8871** (outside U.S. and Canada). **Fax: 1-314-447-8029. E-mail: journalscustomerservice-usa@ elsevier.com (for print support); journalsonlinesupport-usa@elsevier.com (for online support)**.

Reprints. For copies of 100 or more, of articles in this publication, please contact the Commercial Rights Department, Elsevier Inc., 360 Park Avenue South, New York, NY 10010-1710; phone: +1-212-633-3874; fax: +1-212-633-3820; E-mail: reprints@elsevier.com.

Endocrinology and Metabolism Clinics of North America is covered in *MEDLINE/PubMed (Index Medicus)*, *EMBASE/Excerpta Medica, Current Contents/Clinical Medicine, Current Contents/Life Sciences, Science Citation Index, ISI/BIOMED, BIOSIS*, and *Chemical Abstracts*.

Contributors

CONSULTING EDITOR

ADRIANA G. IOACHIMESCU, MD, PhD, FACE
Professor, Departments of Medicine: Endocrinology and Metabolism, and Neurosurgery, Emory University, Emory University School of Medicine, Atlanta, Georgia, USA

EDITOR

NIKI KARAVITAKI, MD, MSc, PhD, FRCP
Senior Clinical Lecturer in Endocrinology, Honorary Consultant Endocrinologist, Institute of Metabolism and Systems Research, College of Medical and Dental Sciences, University of Birmingham, Centre for Endocrinology, Diabetes and Metabolism, Birmingham Health Partners, Department of Endocrinology, Queen Elizabeth Hospital, University Hospitals Birmingham NHS Foundation Trust, Birmingham, United Kingdom

AUTHORS

XIMENE ANTUNES, MD, MSc
Endocrinology Division, Neuroendocrinology Research Center, Medical School and Hospital Universitário Clementino Fraga Filho – Universidade Federal do Rio de Janeiro, Rio de Janeiro, Brazil

SAYKA BARRY, PhD
Centre for Endocrinology, William Harvey Research Institute, Barts and The London School of Medicine, Queen Mary University of London, London, United Kingdom

WAIEL A. BASHARI, MSc, MRCP(UK)
Clinical Research Fellow, Cambridge Endocrine Molecular Imaging Group, Metabolic Research Laboratories, Wellcome Trust-MRC Institute of Metabolic Science, University of Cambridge, National Institute for Health Research, Cambridge Biomedical Research Centre, Addenbrooke's Hospital, Cambridge, United Kingdom

ALBERT BECKERS, MD, PhD
Department of Endocrinology, Centre Hospitalier Universitaire de Liège, Liège Université, Domaine Universitaire Sart-Tilman, Liège, Belgium

NIENKE R. BIERMASZ, MD, PhD
Endocrinologist, Department of Endocrinology, Leiden University Medical Center, Center for Endocrine Tumors Leiden, Leiden, the Netherlands

BEVERLY M.K. BILLER, MD
Neuroendocrine Unit, Neuroendocrine and Pituitary Tumor Clinical Center, Massachusetts General Hospital, Harvard Medical School, Boston, Massachusetts, USA

FELIPE F. CASANUEVA, MD, PhD
Professor, Division of Endocrinology, Complejo Hospitalario Universitario de Santiago (USC/SERGAS), Instituto de Investigacion Sanitaria de Santiago (IDIS), Santiago de

Compostela, A Coruña, Spain; CIBER Fisiopatología de la Obesidad y la Nutrición (CIBERobn), Instituto de Salud Carlos III, Madrid, Spain

MIRJAM CHRIST-CRAIN, MD, PhD
Division of Endocrinology, Diabetes and Metabolism, Departments of Clinical Research, and Endocrinology, University Hospital Basel, University of Basel, Basel, Switzerland

ADRIAN F. DALY, MB, BCh, PhD
Department of Endocrinology, Centre Hospitalier Universitaire de Liège, Liège Université, Domaine Universitaire Sart-Tilman, Liège, Belgium

FRISO DE VRIES, MD
Department of Endocrinology, Leiden University Medical Center, Center for Endocrine Tumors Leiden, Leiden, the Netherlands

STUTI FERNANDES, MD
Fellow, Department of Medicine (Endocrinology, Diabetes and Metabolism), Oregon Health & Science University, Portland, Oregon, USA

MARIA FLESERIU, MD
Professor, Departments of Medicine (Endocrinology, Diabetes and Metabolism) and Neurological Surgery, Pituitary Center, Oregon Health & Science University, Portland, Oregon, USA

ANA M. FORMENTI, MD
Institute of Endocrinology, Università Vita-Salute San Raffaele, Milano, Milan, Italy

ATHANASIOS FOUNTAS, MD, MSc
Clinical Research Fellow, Institute of Metabolism and Systems Research, College of Medical and Dental Sciences, University of Birmingham, Centre for Endocrinology, Diabetes and Metabolism, Birmingham Health Partners, Department of Endocrinology, Queen Elizabeth Hospital, University Hospitals Birmingham NHS Foundation Trust, Birmingham, United Kingdom

STEFANO FRARA, MD
Institute of Endocrinology, Università Vita-Salute San Raffaele, Milano, Milan, Italy

MÔNICA R. GADELHA, MD, PhD
Endocrinology Division, Neuroendocrinology Research Center, Medical School and Hospital Universitário Clementino Fraga Filho – Universidade Federal do Rio de Janeiro, Neuroendocrinology Division, Instituto Estadual do Cérebro Paulo Niemeyer, Neuropatology and Molecular Genetics Laboratory, Instituto Estadual do Cérebro Paulo Niemeyer, Rio de Janeiro, Brazil

DANIEL GILLETT, MSc
Senior Clinical Scientist, Cambridge Endocrine Molecular Imaging Group, Metabolic Research Laboratories, Wellcome Trust-MRC Institute of Metabolic Science, University of Cambridge, National Institute for Health Research, Cambridge Biomedical Research Centre, Addenbrooke's Hospital, Department of Nuclear Medicine, Addenbrooke's Hospital, Cambridge, United Kingdom

ERICA A. GIRALDI, MD
Endocrinology Fellow-in-Training, Department of Medicine: Endocrinology and Metabolism, Emory University, Atlanta, Georgia, USA

ANDREA GIUSTINA, MD
Professor, Institute of Endocrinology, Università Vita-Salute San Raffaele, Milano, Milan, Italy

MARK GURNELL, PhD, FRCP
Professor of Clinical Endocrinology, Cambridge Endocrine Molecular Imaging Group, Metabolic Research Laboratories, Wellcome Trust-MRC Institute of Metabolic Science, University of Cambridge, National Institute for Health Research, Cambridge Biomedical Research Centre, Addenbrooke's Hospital, Cambridge, United Kingdom

MIRELA DIANA ILIE, MD, MSc
Endocrinologist-in-Training, Endocrinology Department VI, "C.I.Parhon" National Institute of Endocrinology, Bucharest, Romania

ADRIANA G. IOACHIMESCU, MD, PhD, FACE
Professor, Departments of Medicine: Endocrinology and Metabolism, and Neurosurgery, Emory University, Emory University School of Medicine, Atlanta, Georgia, USA

EMMANUEL JOUANNEAU, MD, PhD
Professor, Neurosurgery Department, Reference Center for Rare Pituitary Diseases HYPO, "Groupement Hospitalier Est" Hospices Civils de Lyon, "Claude Bernard" Lyon 1 University, Hôpital Pierre Wertheimer, Lyon, Bron, France

NIKI KARAVITAKI, MD, MSc, PhD, FRCP
Senior Clinical Lecturer in Endocrinology, Honorary Consultant Endocrinologist, Institute of Metabolism and Systems Research, College of Medical and Dental Sciences, University of Birmingham, Centre for Endocrinology, Diabetes and Metabolism, Birmingham Health Partners, Department of Endocrinology, Queen Elizabeth Hospital, University Hospitals Birmingham NHS Foundation Trust, Birmingham, United Kingdom

LEANDRO KASUKI, MD, PhD
Endocrinology Division, Neuroendocrinology Research Center, Medical School and Hospital Universitário Clementino Fraga Filho – Universidade Federal do Rio de Janeiro, Neuroendocrinology Division, Instituto Estadual do Cérebro Paulo Niemeyer, Endocrinology Division, Hospital Federal de Bonsucesso, Rio de Janeiro, Brazil

MAARTEN C. KLEIJWEGT, MD
ENT Surgeon, Department of Ear Nose and Throat – Head and Neck Cancer, Leiden University Medical Center, Leiden, the Netherlands

ANGELOS KOLIAS, PhD, FRCS
Division of Neurosurgery, Department of Clinical Neurosciences, University of Cambridge, Addenbrooke's Hospital, Cambridge, United Kingdom

MÁRTA KORBONITS, MD, PhD
Centre for Endocrinology, William Harvey Research Institute, Barts and The London School of Medicine, Queen Mary University of London, London, United Kingdom

OLYMPIA KOULOURI, PhD, MRCP(UK)
Academic Clinical Lecturer, Cambridge Endocrine Molecular Imaging Group, Metabolic Research Laboratories, Wellcome Trust-MRC Institute of Metabolic Science, University of Cambridge, National Institute for Health Research, Cambridge Biomedical Research Centre, Addenbrooke's Hospital, Cambridge, United Kingdom

ELISA BARANSKI LAMBACK, MD
Endocrinology Division, Neuroendocrinology Research Center, Medical School and Hospital Universitário Clementino Fraga Filho – Universidade Federal do Rio de Janeiro, Rio de Janeiro, Brazil

DANIEL J. LOBATTO, MD
Department of Neurosurgery, Leiden University Medical Center, Center for Endocrine Tumors Leiden, Leiden, the Netherlands

M. BEATRIZ S. LOPES, MD, PhD
Professor of Pathology and Neurological Surgery, Department of Pathology, University of Virginia School of Medicine, Charlottesville, Virginia, USA

HERMANN L. MÜLLER, MD
Department of Pediatrics and Pediatric Hematology/Oncology, University Children's Hospital, Klinikum Oldenburg AöR, Oldenburg, Germany

JAMES MACFARLANE, MRCP(UK)
Academic Clinical Fellow, Cambridge Endocrine Molecular Imaging Group, Metabolic Research Laboratories, Wellcome Trust-MRC Institute of Metabolic Science, University of Cambridge, National Institute for Health Research, Cambridge Biomedical Research Centre, Addenbrooke's Hospital, Cambridge, United Kingdom

MIGUEL A. MARTINEZ-OLMOS, MD
Division of Endocrinology, Complejo Hospitalario Universitario de Santiago (USC/SERGAS), Instituto de Investigacion Sanitaria de Santiago (IDIS), Santiago de Compostela, A Coruña, Spain; CIBER Fisiopatología de la Obesidad y la Nutrición (CIBERobn), Instituto de Salud Carlos III, Madrid, Spain

SHIRLEY McCARTNEY, PhD
Associate Professor, Department of Neurological Surgery, Oregon Health & Science University, Portland, Oregon, USA

ALBERTO M. PEREIRA, MD, PhD
Endocrinologist, Department of Endocrinology, Leiden University Medical Center, Center for Endocrine Tumors Leiden, Leiden, the Netherlands

ANDREW S. POWLSON, MRCP(UK)
Consultant Endocrinologist, Cambridge Endocrine Molecular Imaging Group, Metabolic Research Laboratories, Wellcome Trust-MRC Institute of Metabolic Science, University of Cambridge, National Institute for Health Research, Cambridge Biomedical Research Centre, Addenbrooke's Hospital, Cambridge, United Kingdom

GÉRALD RAVEROT, MD, PhD
Professor, Endocrinology Department, Reference Center for Rare Pituitary Diseases HYPO, "Groupement Hospitalier Est" Hospices Civils de Lyon, "Claude Bernard" Lyon 1 University, Hôpital Louis Pradel, Lyon, Bron, France

JULIE REFARDT, MD
Division of Endocrinology, Diabetes and Metabolism, Departments of Clinical Research, and Endocrinology, University Hospital Basel, University of Basel, Basel, Switzerland

GEMMA RODRIGUEZ-CARNERO, MD
Division of Endocrinology, Complejo Hospitalario Universitario de Santiago (USC/SERGAS), Instituto de Investigacion Sanitaria de Santiago (IDIS), Santiago de Compostela, A Coruña, Spain

PIETER J. SCHUTTE, MD
Neurosurgeon, Department of Neurosurgery, Leiden University Medical Center, Center for Endocrine Tumors Leiden, Leiden, the Netherlands

RUSSELL SENANAYAKE, MSc, MRCP(UK)
Clinical Research Fellow, Cambridge Endocrine Molecular Imaging Group, Metabolic Research Laboratories, Wellcome Trust-MRC Institute of Metabolic Science, University of Cambridge, National Institute for Health Research, Cambridge Biomedical Research Centre, Addenbrooke's Hospital, Cambridge, United Kingdom

NICHOLAS A. TRITOS, MD, DSc
Neuroendocrine Unit, Neuroendocrine and Pituitary Tumor Clinical Center, Massachusetts General Hospital, Harvard Medical School, Boston, Massachusetts, USA

MEREL VAN DER MEULEN, BSc
PhD Student, Cambridge Endocrine Molecular Imaging Group, Metabolic Research Laboratories, Wellcome Trust-MRC Institute of Metabolic Science, University of Cambridge, National Institute for Health Research, Cambridge Biomedical Research Centre, Addenbrooke's Hospital, Cambridge, United Kingdom

WOUTER R. VAN FURTH, MD, PhD
Neurosurgeon, Department of Neurosurgery, Leiden University Medical Center, Center for Endocrine Tumors Leiden, Leiden, the Netherlands

ELENA V. VARLAMOV, MD
Assistant Professor, Departments of Medicine (Endocrinology, Diabetes and Metabolism) and Neurological Surgery, Pituitary Center, Oregon Health & Science University, Portland, Oregon, USA

MARCO J.T. VERSTEGEN, MD
Neurosurgeon, Department of Neurosurgery, Leiden University Medical Center, Center for Endocrine Tumors Leiden, Leiden, the Netherlands

BETTINA WINZELER, MD
Division of Endocrinology, Diabetes and Metabolism, Departments of Clinical Research, and Endocrinology, University Hospital Basel, University of Basel, Basel, Switzerland

Contents

Foreword: Pituitary Endocrinology in 2020: An Update   xv

Adriana G. Ioachimescu

Preface: Pituitary Disorders: Striving for Excellence   xvii

Niki Karavitaki

The Epidemiology of Pituitary Adenomas   347

Adrian F. Daly and Albert Beckers

Pituitary adenomas are usually nonmalignant, but have a heavy burden on patients and health care systems. Increased availability of MRI has led to an increase in incidentally found pituitary lesions and clinically relevant pituitary adenomas. Epidemiologic studies show that pituitary adenomas are increasing in incidence (between 3.9 and 7.4 cases per 100,000 per year) and prevalence (76 to 116 cases per 100,000 population) in the general population (approximately 1 case per 1000 of the general population). Most new cases diagnosed are prolactinomas and nonsecreting pituitary adenomas. Most clinically relevant pituitary adenomas occur in females, but pituitary adenomas are clinically heterogeneous.

Advances in the Imaging of Pituitary Tumors   357

James MacFarlane, Waiel A. Bashari, Russell Senanayake, Daniel Gillett, Merel van der Meulen, Andrew S. Powlson, Angelos Kolias, Olympia Koulouri, and Mark Gurnell

In most patients with pituitary adenomas magnetic resonance imaging (MRI) is essential to guide effective decision-making. T1- and T2-weighted sequences allow the majority of adenomas to be readily identified. Supplementary MR sequences (e.g. FLAIR; MR angiography) may also help inform surgery. However, in some patients MRI findings are 'negative' or equivocal (e.g. with failure to reliably identify a microadenoma or to distinguish postoperative change from residual/recurrent disease). Molecular imaging [e.g. ^{11}C-methionine PET/CT coregistered with volumetric MRI (Met-PET/MR[CR])] may allow accurate localisation of the site of de novo or persistent disease to guide definitive treatment (e.g. surgery or radiosurgery).

World Health Ozganization 2017 Classification of Pituitary Tumors   375

M. Beatriz S. Lopes

The 2017 (fourth edition) World Health Organization Classification of Endocrine Tumors has recommended major changes in classification of tumors of the pituitary gland and region. In addition to the accurate tumor subtyping, assessment of the tumor proliferative potential (mitotic and/or Ki-67 index) and other clinical parameters such as tumor invasion is strongly recommended in individual cases for consideration of clinically aggressive adenomas. It is expected that this new WHO classification will establish more uniform biologically and clinically groups of pituitary tumors and contribute to understanding of clinical outcomes for patients harboring pituitary tumors.

A Novel Etiology of Hypophysitis: Immune Checkpoint Inhibitors   387

Stuti Fernandes, Elena V. Varlamov, Shirley McCartney, and Maria Fleseriu

Checkpoint inhibitors trigger an immune process against cancer cells while causing cytotoxicity and self-antibody production against normal cells. Hypophysitis is a common endocrine toxicity. Hypophysitis may occur at any time during and after therapy, necessitating close clinical monitoring and screening for pituitary deficiencies. Treatment with high-dose glucocorticoids and temporary cessation of immunotherapy is indicated for severe hypophysitis with intractable headaches and vision changes, and for adrenal crisis. Increased awareness about this novel hypophysitis and multidisciplinary collaboration are needed to improve outcomes. This article reviews the function of immune checkpoint inhibitors and pituitary adverse effects with immune checkpoint inhibitor use.

Advances in the Medical Treatment of Cushing Disease   401

Nicholas A. Tritos and Beverly M.K. Biller

Medical therapy has an adjunctive role in management of Cushing disease. Medical therapy is recommended for patients who received pituitary radiotherapy and are awaiting its salutary effects. Medications are used preoperatively to stabilize the condition of seriously ill patients before surgery. Medical therapy is used to control hypercortisolism in patients with uncertain tumor location. Medical therapies available for management of patients with Cushing disease include steroidogenesis inhibitors, centrally acting agents, and glucocorticoid receptor antagonists. All agents require careful monitoring to optimize clinical effectiveness and manage adverse effects. Novel agents in development may expand the armamentarium for management of this condition.

Nelson's Syndrome: An Update   413

Athanasios Fountas and Niki Karavitaki

Nelson's syndrome (NS) is a condition which may develop in patients with Cushing's disease after bilateral adrenalectomy. Although there is no formal consensus on what defines NS, corticotroph tumor growth and/or gradually increasing ACTH levels are important diagnostic elements. Pathogenesis is unclear and well-established predictive factors are lacking; high ACTH during the first year after bilateral adrenalectomy is the most consistently reported predictive parameter. Management is individualized and includes surgery, with or without radiotherapy, radiotherapy alone, and observation; medical treatments have shown inconsistent results. A subset of tumors demonstrates aggressive behavior with challenging management, malignant transformation and poor prognosis.

Update on the Genetics of Pituitary Tumors   433

Sayka Barry and Márta Korbonits

Pituitary adenomas are common intracranial neoplasms, with diverse phenotypes. Most of these tumors occur sporadically and are not part of genetic disorders. Over the last decades numerous genetic studies have led to identification of somatic and germline mutations associated with pituitary tumors, which has advanced the understanding of pituitary tumorigenesis. Exploring the genetic background of pituitary neuroendocrine tumors can lead to early diagnosis associated with better outcomes, and their molecular mechanisms should lead to novel targeted therapies even for sporadic tumors. This article summarizes the genes and the syndromes associated with pituitary tumors.

The Role of Dopamine Agonists in Pituitary Adenomas 453

Erica A. Giraldi and Adriana G. Ioachimescu

Dopamine agonist therapy is the primary therapy for prolactin-secreting adenomas and usually results in normoprolactinemia, eugonadism, and tumor reduction. Cabergoline is superior to bromocriptine with regard to efficacy and tolerance. Withdrawal of cabergoline can be attempted in patients with normal prolactin levels on low doses of medication and evidence of radiographic tumor involution. Dopamine agonists have been used off label in patients with acromegaly, Cushing disease, and nonfunctioning adenomas. A trial of cabergoline monotherapy can be effective in patients with biochemically mild acromegaly. Cabergoline combination with somatostatin receptor ligands or pegvisomant improves insulin-like growth factor level 1 in majority of patients.

Acromegaly: Update on Management and Long-Term Morbidities 475

Leandro Kasuki, Ximene Antunes, Elisa Baranski Lamback, and Mônica R. Gadelha

Acromegaly is a systemic disease associated with great morbidity and increased mortality if not adequately treated. In the past decades much improvement has been achieved in its treatment and in the knowledge of its comorbidities. We provide an update of acromegaly management with current recommendations. We also address long-term comorbidities emphasizing the changing face of the disease in more recent series, with a decrease of cardiovascular disease severity and an increased awareness of comorbidities like bone disease, manifested mainly as vertebral fractures and the change in the main cause of death (from cardiovascular disease to cancer in more recent series).

Endoscopic Surgery for Pituitary Tumors 487

Wouter R. van Furth, Friso de Vries, Daniel J. Lobatto, Maarten C. Kleijwegt, Pieter J. Schutte, Alberto M. Pereira, Nienke R. Biermasz, and Marco J.T. Verstegen

 Video content accompanies this article at http://www.endo.theclinics.com.

Endoscopic transsphenoidal surgery for pituitary adenomas is a safe and highly effective first-line treatment that is well tolerated by patients. There are many potential complications, and there is a large variation in complexity of surgery. This article presents the philosophy, surgical techniques, and outcomes of a high-volume pituitary adenoma center. Three surgical videos illustrate some procedures. The experience has reinforced the authors' belief that experience and surgical volume are key to high quality of care.

Aggressive Pituitary Adenomas and Carcinomas   505

Mirela Diana Ilie, Emmanuel Jouanneau, and Gérald Raverot

A subset of pituitary tumors present an aggressive behavior that remains difficult to predict, and in rare cases they metastasize. The current European Society for Endocrinology (ESE) guidelines for the management of aggressive pituitary tumors and carcinomas provide valuable guidance, but several issues remain unaddressed because of the scarcity of data in the literature. This article presents key clinical aspects regarding aggressive pituitary tumors and carcinomas, and also discusses some of the unanswered questions of the ESE guidelines, focusing on both diagnosis and treatment.

Diabetes Insipidus: An Update   517

Julie Refardt, Bettina Winzeler, and Mirjam Christ-Crain

The differential diagnosis of diabetes insipidus involves the distinction between central or nephrogenic diabetes insipidus and primary polydipsia. Differentiation is important because treatment strategies vary; the wrong treatment can be dangerous. Reliable differentiation is difficult especially in patients with primary polydipsia or partial forms of diabetes insipidus. New diagnostic algorithms are based on the measurement of copeptin after osmotic stimulation by hypertonic saline infusion or after nonosmotic stimulation by arginine and have a higher diagnostic accuracy than the water deprivation test. Treatment involves correcting preexisting water deficits, but is different for central diabetes insipidus, nephrogenic diabetes insipidus, and primary polydipsia.

Management of Hypothalamic Obesity   533

Hermann L. Müller

Energy homeostasis, appetite, and satiety are modulated by a complex neuroendocrine system regulated by the hypothalamus. Dysregulation of this system resulting in hypothalamic obesity (HO) is caused by brain tumors, neurosurgery, and/or cranial irradiation. Craniopharyngioma (CP) is a paradigmatic disease with regard to the development of HO. Initial hypothalamic involvement of CP and/or treatment-related damage to hypothalamic-pituitary axes result in HO. Attempts to control HO with lifestyle interventions have not been satisfactory. No generally accepted pharmacologic or bariatric therapy for HO in CP has been effective in randomized controlled trials. Accordingly, prevention of HO is recommended.

Pituitary Tumors Centers of Excellence   553

Stefano Frara, Gemma Rodriguez-Carnero, Ana M. Formenti, Miguel A. Martinez-Olmos, Andrea Giustina, and Felipe F. Casanueva

Pituitary tumors are common and require complex and sophisticated procedures for both diagnosis and therapy. To maintain the highest standards of quality, it is proposed to manage patients in pituitary tumors centers of excellence (PTCOEs) with patient-centric organizations, with expert clinical endocrinologists and neurosurgeons forming the core. That core needs to be supported by experts from different disciplines such as neuroradiology, neuropathology, radiation oncology, neuro-ophthalmology, otorhinolaryngology, and trained nursing. To provide high-level medical care to patients with pituitary tumors, PTCOEs further pituitary science through research publication, presentation of results at meetings, and performing clinical trials.

ENDOCRINOLOGY AND METABOLISM CLINICS OF NORTH AMERICA

FORTHCOMING ISSUES

December 2020
Pediatric Endocrinology
Andrea Kelly, *Editor*

March 2021
Androgens in Women: Too Much, Too Little, Just Right
Margaret E. Wierman, *Editor*

June 2021
Updates on Osteoporosis
Pauline M. Camacho, *Editor*

RECENT ISSUES

June 2020
Obesity
Michael D. Jensen, *Editor*

March 2020
Technology in Diabetes
Grazia Aleppo, *Editor*

December 2019
Endocrine Hypertension
Amir H. Hamrahian, *Editor*

SERIES OF RELATED INTEREST

Medical Clinics
https://www.medical.theclinics.com
Primary Care: Clinics in Office Practice
https://www.primarycare.theclinics.com/

VISIT THE CLINICS ONLINE!
Access your subscription at:
www.theclinics.com

Foreword

Pituitary Endocrinology in 2020: An Update

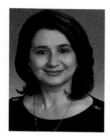

Adriana G. Ioachimescu, MD, PhD, FACE
Consulting Editor

The "Pituitary Disorders" issue of the *Endocrinology and Metabolism Clinics* features current best standards of practice and the important advances in recent years. The guest editor is Dr Niki Karavitaki, Senior Lecturer of Endocrinology at University of Birmingham, United Kingdom and Honorary Consultant Endocrinologist at the Queen Elizabeth Hospital Birmingham, where she codirects the pituitary multidisciplinary team. Dr Karavitaki, a distinguished pituitary clinician and researcher, gathered an international group of authors to deliver a clinically meaningful pituitary update.

Detection of pituitary masses increased in the past 2 decades with widespread use of MRI. Studies indicate a higher prevalence of both clinically relevant and asymptomatic adenomas, which is relevant not only for endocrinologists but also for primary care physicians and other specialists. Radiology techniques made significant progress, allowing clinical correlations between tumor appearance and clinical course. The classification of pituitary tumors changed in 2017 according to adenohypophyseal cell lineages; also, the interpretation of tumor proliferation markers was altered to reflect clinical-pathologic correlations. New discoveries of somatic and germline mutations in patients with pituitary tumors enhanced our understanding for pituitary tumorigenesis and opened pathways for novel treatments.

The clinical spectrum of pituitary and hypothalamic diseases is wide, reflecting the widespread pathologic effects on endocrine and other systems and organs. Therefore, the diagnosis and management of pituitary patients entail multiple aspects, including endocrine, neurologic, and quality of life. Reports from multidisciplinary pituitary centers with dedicated endocrinologists and neurosurgeons working together with neuropathologists, neuroradiologists, and neuroophthalmologists indicate that a patient-centered standardized approach is the key for optimizing outcomes. Hence, the concept of pituitary center excellence has been refined in recent years.

Endocrinol Metab Clin N Am 49 (2020) xv–xvi
https://doi.org/10.1016/j.ecl.2020.06.003
0889-8529/20/© 2020 Published by Elsevier Inc.

The first line of treatment for nonfunctioning and most functioning pituitary tumors with the exception of prolactinomas is transsphenoidal surgery. In recent years, the surgical approach for pituitary tumors has shifted from microscopic to endoscopic. Reports of hormonal and neurosurgical outcomes and more recent patient-reported outcomes have increased, emphasizing the importance of experienced neurosurgeons and multidisciplinary evaluation and surveillance.

Significant progress has occurred regarding medical therapy for pituitary adenomas, with multiple clinical trials completed or underway. New classes of medications have been developed for treatment of Cushing disease, which require a thorough understanding of disease pathophysiology and mechanism of action for specific medications. Dopamine agonists remain the mainstay of treatment for prolactinomas; in recent years, literature has also accumulated regarding their off-label use in other types of pituitary adenomas. In acromegaly, recent studies have unveiled a more personalized approach to patient care by considering the effects of different therapies on hormonal and radiologic aspects as well as comorbidities.

Pituitary conditions, such as pituitary adenomas resistant to conventional therapies, pituitary carcinomas, and Nelson syndrome, are rare but potentially devastating. These are challenging cases, which emphasize the importance of expert management and access to the latest therapies and research trials.

As biological treatments have become increasingly used in various cancers, hypophysis induced by the checkpoint inhibitors has been recognized. Anterior pituitary hormone perturbations, especially cortisol deficiency, as well as mass effect symptoms, have significant implications for clinical care and disease prognosis.

Diabetes insipidus and hypothalamic obesity are not often encountered in the general endocrine practice. Their management requires a thorough understanding of pathophysiologic mechanisms as well as diagnostic and current therapeutic modalities, which have expanded in recent years.

I hope you find this issue of the *Endocrinology and Metabolism Clinics* interesting and helpful in your practice. I thank the guest editor, Dr Karavitaki, for compiling a collection of articles that nicely reflects the progress in the field. I thank the authors for their important contributions and the Elsevier editorial staff for their support.

Adriana G. Ioachimescu, MD, PhD, FACE
Emory University School of Medicine
1365 B Clifton Road, Northeast, B6209
Atlanta, GA 30322, USA

E-mail address:
aioachi@emory.edu

Preface

Pituitary Disorders: Striving for Excellence

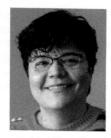

Niki Karavitaki, MD, MSc, PhD, FRCP
Editor

Pituitary disease remains a vibrant, fascinating, and often challenging field throughout the whole patient journey: from presentation and diagnosis to treatment and long-term outcomes. Over the last several years, we have witnessed advances in this arena opening exciting perspectives in research and guiding optimal patient care. Just to name a few: elucidation of the burden of pituitary disease; development of elegant diagnostic approaches; progress in the genetics, pathologic classification, and management of pituitary tumors and their related morbidities; insights on rare entities; crosstalk with other disciplines; and systematic efforts to achieve outstanding clinical care.

Thus, this *Endocrinology and Metabolism Clinics* issue aims to provide an update on pituitary disorders with particular emphasis on research outputs informing optimal practice and facilitating delivery of best care.

Daly and Beckers delineate the epidemiology of incidentally found and of clinically relevant pituitary adenomas. They confirm that both incidence and prevalence are rising with a wide range of disease severity, and they highlight the need for comprehensive diagnostic and therapeutic measures in order to achieve optimal outcomes. MacFarlane, Bashari, Senanayake, Gillett, van der Meulen, Powlson, Kolias, Koulouri, and Gurnell take us through advances in imaging of pituitary tumors, and how these can inform treatment strategies. Lopes underlines the changes introduced in the 2017 (4th edition) World Health Organization classification of pituitary tumors (use of adenohypophyseal cell lineages, modifications in histological grading, introduction of new entities) and the basis for characterizing clinically aggressive pituitary neuroendocrine tumors. Fernandes, Varlamov, McCartney, and Fleseriu expand on the hot topic of immune checkpoint inhibitors and hypophysitis, emphasizing the key role of multidisciplinary communication for improving outcomes. Tritos and Biller review the clinical effectiveness and the safety profile of medical treatments for

Endocrinol Metab Clin N Am 49 (2020) xvii–xviii
https://doi.org/10.1016/j.ecl.2020.06.001
0889-8529/20/© 2020 Published by Elsevier Inc.

Cushing, an as ever-demanding condition, and update us on the novel agents under development that may eventually expand our therapeutic potential. Fountas and Karavitaki portray Nelson syndrome and address the plethora of areas requiring enlightenment (diagnostic criteria, optimal management and follow-up, aggressive tumor behavior). Barry and Korbonits overview the expanding landscape of somatic and germline mutations associated with pituitary tumors and address the challenges and implications of these findings in current practice. Giraldi and Ioachimescu appraise the published literature on the place of dopamine agonists in the management of various adenoma subtypes offering grounds for evidence-based treatment strategies. Kasuki, Antunes, Baranski Lamback, and Gadelha discuss the current recommendations on the management of acromegaly and shed light on the evolving face of this disease over the last years. Van Furth, de Vries, Lobatto, Schutte, Pereira, Kleijwegt, Biermasz, and Verstegen outline the fundamentals of endoscopic pituitary surgery and its contributions in the management of pituitary tumors. Ilie, Jouanneau, and Raverot explore the enigmatic entity of aggressive pituitary adenomas and carcinomas and the dilemmas surrounding these often-ominous tumors. Refardt, Winzeler, and Christ-Crain inform us on advances in the scenery of posterior lobe disorders with new diagnostic algorithms for problems in water balance, changing our practice. Müller synopsizes the daunting entity of hypothalamic obesity and the pros and cons of available management options. And, last but not least, Frara, Rodriguez-Carnero, Formenti, Martinez-Olmos, Giustina, and Casanueva epitomize the concept and the multidimensional missions Pituitary Tumors Centers of Excellence (PTCOE), the future organizational "gold standard" to provide high-level medical care and promote patient-centered clinical and research excellence.

I am extremely grateful to all authors and esteemed colleagues for their generous and truly valuable contributions featuring the, as ever, elegant world of the Master Gland. Also, my sincere thanks to the Elsevier editorial staff for their continuous support during the preparation of this issue.

Finally, I very much hope this piece of work will be an informative and useful addition for all those striving for excellence in pituitary patient care.

Niki Karavitaki, MD, MSc, PhD, FRCP
Institute of Metabolism and Systems Research
College of Medical and Dental Sciences
University of Birmingham
IBR Tower, Level 2
Birmingham, B15 2TT, UK

E-mail address:
n.karavitaki@bham.ac.uk

The Epidemiology of Pituitary Adenomas

Adrian F. Daly, MB BCh, PhD*, Albert Beckers, MD, PhD*

KEYWORDS

- Pituitary adenoma • Epidemiology • Prevalence • Incidence • Acromegaly
- Prolactinoma • Cushing's disease • Nonfunctioning pituitary adenoma

KEY POINTS

- Pituitary adenomas are an important cause of morbidity and are increasingly encountered in the diagnostic and clinical settings, particularly owing to increased availability of MRI.
- Incidentally found pituitary adenomas are generally small, expand infrequently, and rarely cause clinical symptoms.
- Prolactinomas and nonfunctioning pituitary adenomas are the most frequent subtypes of clinically relevant adenomas, followed by acromegaly and Cushing's disease.
- The incidence of pituitary adenomas is 3.9 to 7.4 cases per 100,000 and the prevalence of clinically-relevant pituitary adenomas is about 1 per 1000 of the general population. Most new cases diagnosed annually are prolactinomas and nonfunctioning pituitary adenomas.
- The incidence and prevalence of is increasing; the largest patient subgroup is young females with microprolactinomas.

INTRODUCTION

Pituitary adenoma form via a process that is thought to be derived from the clonal expansion of single abnormal cells owing to somatic genetic mutations or chromosomal abnormalities.[1,2] In a minority of cases (approximately 5%), familial or heritable diseases often related to known germline genetic mutations are associated with pituitary adenoma formation; these include familial isolated pituitary adenomas (FIPA), multiple endocrine neoplasia types 1 and 4 and X-linked acrogigantism, among others.[3] At the tissue level, the occurrence of molecular genetic abnormalities leading to pituitary tumorigenesis is probably a constant process that is addressed by repair or apoptotic pathways, like in other tissues. Pituitary adenomas, when they occur, can be discovered by specific investigation of suggestive signs and symptoms owing to either hormonal dysregulation, or tumor expansion, such as compression by the adenoma of

Department of Endocrinology, Centre Hospitalier Universitaire de Liège, Liège Université, Domaine Universitaire Sart-Tilman, Liège 4000, Belgium
* Corresponding authors.
E-mail addresses: Adrian.daly@uliege.be (A.F.D.); albert.beckers@chu.ulg.ac.be (A.B.)
Twitter: @HomeofFIPA (A.F.D.)

Endocrinol Metab Clin N Am 49 (2020) 347–355
https://doi.org/10.1016/j.ecl.2020.04.002
0889-8529/20/© 2020 Elsevier Inc. All rights reserved.

endo.theclinics.com

the optic chiasm or surrounding structures. In addition, pituitary adenomas are increasingly being identified incidentally during imaging investigations for unrelated causes (headaches, head injury). As discussed elsewhere in this article, only a limited proportion of pituitary adenomas that occur actually cause symptoms, and it is important to focus on the epidemiology of clinically relevant pituitary adenomas, when considering the burden of disease on patients and health system resources.

PITUITARY INCIDENTALOMA VERSUS CLINICALLY RELEVANT PITUITARY ADENOMAS
Incidentaloma

The practice guideline of the Endocrine Society and the European Society of Endocrinology define a pituitary incidentaloma as "a previously unsuspected pituitary lesion that is discovered on an imaging study performed for an unrelated reason."[4] Adenomas form frequently in the anterior pituitary, but have a size and natural history that means that the overwhelming majority of them are asymptomatic and rarely clinically relevant. Histologic autopsy studies on pituitaries from otherwise normal individuals who died of non–pituitary-related causes first began as far back as Costello's work in the 1930s.[5] Taken together, these studies have shown that asymptomatic pituitary adenomas occur in about 10.7% to 14.4% of individuals.[6,7] Importantly, most of these unsuspected pituitary adenomas are tiny in size. For instance, Buurman and Saeger[8] found pituitary adenomas in 316 of 3048 individuals at autopsy (10.4%), with an equal sex distribution; overall, the median diameter was 1.5 mm. In that and other autopsy series, these very small microadenomas were most frequently derived from lactotrope cells.[6-8] The occurrence of unsuspected macroadenomas in autopsy series is, in contrast, very infrequent (0.35% of adenomas) and these are usually gonadotropin positive or plurihormonal.[6,8] As noted by Molitch,[7] the very low rate of macroadenomas strongly suggests that progression from tiny microadenoma to larger tumors only occurs in exceptional circumstances. Taken together, autopsy studies indicate that incidentally occurring pituitary adenomas are usually tiny in size, and owing to this and their hormonal staining characteristics, the vast majority are unlikely to provoke clinical symptoms.

Another approach to understanding the underlying rate of pituitary adenoma formation in the general population comes from analyses of radiologic imaging studies. MRI has become widely available in developed countries and is an integral part of the investigation of diverse conditions such as headache, seizure, or loss of consciousness and is used for assessments after head injury. Also, the resolution of MRI has improved over the last few decades, so that brain MRI has moved in many settings to 3T equipment thereby providing resolution at around 1 mm. These increases in the availability, use, and resolution of MRI have contributed to an increase in the number of pituitary lesions being identified in those undergoing brain MRI for other reasons. These incidental lesions include pituitary adenomas, but also a vast range of other potential abnormalities, from Rathke's cleft cysts, to benign (meningioma) and malignant tumors (germ cell tumors, metastases), including vascular lesions and artifacts. The potential pitfalls in the assessment of pituitary incidentalomas identified on radiologic imaging are discussed in depth by Vasilev and colleagues.[9] It is important to note that some of these incidentally discovered pathologies are themselves clinically relevant. For instance, in a series of 282 incidental pituitary masses noted among 2598 patients undergoing pituitary imaging from 1999 to 2009, important diagnoses, including malignancies, metastases, apoplexy, and active pituitary adenomas, were later established.[10] The best approach to the assessment of the clinical relevance of incidentally found pituitary masses is one that combines clinical endocrine and neuroimaging expertise and follows practical guidelines.[4,9]

MRI (and computed tomography) studies undertaken in those not known to have pituitary disease showed a prevalence of pituitary adenomas of about 22.5% in a systematic review undertaken by Ezzat and colleagues.[6] As is the case with autopsy studies, radiologically discovered incidental pituitary adenomas are usually very small in size.[4,6,9] Incidentally discovered macroadenomas or tumors that were subsequently found to produce hormonal or mass effects are identified infrequently in radiologic series.[11–13] Because most small pituitary incidentalomas (<10 mm diameter) that are asymptomatic at baseline do not grow further, the joint guidelines from the Endocrine Society and European Society of Endocrinology suggest that follow-up should comprise a repeat MRI after 12 months and more infrequently thereafter if no growth has occurred.[4] Incidentally discovered macroincidentalomas often require active management, because they are far more likely to cause symptoms and grow over time than microadenomas.[14] The guidelines recommend follow-up imaging initially every 6 months for macroadenomas that do not need immediate surgery; this schedule is in addition to complete a clinical and hormonal workup to identify mass effects and hormone hypersecretion or deficiency.[4] Recent radiology guidelines have taken a similar approach to follow-up based on the size of the pituitary incidentaloma on the initial MRI.[15]

Clinically Relevant Pituitary Adenomas

Broadly speaking, a clinically relevant pituitary adenoma is one that causes or has caused signs and symptoms and that has been confirmed by imaging and hormonal testing; surgical and pathologic confirmation should be available in operated cases. This clinically relevant class of pituitary adenomas can include all subtypes, irrespective of size, expansion, molecular genetics, pathologic features, and secretory patterns. In addition, these are the pituitary adenomas that place a clinical burden on patients, and require specialized infrastructure and personnel for diagnosis, treatment, and long-term management. The importance of the pituitary gland in regulating multiple physiologic systems and the high level of training and expertise needed for surgery, radiology, and medical management means that accurate epidemiologic assessments of clinically relevant pituitary adenomas provide valuable information for health resource expenditure in endocrinology.

The identification of pituitary adenomas has been aided by the more widespread availability of MRI and reliable hormonal testing over the past few decades. In parallel, effective treatment of pituitary adenomas has improved morbidity and, in some diseases like acromegaly, disease-related mortality has been brought closer to that of the normal population. Improved detection increases the incident number of cases diagnosed per year. This finding, in conjunction with longer survival, leads to an increase in the number of prevalent cases of pituitary adenomas at any given time.

Incidence studies

The largest database reporting incidence statistics for pituitary tumors is the Central Brain Tumor Registry of the US, which collects, analyses and publishes reports on all central nervous system tumors by site and histology. The most recent report of the Central Brain Tumor Registry of the US covers the years 2012 to 2016.[16] Among central nervous system tumors, pituitary lesions comprise a sizable proportion of new tumors diagnosed annually and have an incidence of 4.07 cases per 100,000 per year. Histologically confirmed pituitary adenomas have an incidence of 3.23 and 3.84 cases per 100,000 per year in males and females, respectively. Importantly, there is a statistically significant higher incidence of pituitary tumors (including adenomas) in blacks as compared with whites, a finding that requires further investigation. Tumors of the pituitary region also represent the highest proportion of central nervous system tumors occurring in children, adolescents and young adults (15–39 years). These results underline that pituitary adenomas represent an important burden on health in the community in the United States, and particularly among young patients, females, and racial minorities.

A series of local and regional incidence studies have been published in recent years covering populations from Europe, Canada and Argentina.[17–22] Most have used similar calculation methodologies to express incidence as standard incidence rates (SIR) based on the World Health Organisation 2000 standards.[23] These studies document an increasing incidence of pituitary adenomas over recent decades, particularly since the introduction of MRI. Overall, pituitary adenomas occur with a mean incidence of approximately 5.1 cases per 100,000 per year (range 3.9–7.4 cases per 100,000 per year). The rank order of mean SIR of the various pituitary adenoma subtypes is: prolactinoma > nonfunctioning pituitary adenoma > acromegaly > Cushing's disease > thyroid-stimulating hormone–secreting adenoma. There is some heterogeneity among the data, with studies from Sweden and Canada reporting equal SIR for prolactinoma and nonfunctioning pituitary adenoma.[19,22] In general, more recent data indicate that prolactinomas constitute an increasing proportion of all new pituitary adenomas. With an SIR ranging from 1.6 to 5.4 cases per 100,000 per year, overall prolactinomas comprise approximately 50% of new pituitary adenomas diagnosed annually. When analyzed be gender and age, incidence data indicate that pituitary adenomas are diagnosed at a younger age in women than in men owing to the high frequency of prolactinomas in females of childbearing age.

Prevalence studies

A useful methodology to measure the true prevalence of clinically relevant pituitary adenomas is by performing comprehensive case identification in a geographically delimited region in which a full range of hospital- and community-based medical practitioners can be included. This approach avoids the weakness of other study methods that include patients from outside the geographic region of the site or having incomplete inclusion of patients. The geographic delimitation can be achieved using political boundaries, such as county or city limits, or using newer mapping methods like geolocalization.[24,25] National datasets from smaller countries with clearly demarcated national borders such as Malta or Iceland can also be assessed in a similar manner. Expansion of the population studied to larger countries comes at the expense of verification steps using patient records (eg, MRI, hormonal levels) and usually cannot provide a data-rich, comprehensive analysis set of clinical, radiologic, hormonal, and therapeutic information.

We initially analyzed the prevalence of pituitary adenomas in a community-based population sample in the Province of Liège, Belgium, in 2006.[26] That study included 3 defined sampling areas with rural, suburban, and urban characteristics, and boundaries were defined by postal codes of residence. Case identification and inclusion was performed at the community level in collaboration with general practitioners and other relevant doctors, including gynecologists and private physicians. After inclusion, all patients had to have confirmatory results of a pituitary adenoma on imaging, hormonal tests, and clinical data confirming signs and symptoms related to the pituitary adenoma. All incidental pituitary tumors or cases of hormonal abnormalities without a visualized adenoma (eg, hyperprolactinemia) were excluded. Among the population of 71,972, there were 68 patients with clinically relevant pituitary adenomas (mean 1:1064 of the 3 sample regions of the population). Patients were mostly suffering from prolactinomas (66.2%), followed by nonfunctioning pituitary adenomas

Table 1
Prevalence studies of clinically relevant pituitary adenomas in the general population

Reference, Year	Region	Population (n)	Number of PA	Prevalence	Prevalence/100,000	Female (%)	Macro (%)	Prolactinoma (%)	NFPA (%)	GH (%)	CD (%)	Other (%)
Cross-sectional studies												
Daly et al,[26] 2006	Liège, Belgium	71,972	68	1/1064[a]	94.0	67.6	42.6	66.2	14.7	13.2	5.9	
Fontana & Gaillard,[28] 2009	Fribourg, Switzerland	54,607	44	1/1241	80.6	73.0	N/A	56.0	30.0	9.0	5.0	
Fernandez et al,[27] 2010	Oxfordshire, UK	81,149	63	1/1288	77.6	66.7	41.3	57.1	28.6	11.1	1.6	1.6
National case finding studies												
Gruppetta et al,[18] 2013	Malta	417608	316	1/1322	75.7	69.6	43.4	46.2	34.2	16.5	2.2	0.94
Agustsson et al,[20] 2015	Iceland	321857	372	1/865	115.6	62.4	54.8	47.1	35.8	11.8	5.4	
Regional database studies												
Al-Dahmani et al,[19] 2015	Nova Scotia, Canada	945061	838	1/1128	82.2	62.2	56.9	41.0	48.0	6.5	4.5	
Fainstein-Day et al,[17] 2016	Buenos Aires, Argentina	135019	132	1/1023	97.8	77.3	48.0	57.5	21.9	14.5	6.1	
Overall				1/1106	89.1	68.4	47.8	53.0	30.5	11.8	4.4	1.3[b]

Abbreviations: CD, Cushing's disease; GH, acromegaly; Macro, macroadenoma (>10 mm diameter); NFPA, nonfunctioning pituitary adenoma; Other, thyroid-stimulating hormone–secreting or unclassified pituitary adenomas; PA, pituitary adenoma.
[a] Mean prevalence across sampling localities.
[b] Percentages may add up to >100% due to rounding.
Data from Refs.[17–20,26–28]

(14.7%), acromegaly (13.2%) and Cushing's disease (5.9%). The predominant sub-group overall consisted of premenopausal female patients with microprolactinomas who were successfully controlled with dopamine agonists.

Since that work in 2006, a number of other study populations in different countries have been assessed using largely similar methodologies (**Table 1**). These include community-based cross-sectional studies in the UK and Switzerland, a regional database in Argentina and a sellar mass registry in Canada, in addition to national collections in Malta and Iceland.[17–20,27,28] Together, these data in a geographically diverse population of more than 2 million people, validate and expand on the initial findings. Clinically relevant pituitary adenomas occur with a mean prevalence of 89.1 per 100,000 (range, 75.7–115.6 per 100,000) and the majority of pituitary adenoma patients are female (68.4%; range, 62.2%–77.3%). Macroadenomas are seen at diagnosis in 47.8% of patients (range, 41.3%–56.9%). Among the pituitary adenoma subtypes, prolactinomas are the most commonly diagnosed clinically relevant pituitary adenomas, comprising just more than one-half of the total (53.0%; range, 41.0%–66.2%). In descending order, they are followed by nonfunctioning pituitary adenomas (30.5%), somatotropinomas causing acromegaly (11.8%), and Cushing's disease (4.4%). Individual studies have reported rare thyroid-stimulating hormone–secreting pituitary adenomas. In general, women presented at a younger age than men, which is likely to be driven by the sizable group of young women with

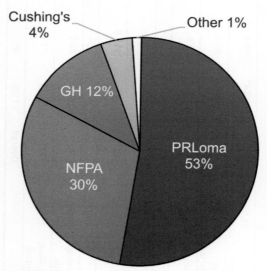

Fig. 1. The prevalence of pituitary adenomas in the general population. The most extensive autopsy studies indicate that about 1 in 10 anterior pituitary glands from individuals without known pituitary disease harbors a pituitary adenoma. The vast majority of these histologic incidentalomas are tiny (median diameter, 1.5 mm) prolactin-positive adenomas that very rarely expand in size. Among the general population, prevalence studies across various countries have demonstrated that clinically relevant pituitary adenomas occur with a prevalence of about 1 case per 1000. These clinically confirmed symptomatic pituitary adenomas are most frequently prolactinomas (53%) or nonfunctioning PA (30%), whereas GH secreting tumors comprise just under 12% and Cushing's disease approximately 4%. CD, Cushing's disease; GH, acromegaly; NFPA, nonfunctioning pituitary adenoma; PA, pituitary adenoma.

symptomatic microprolactinomas affecting their menstrual cycles and reproductive health. Taken together, the reported data across all series indicate that there is 1 clinically relevant pituitary adenoma case in every 1106 members of the general population. In Iceland, the prevalence has risen markedly owing to a greater number of nonfunctioning pituitary adenomas and prolactinomas being identified, probably -as the authors suggest- owing to improved availability of radiologic and hormonal diagnostics from about 1990 onwards.[20]

SUMMARY

The epidemiology data on clinically relevant pituitary adenomas show the wide range of presentations and potential therapeutic pathways that need to be followed by patients (**Fig. 1**, see **Table 1**). For example, the largest individual group of patients are those with prolactinomas, and from a treatment perspective, many female patients with microprolactinomas can likely be managed with dopamine agonists alone. The situation for males with prolactinomas is much more complex, because they tend to be older and have larger tumors that may be resistant to dopamine agonists.[29] Even within each tumor subtype, the epidemiology data underline that a full range of therapeutic pathways must be available to patients, particularly to manage those with greater need for multimodal therapy owing to disease severity and treatment resistance. Increasing access to MRI will continue to highlight pituitary incidentalomas, which require a careful approach to identify the cases that progress to produce clinically relevant symptoms.

DISCLOSURE

The work was supported in part by grants from the FIRS funds of the CHU de Liège and by the JABBS Foundation, UK.

REFERENCES

1. Melmed S. Mechanisms for pituitary tumorigenesis: the plastic pituitary. J Clin Invest 2003;112(11):1603–18.
2. Asa SL, Ezzat S. The pathogenesis of pituitary tumors. Annu Rev Pathol 2009;4: 97–126.
3. Vandeva S, Daly AF, Petrossians P, et al. GENETICS IN ENDOCRINOLOGY: somatic and germline mutations in the pathogenesis of pituitary adenomas. Eur J Endocrinol 2019. https://doi.org/10.1530/EJE-19-0602.
4. Freda PU, Beckers AM, Katznelson L, et al. Pituitary incidentaloma: an endocrine society clinical practice guideline. J Clin Endocrinol Metab 2011;96(4):894–904.
5. Costello RT. Subclinical Adenoma of the Pituitary Gland. Am J Pathol 1936;12(2): 205–16. Available at: http://www.ncbi.nlm.nih.gov/pubmed/19970261. Accessed January 20, 2020.
6. Ezzat S, Asa SL, Couldwell WT, et al. The prevalence of pituitary adenomas: a systematic review. Cancer 2004;101(3):613–9.
7. Molitch ME. Pituitary incidentalomas. Best Pract Res Clin Endocrinol Metab 2009; 23(5):667–75.
8. Buurman H, Saeger W. Subclinical adenomas in postmortem pituitaries: classification and correlations to clinical data. Eur J Endocrinol 2006;154(5):753–8.
9. Vasilev V, Rostomyan L, Daly AF, et al. Management of endocrine disease: pituitary "incidentaloma": neuroradiological assessment and differential diagnosis. Eur J Endocrinol 2016;175(4):R171–84.

10. Famini P, Maya MM, Melmed S. Pituitary magnetic resonance imaging for sellar and parasellar masses: ten-year experience in 2598 patients. J Clin Endocrinol Metab 2011;96(6):1633–41.
11. Yue NC, Longstreth WT, Elster AD, et al. Clinically serious abnormalities found incidentally at MR imaging of the brain: data from the Cardiovascular Health Study. Radiology 1997;202(1):41–6. https://doi.org/10.1148/radiology.202.1.8988190.
12. Haberg AK, Hammer TA, Kvistad KA, et al. Incidental intracranial findings and their clinical impact; The HUNT MRI Study in a general population of 1006 participants between 50-66 Years. PLoS One 2016;11(3). https://doi.org/10.1371/journal.pone.0151080.
13. Sandeman EM, Hernandez Mdel CV, Morris Z, et al. Incidental findings on brain MR imaging in older community-dwelling subjects are common but serious medical consequences are rare: a cohort study. PLoS One 2013;8(8). https://doi.org/10.1371/journal.pone.0071467.
14. Karavitaki N, Collison K, Halliday J, et al. What is the natural history of nonoperated nonfunctioning pituitary adenomas? Clin Endocrinol (Oxf) 2007;67(6):938–43.
15. Hoang JK, Hoffman AR, González RG, et al. Management of incidental pituitary findings on CT, MRI, and 18 F-fluorodeoxyglucose PET: a white paper of the ACR Incidental Findings Committee. J Am Coll Radiol 2018;15(7):966–72.
16. Ostrom QT, Cioffi G, Gittleman H, et al. CBTRUS statistical report: primary brain and other central nervous system tumors diagnosed in the United States in 2012–2016. Neuro Oncol 2019;21(Supplement_5):v1–100.
17. Fainstein Day P, Loto MG, Glerean M, et al. Incidence and prevalence of clinically relevant pituitary adenomas: retrospective cohort study in a health management organization in Buenos Aires, Argentina. Arch Endocrinol Metab 2016;60(6):554–61.
18. Gruppetta M, Mercieca C, Vassallo J. Prevalence and incidence of pituitary adenomas: a population based study in Malta. Pituitary 2013;16(4):545–53.
19. Al-Dahmani K, Mohammad S, Imran F, et al. Sellar masses: an epidemiological study from the department of medicine, Tawam Hospital in affiliation with. Can J Neurol Sci 2016;43:291–7.
20. Agustsson TT, Baldvinsdottir T, Jonasson JG, et al. The epidemiology of pituitary adenomas in Iceland, 1955-2012: a nationwide population-based study. Eur J Endocrinol 2015;173(5):655–64.
21. Raappana A, Koivukangas J, Ebeling T, et al. Incidence of pituitary adenomas in Northern Finland in 1992-2007. J Clin Endocrinol Metab 2010;95(9):4268–75.
22. Tjörnstrand A, Gunnarsson K, Evert M, et al. The incidence rate of pituitary adenomas in western Sweden for the period 2001-2011. Eur J Endocrinol 2014;171(4):519–26.
23. Ahmad OB, Boschi-Pinto C, Lopez Christopher AD, et al. Age standardization of rates: a new WHO standard 2001. World Health Organization Discussion Paper Series 31. Available at: https://www.who.int/healthinfo/paper31.pdf.
24. Naves LA, Porto LB, Rosa JWC, et al. Geographical information system (GIS) as a new tool to evaluate epidemiology based on spatial analysis and clinical outcomes in acromegaly. Pituitary 2015;18(1):8–15.
25. Zakir JC, Casulari LA, Rosa JWC, et al. Prognostic value of invasion, markers of proliferation, and classification of giant pituitary tumors, in a georeferred cohort in Brazil of 50 patients, with a long-term postoperative follow-up. Int J Endocrinol 2016;2016:7964523.

26. Daly AF, Rixhon M, Adam C, et al. High prevalence of pituitary adenomas: a cross-sectional study in the province of Liège, Belgium. J Clin Endocrinol Metab 2006;91(12):4769–75.
27. Fernandez A, Karavitaki N, Wass JA. Prevalence of pituitary adenomas: a community-based, cross-sectional study in Banbury (Oxfordshire, UK). Clin Endocrinol 2010;72(3):377–82.
28. Fontana Gaillard RE. Epidemiology of pituitary adenoma: results of the first Swiss study. Rev Med Suisse 2009;5(223):2172–4.
29. Vroonen L, Daly AF, Beckers A. Epidemiology and management challenges in prolactinomas. Neuroendocrinology 2019;109(1):20–7.

Advances in the Imaging of Pituitary Tumors

James MacFarlane, MRCP(UK)[a,1], Waiel A. Bashari, MSc, MRCP(UK)[a,1],
Russell Senanayake, MSc, MRCP(UK)[a,1], Daniel Gillett, MSc[a,b],
Merel van der Meulen, BSc[a], Andrew S. Powlson, MRCP(UK)[a],
Angelos Kolias, PhD, FRCS[c], Olympia Koulouri, PhD, MRCP(UK)[a],
Mark Gurnell, PhD, FRCP[a,*]

KEYWORDS

- Pituitary adenoma • MRI • PET/CT • ^{11}C-methionine • Met-PET/MR[CR]

KEY POINTS

- MRI remains the primary modality for imaging pituitary tumors (pituitary adenomas [PA]).
- Conventional magnetic resonance (MR) sequences provide sufficient information to guide management in most patients, but can lack sensitivity and specificity for (i) detection of microadenomas; or (ii) identification of the site or sites of residual/recurrent disease following primary therapy.
- Alternative MR sequences may aid characterization of specific tumor traits (eg, tumoral consistency; presence of apoplexy; invasion of surrounding structures).
- Several different radiotracers have been investigated for molecular imaging of pituitary tumors with varying success.
- ^{11}C-methionine PET coregistered with volumetric (1-mm slice) MRI (Met-PET/MR[CR]) can aid accurate localization of microadenomas/picoadenomas of all PA subtypes, identify sites of recurrent or incompletely resected disease, and distinguish from postoperative change (eg, acromegaly, Cushing disease), and augment radiotherapy planning in selected cases.

Funding sources: J. MacFarlane, W.A. Bashari, R. Senanayake, D. Gillett, A. Kolias, O. Koulouri, and M. Gurnell are supported by the Cambridge NIHR Biomedical Research Centre; this work was also supported by a project grant from the Evelyn Trust (W.A. Bashari, O. Koulouri, M. Gurnell).
[a] Cambridge Endocrine Molecular Imaging Group, Metabolic Research Laboratories, Wellcome Trust-MRC Institute of Metabolic Science, University of Cambridge, National Institute for Health Research, Cambridge Biomedical Research Centre, Addenbrooke's Hospital, Hills Road, Cambridge CB2 0QQ, UK; [b] Department of Nuclear Medicine, Addenbrooke's Hospital, Hills Road, Cambridge CB2 0QQ, UK; [c] Division of Neurosurgery, Department of Clinical Neurosciences, University of Cambridge & Addenbrooke's Hospital, Cambridge CB2 0QQ, UK
[1] These authors contributed equally to this work.
* Corresponding author.
E-mail address: mg299@medschl.cam.ac.uk

INTRODUCTION

Pituitary adenomas (PA) are typically benign, slow-growing tumors of the adenohypophysis, which come to attention because of associated endocrine dysfunction (eg, hyperprolactinemia, hypercortisolism, acromegaly/gigantism, hypopituitarism) or mass effect (eg, compression of the optic chiasm or cranial nerves in the wall of the cavernous sinus), or when they are discovered incidentally during cross-sectional imaging of the brain performed for a separate indication.[1]

Pituitary incidentalomas are a relatively common finding in the general population, with a large metaanalysis of autopsy series suggesting a mean prevalence of 10.7% (range 1.5%–31%).[2] These findings are broadly consistent with MRI studies of the sella and parasellar regions, which identify abnormalities in as many as 10% to 38% of subjects in unselected cohorts.[3,4] Most of these are microadenomas, and most do not result in endocrine dysfunction.[5] In contrast, clinically relevant PA have been estimated to affect between 1:1064 and 1:1200 of the general population.[6,7]

Modern management of PA is ideally overseen by a specialist multidisciplinary team comprising neuroendocrinology, neurosurgery, otolaryngology, neuroradiology, neuropathology, neuroophthalmology and neurooncology.[8] Cross-sectional imaging (MRI and/or computed tomography [CT]) of the sella and parasellar regions is central to effective decision making and may be the major determinant of whether a patient is offered surgery, radiotherapy, medical therapy, or surveillance. For most cases, MRI remains the primary imaging modality and distinguishes the adenoma from normal pituitary tissue and adjacent structures.[9,10] However, in a small but important subgroup of patients, conventional pituitary imaging is not informative. For example, although incidentalomas are a common finding in the general population, paradoxically some functioning microadenomas (including 30%–40% of corticotroph adenomas) are not readily visualized on standard pituitary magnetic resonance (MR) sequences.[11] Similarly, following transsphenoidal surgery (TSS), sites of residual or recurrent disease may not be evident or readily distinguished from posttreatment changes.[12] In these contexts, the decision then lies between "blind" surgical (re-)exploration, long-term (in some cases life-long) medical therapy, radiotherapy, or even a combination of approaches, each with their own limitations with respect to the likelihood and time to achieving disease control, risk of inducing hypopituitarism, and causation of other adverse effects.

Accordingly, several novel approaches to pituitary imaging have been proposed, largely based on the deployment of alternative MR sequences or novel techniques for image analysis, with the aims of (i) improving diagnostic resolution, (ii) informing pretreatment planning, and (iii) predicting likely responses to different therapeutic strategies. In addition, a role for molecular imaging, with its ability to confirm/localize sites of functioning active tumor, is gaining prominence and may be particularly valuable when cross-sectional imaging remains equivocal. Here, the authors consider how these advances might be integrated into modern imaging algorithms to better inform the management of patients with PA.

MRI

In a patient in whom a PA is suspected, dedicated MRI of the sella and parasellar regions should be performed to confirm the site and size of the tumor and its relationship to surrounding important structures. CT may offer important supplementary information in some cases (eg, defining the extent of bony erosion with larger tumors; confirming/excluding the presence of calcification), and modern thin-slice CT is a reasonable alternative for those unable or unwilling to undergo MRI.[10]

Standard Clinical Pituitary MRI

Spin-echo (SE) pulse sequences are one of the earliest developed and still widely used of all MRI pulse sequences and remain a cornerstone of modern pituitary imaging. Although practice varies from center to center, routine clinical pituitary MRI protocols (using a 1.5 Tesla [1.5 T] or 3 T scanner) typically include the following:

- Precontrast T1-weighted SE and T2-weighted fast SE (FSE) coronal and sagittal sections with thin slices (typically 2–3 mm)
- Postcontrast T1-weighted SE coronal and sagittal sections with thin slices

The addition of axial images may also be helpful in some cases and allows for more complete evaluation of the posterior pituitary gland.[13]

The normal anterior pituitary gland is isointense to gray matter on noncontrast T1- and T2-weighted SE/FSE sequences; the posterior lobe demonstrates high T1 signal, but is hypointense on T2. Following injection of contrast, the infundibulum and gland progressively enhance (homogeneously). Contrast uptake by PA is typically slower, resulting in delayed enhancement and washout.[10,14]

For cases without a clear abnormality on MRI, but in whom a lesion is strongly suspected on clinical grounds (eg, ACTH-dependent Cushing syndrome with biochemical and/or petrosal sinus catheter evidence of a central origin), dynamic contrast-enhanced MRI (using T1-weighted sequences precontrast and immediately postcontrast administration) may help identify the site of a microadenoma. However, gradient echo (for example, spoiled gradient echo, [fast] spoiled gradient recalled echo [FSPGR/SPGR]), which allows imaging with a 1-mm-slice interval, has been suggested to offer greater sensitivity for localizing microadenomas in the context of Cushing disease.[15,16]

The most commonly used contrast agent for pituitary imaging is gadolinium, a naturally occurring lanthanide with strong paramagnetic properties (owing to 7 unpaired electrons). In its free form, gadolinium is toxic and must therefore be chelated to a carrier ligand to permit safe clinical use. Recently, however, concern has arisen regarding the potential for gadolinium deposition in the central nervous system even in patients with normal renal function,[17,18] which presents a particular challenge for pituitary endocrinologists and their patients given the often long-term requirement for periodic surveillance imaging.[19] It is therefore important that the need for contrast enhancement is carefully considered whenever imaging of the sella and parasellar regions is requested. For example, in a patient with a well-defined intrasellar tumor remnant following primary surgery for a nonfunctioning PA, and which is well visualized on noncontrast MRI, the inclusion of postgadolinium sequences is likely to add little to the clinical decision-making process; if there are concerns regarding tumor enlargement on noncontrast T1- and T2-weighted images, the patient can be recalled for further assessment.

Similarly, attention has recently been drawn to those clinical settings in which T2-weighted MRI can afford comparable or even superior information to that provided by T1-weighted postcontrast imaging,[20] thus potentially avoiding the need for initial and/or repeat gadolinium administration (**Fig. 1, Table 1**).

Alternative Pituitary Magnetic Resonance Sequences/Techniques

An increasing array of MR sequences has been adapted for use in pituitary disease. In addition, as the availability of higher-field-strength MRI systems (eg, 7 T) increases, potential applications in patients with PA are being increasingly explored. Currently, most of these approaches remain outside standard clinical protocols for imaging of

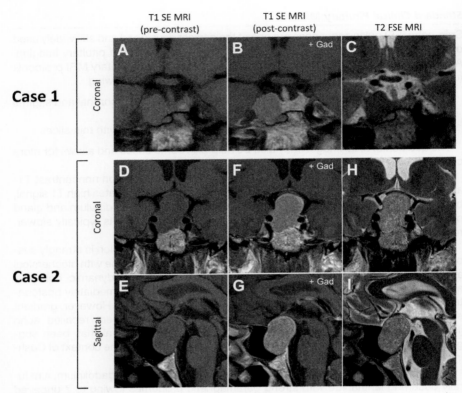

Fig. 1. Prediction of pituitary tumor phenotype based on T2-weighted MRI appearances. (*A–C*) T1 SE (precontrast and postcontrast) and T2 FSE MRI in a patient with acromegaly, demonstrating a right-sided macroadenoma; the tumor is hypointense on T2 sequences when compared with the adjacent temporal lobe, which has been linked with somatostatin analogue responsiveness and a densely granulated appearance on histology. (*D–I*) T1 SE (precontrast and postcontrast) and T2-weighted FSE MRI showing a macroadenoma with suprasellar extension in a patient who presented with visual loss, but no clinical or biochemical features of hypercortisolism; the tumor exhibits multiple microcysts (focal small areas of high intensity) on the T2 images. Gad, gadolinium; T1, T1 weighted; T2, T2 weighted.

the sella and parasellar regions, but may be requested when conventional sequences leave important questions unanswered. These sequences can be broadly considered under the following 3 indications (**Table 2**):

A. To aid a diagnosis
B. To help inform preoperative assessment
C. To predict likely treatment outcomes

Advances in Image Analysis

Novel approaches to image analysis are also being translated from other disease areas, allowing additional information to be derived from existing pituitary MR protocols. For example, in a study of 89 patients who had undergone TSS, and for whom the tumor Ki-67 proliferation index was available, machine learning analysis of texture-derived parameters from preoperative T2-weighted MRI allowed prediction of which tumors would

Table 1
Utility of T2-weighted magnetic resonance sequences in pituitary imaging

T2-weighted MRI Appearance	Differential Diagnosis	References
Hypointense	Rathke cleft cyst Hypointensity observed in one-third of cases, although hypointense intracystic nodules are present in up to 70% of cases, which are virtually pathognomonic	20

	GH-secreting PA (>50%)
	    Hypointensity typically associated with:
	    • Smaller tumors
	    • Lower tendency to CSI
	    • Greater SSA responsiveness
		20,59,60

	Prolactinoma Hypointensity seen in a subset of cases (up to 20%, especially in men); unclear whether this predicts resistance to DA therapy; may indicate greater likelihood of growth during pregnancy	61
Hyperintense (often strongly)	Hypophysitis For example, lymphocytic/autoimmune, immunotherapy-related or IgG4 disease	20
Hyperintense	Rathke cleft cyst Hyperintensity observed in 70% of cases	20
Hyperintense (mild-moderate)	Prolactinoma (especially microadenomas) In general, degree of hyperintensity does not reliably predict response to DA therapy; accentuation of hyperintensity may occur following DA therapy	61

Hyperintense/ isointense	GH-secreting PA
	    Hyperintensity/isointensity associated with:
	    • Larger tumors
	    • Greater tendency to CSI
	    • Less SSA responsiveness
		20,59,60

Microcystic pattern	Silent corticotroph (macro)adenoma Multiple microcysts (small areas of high-intensity signal covering at least 25% of the tumor) observed in 50%–75% of cases	20,62

Abbreviations: CSI, cavernous sinus invasion; GH, growth hormone; IgG4, immunoglobulin subtype 4.
Data from Refs.[20,59–62]

exhibit a high Ki-67 labeling index.[21] The adoption of a machine learning approach to the analysis of T2-weighted MRI has also been proposed as a means of evaluating macroadenoma consistency (and hence potential ease of resection) before surgery.[22] If substantiated in larger studies, wider rollout of automated image analysis techniques could enable a more personalized approach to initial management and follow-up, using protocols for image acquisition that are already well established in most centers.

MOLECULAR (FUNCTIONAL) IMAGING

Molecular (functional) imaging is an important diagnostic pathway for several endocrine disorders: for example, technetium 99m (^{99m}Tc)-pertechnetate scintigraphy in hyperthyroidism; ^{99m}Tc-sestamibi scintigraphy/single-photon emission computed tomography (SPECT) in hyperparathyroidism; indium-111 (^{111}In)-pentetreotide or (^{99m}Tc)-HYNIC-Ty3-octreotide scintigraphy/SPECT, or Gallium-68 (^{68}Ga)-DOTATATE positron emission tomography (PET)/CT in neuroendocrine tumours (NETs). In addition to identifying the cause/localizing sites of abnormal functioning tissue, in some instances, it can also inform treatment decisions (for example, use of lutetium-177-DOTATATE therapy in patients with metastatic NETs).

In contrast, molecular imaging has not traditionally been considered part of the diagnostic armamentarium for de novo or recurrent PA. Although several groups have explored tracers targeting different cellular pathways and receptor expression, the limitations associated with imaging the sella and parasellar regions using scintigraphy or CT have proved a significant challenge for both accurate PA localization and discrimination of tumor from remaining normal pituitary tissue. However, several recent advances, including coregistration of high-resolution PET-CT with volumetric (1-mm slice) MRI (PET/MR^{CR}) and the advent of PET/MR scanners, have allowed for more accurate localization of the site or sites of tracer uptake and differentiation from physiologic uptake by the remaining normal pituitary gland.

Somatostatin Receptor Imaging

Earlier attempts at imaging PA using tracers targeting somatostatin receptors faltered on several counts, including the relatively poor spatial resolution of scintigraphy (even when combined with CT), variable somatostatin receptor expression of individual tumors, and competing background uptake by normal pituitary tissue. More recently, studies using ^{68}Ga-DOTATATE and ^{68}Ga-DOTATOC have shown greater promise, benefiting from the significantly improved spatial resolution offered by PET. Intriguingly, in 1 study, lower tracer uptake was observed in clinically nonfunctioning PA (7 SF-1 and 2 T-Pit staining tumors) when compared with normal pituitary gland.[23] Moreover, comparing and contrasting appearances from ^{68}Ga-DOTATATE PET with those of ^{18}F-fluorodeoxyglucose (^{18}F-FDG)-PET has been proposed as a means of differentiating recurrent/residual PA from normal pituitary tissue[24,25] and may also inform decision making for aggressive pituitary tumors.[26,27]

Dopamine Receptor Imaging

Prolactin secretion from normal lactotrophs is subject to tonic dopaminergic inhibition, which is predominantly mediated by the dopamine receptor subtype 2.[28] Although several high-affinity ligands for the D2 receptor, which have been used for PET imaging in other clinical contexts (eg, psychiatric disorders), have been deployed for imaging PA,[29,30] to date they have failed to find a role in routine pituitary practice. In part, this likely reflects the relatively limited utility of functional imaging in tumors that are predominantly managed medically, with a high expectation of dopamine agonist (DA) sensitivity. In contrast, in acromegaly, where only approximately 1 in 4 somatotroph adenomas respond to DA therapy, a functional imaging modality capable of predicting response to treatment (as reflected by focal PET tracer uptake) could represent a useful addition to the diagnostic algorithm when considering which patients might benefit from a trial of DA for persistent residual disease.

Fluorine-18-Fluorodeoxyglucose PET

^{18}F-FDG is a well-established PET tracer that finds widespread use in clinical oncology. Importantly, in a large retrospective study, which assessed pituitary uptake in 40,967 subjects undergoing ^{18}F-FDG PET/CT for other indications, focal increased tracer uptake in the pituitary fossa was observed in just 0.073% of cases, several of

Table 2
Alternative magnetic resonance sequences/techniques for pituitary imaging

Indications	MR Sequence/Technique	References
A: Aid to diagnosis		
Distinguish normal pituitary gland from PA or cyst	Magnetic resonance spectroscopy (MRS) Golden-angle radial sparse parallel MRI (GRASP)	63–65
Distinguish PA from vascular lesions (eg, aneurysm, meningioma)	Magnetic resonance angiography (MRA) Perfusion-weighted imaging (PWI)	66 67,68
Detection of apoplexy and cystic lesions	Diffusion-weighted imaging (DWI)	69,70
Localization of corticotroph tumors	7 T (ultra-high field) MRI Fluid-attenuation inversion recovery (FLAIR) Constructive interference in steady state (CISS[a])	71–74
B: Preoperative assessment		
Assessment of tumor consistency	Contrast-enhanced fast imaging employing steady-state acquisition (FIESTA) Magnetic resonance elastography (MRE) Apparent diffusion coefficient (ADC, a subtype of DWI)	75 76 77–83
Assessment of tumor vascularity	PWI	84
Delineation of cavernous sinus structures/tumor invasion	MRA	85,86
Delineation of visual pathways (including optic nerve tractography)	Contrast-enhanced FIESTA 3-Dimensional CISS[a] Diffusion tensor imaging (DTI, an extension of DWI)	87 88 89–91
C: Prediction of treatment outcome		
Response to SSA therapy	MRS	92
Visual outcomes following pituitary surgery	DTI	91
Successful tumor resection at TSS	Apparent diffusion coefficient (ADC, a subtype of DWI)	80,93

[a] CISS denotes a T2 gradient echo sequence.
Data from Refs.[63–93]

whom were subsequently shown to have PA [31]; in a second study with a smaller sample size (13,145 subjects), incidental pituitary uptake was noted in 0.8% of subjects, although a significant proportion of these were not confirmed to represent pathologic uptake on subsequent assessment.[32] Together, these studies point to a likely low risk of false positive scans (<1%) and highlight the importance of referral for endocrine assessment in any patient with incidentally detected pituitary ^{18}F-FDG uptake. In keeping with this, the literature contains numerous examples of different PA subtypes discovered incidentally during ^{18}F-FDG PET/CT (nonfunctioning PA,[33–35] prolactinoma,[36] gonadotropinoma,[37] somatotropinoma,[38,39] and corticotropinoma[40]).

A role for ^{18}F-FDG PET in the detection of de novo and residual/recurrent PA has been explored by several groups. In a prospective study of 24 patients with different subtypes of PA, all macroadenomas (n = 14) and half of microadenomas (n = 5) demonstrated increased tracer uptake.[41] As outlined previously, ^{18}F-FDG PET may also help distinguish residual or recurrent adenoma from remaining normal pituitary tissue following TSS when combined with ^{68}Ga-DOTATATE PET.[24]

However, perhaps the greatest interest in the application of [18]FDG PET in the management of pituitary disease has been in Cushing disease, whereby 30% to 40% of microadenomas may go unidentified on standard clinical MRI. In a study of 12 patients with pituitary Cushing, ^{18}F-FDG PET was found to be comparable to MRI for the localization of corticotroph adenomas with a detection rate of approximately 60%, albeit without complete overlap between the 2 imaging modalities.[42] In a prospective study of 10 patients with Cushing disease, Chittiboina and colleagues[43] were able to show slight superiority of ^{18}F-FDG PET in comparison with conventional SE MRI but, in the same cohort, SPGR MRI was superior to [18]FDG PET. However, more recently the same group has shown that prior stimulation with corticotropin-releasing hormone may enhance the ability of ^{18}F-FDG PET to detect corticotropinomas.[44]

Nitrogen-13-Ammonia PET

[13]N-ammonia has previously been proposed as a marker of pituitary gland perfusion and metabolism, which allows the localization of normal functioning tissue, with reduced/absent uptake following pituitary injury.[45] Perhaps mirroring this, in a single study of ^{13}N-ammonia PET/CT in 48 patients with different PA subtypes (22 non-functioning PA (NFPA), 12 acromegaly, 10 Cushing disease, 4 prolactinomas), higher tracer uptake was observed in normal residual pituitary tissue compared with adenoma (which contrasted with findings on ^{18}F-FDG PET/CT).[46] However, the ability of ^{13}N-ammonia PET/CT to identify the site of normal pituitary tissue was diminished when the maximal tumor diameter exceeded 2 cm.[46]

Fluorine-18-Choline PET

[18]F-Choline, a PET tracer used in the staging and restaging of prostate cancer, is taken up by the normal pituitary gland,[47,48] raising the possibility of a role in imaging PA. However, to date, support for such a role is limited to a small number of case reports of incidentally detected pituitary macroadenomas.[49,50] It is also unclear whether uptake in PA is dependent on cellular proliferation (with incorporation into cell membranes) or reflects other aspects of choline transport/metabolism, as has been proposed for other well-differentiated endocrine tumors.[51]

Carbon-11-Methionine PET

The hallmark of PA is inappropriate peptide synthesis, even in clinically nonfunctioning tumors of the gonadotrope (SF-1) lineage. Accordingly, molecular imaging using a labeled amino acid PET tracer has the immediate attraction of potentially finding application in all PA subtypes. To date, the most studied amino acid tracer in PA is ^{11}C-methionine, which benefits from considerably lower brain uptake (producing a more favorable target-to-background ratio), and increased sensitivity for the detection of PA, when compared with ^{18}F-FDG.[52–54]

Perhaps the single most important recent advance in pituitary imaging using ^{11}C-methionine has been the move to routine coregistration of PET/CT and MRI images

(Met-PET/MRI[CR]), which allows (i) more accurate (anatomic) localization of the site or sites of methionine uptake, and (ii) more reliable distinction between tumoral and normal pituitary tissue tracer uptake[12,54–56]; the advent of PET/MR hybrid scanners will likely further capitalize on these advances.

As with other functional imaging modalities, biochemical assessment of disease status should be performed on the day of the ^{11}C-methionine scan. In addition, patients treated with agents that suppress tumor function require a period of medication washout before imaging (eg, 3 months for somatostatin analogue therapy [SSA] therapy; 4 weeks for DA therapy).

Currently, there are 2 main clinical scenarios when Met-PET/MRI[CR] should be considered:

A. In de novo pituitary disease when targeted intervention (eg, TSS or stereotactic radiosurgery) is being considered, but MRI is either "negative" or equivocal.
B. In patients with persistent/recurrent disease following previous intervention (surgery ± radiotherapy/radiosurgery ± medical therapy), when further targeted intervention would be considered but MRI is unable to reliably identify the site or sites of residual/recurrent disease and/or distinguish from posttreatment change.

Patients in group A include up to 30% of patients with Cushing disease (**Fig. 2**), occasional patients with acromegaly owing to an occult microadenoma (**Fig. 3**), some thyrotropinomas, and a small group of prolactinomas with DA resistance and/or intolerance.[56,57]

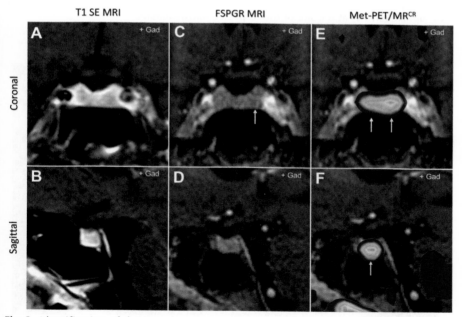

Fig. 2. Identification of the site of an occult microadenoma in Cushing disease. (*A, B*) T1 SE MRI is unable to identify a discrete adenoma. (*C, D*) Volumetric (FSPGR) MRI is also equivocal, but raises the possibility of a subtle area of hypoattenuation in the left side of the gland (*yellow arrow*). (*E, F*) Met-PET/MR[CR] demonstrates focal increased tracer uptake (*yellow arrow*) corresponding to the area seen on volumetric MRI (and subsequently confirmed at TSS); normal physiologic tracer uptake is seen in the right side of the gland (*white arrow*).

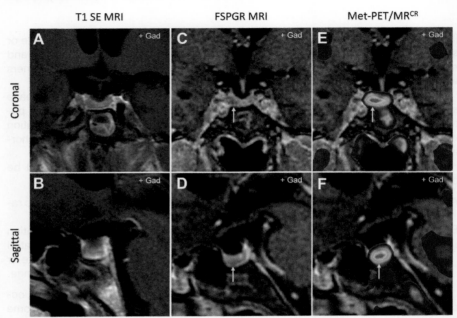

Fig. 3. Identification of the site of an occult microadenoma in acromegaly. (*A, B*) T1 SE MRI demonstrates equivocal findings with no discrete adenoma visualized. (*C, D*) Volumetric (FSPGR) MRI identifies a 5-mm focal hypointensity in the right inferior aspect of the gland (*arrow*) suggestive of a microadenoma. (*E, F*) Met-PET/MR^CR reveals an area of focal high tracer uptake (*arrow*) at the site of the suspected microadenoma.

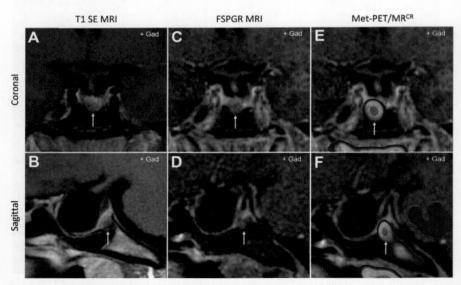

Fig. 4. Localization of the site of early recurrence (at 8 months) following primary surgery in a patient with acromegaly (sparsely granulated tumor; MIB-1 proliferation index = 15%). (*A, B*) T1 SE MRI shows a largely empty sella, but with a possible area of abnormal tissue posterior to the site of insertion of the infundibulum (*arrow*). (*C, D*) Volumetric (FSPGR) MRI demonstrates a similar appearance. (*E, F*) Met-PET/MR^CR shows focal high tracer uptake at the suspected site of recurrence (confirmed at repeat TSS).

T1 SE MRI   FSPGR MRI   Met-PET/MR^{CR}

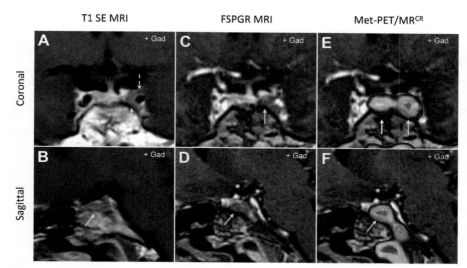

Fig. 5. Localization of the site of late recurrence (at 48 months) following primary surgery in a patient with Cushing disease. (*A, B*) T1 SE MRI demonstrates an area of hypointensity adjacent to (*yellow arrow*), and possibly invading (*yellow dashed arrow*), the left cavernous sinus. (*C, D*) Volumetric (FSPGR) MRI suggests the area of abnormal signal lies medial to the cavernous sinus. (*E, F*) Met-PET/MR^{CR} shows focal high tracer uptake that corresponds with the findings of FSPGR MRI (confirmed at repeat TSS with complete postoperative biochemical remission); normal physiologic tracer uptake is seen in the right side of the gland (*white arrow*).

Although all PA subtypes may be represented in group B, persistence or recurrence of hypercortisolism or acromegaly is the most common reason for referral to the authors' center for Met-PET/MRI^{CR} (**Figs. 4** and **5**).[12,56] Importantly, a significant proportion of patients with acromegaly who were previously deemed unsuitable for further surgical intervention can be offered a repeat transsphenoidal approach following Met-PET/MRI^{CR} with the expectation of achieving full remission or a significant improvement in disease control.[12] More recently, the authors have also shown that subjects with suspected lateral sellar/parasellar disease may derive particular benefits from such an approach.[58]

SUMMARY

For most patients diagnosed with a PA, good-quality T1- ($\pm$ contrast enhancement) and T2-weighted MRI sequences will provide all of the information that is required to facilitate effective and timely decision making. However, imaging of pituitary tumors is an evolving field, both in response to and as a driver of, developments in surgical, radiotherapeutic, and pharmacologic management strategies. Increasing use of alternative MR sequences may aid localization of small functional tumors. Advances in analysis of MRI characteristics have the potential to predict tumor type and response to medical treatment. Molecular (functional) imaging, most clearly demonstrated to date with ¹¹C-methionine PET (Met-PET/MR^{CR}), is potentially able to facilitate curative surgery/radiotherapy (with minimum disruption of normal pituitary function) in an increasing number of scenarios, in both de novo and residual/recurrent pituitary disease. Molecular imaging may also be an aid in predicting response to specific medical therapies. In an era of personalized, precision medicine, imaging has an important and increasing role in decision making in pituitary disease.

DISCLOSURE

The authors have nothing to disclose.

REFERENCES

1. Melmed S. Pituitary-tumor endocrinopathies. N Engl J Med 2020;382(10):937–50. Longo DL, ed.
2. Molitch ME. Pituitary incidentalomas. Best Pract Res Clin Endocrinol Metab 2009; 23(5):667–75.
3. Hall WA. Pituitary magnetic resonance imaging in normal human volunteers: occult adenomas in the general population. Ann Intern Med 1994;120(10):817.
4. Chong BW, Kucharczyk W, Singer W, et al. Pituitary gland MR: a comparative study of healthy volunteers and patients with microadenomas. Am J Neuroradiol 1994;15(4):675–9. Available at: http://www.ncbi.nlm.nih.gov/pubmed/8010269.
5. Vasilev V, Rostomyan L, Daly AF, et al. Pituitary "incidentaloma": neuroradiological assessment and differential diagnosis. Eur J Endocrinol 2016;175(4):R171–84.
6. Daly AF, Rixhon M, Adam C, et al. High prevalence of pituitary adenomas: a cross-sectional study in the province of Liège, Belgium. J Clin Endocrinol Metab 2006;91(12):4769–75.
7. Fernandez A, Karavitaki N, Wass JAH. Prevalence of pituitary adenomas: a community-based, cross-sectional study in Banbury (Oxfordshire, UK). Clin Endocrinol (Oxf) 2010. https://doi.org/10.1111/j.1365-2265.2009.03667.x.
8. Casanueva FF, Barkan AL, Buchfelder M, et al. Criteria for the definition of pituitary tumor centers of excellence (PTCOE): a pituitary society statement. Pituitary 2017;20(5):489–98.
9. Pressman BD. Pituitary imaging. Endocrinol Metab Clin North Am 2017;46(3): 713–40.
10. Bashari WA, Senanayake R, Fernández-Pombo A, et al. Modern imaging of pituitary adenomas. Best Pract Res Clin Endocrinol Metab 2019;33(2):101278.
11. Erickson D, Erickson B, Watson R, et al. 3 Tesla magnetic resonance imaging with and without corticotropin releasing hormone stimulation for the detection of microadenomas in Cushing's syndrome. Clin Endocrinol (Oxf) 2010;72(6):793–9.
12. Koulouri O, Kandasamy N, Hoole AC, et al. Successful treatment of residual pituitary adenoma in persistent acromegaly following localisation by 11C-methionine PET co-registered with MRI. Eur J Endocrinol 2016;175(5):485–98.
13. Bonneville J-F. Magnetic resonance imaging of pituitary tumors. Front Horm Res 2016;45:97–120.
14. Bonneville JF, Bonneville F, Cattin F. Magnetic resonance imaging of pituitary adenomas. Eur Radiol 2005;15(3):543–8.
15. Kasaliwal R, Sankhe SS, Lila AR, et al. Volume interpolated 3D-spoiled gradient echo sequence is better than dynamic contrast spin echo sequence for MRI detection of corticotropin secreting pituitary microadenomas. Clin Endocrinol (Oxf) 2013;78(6):825–30.
16. Grober Y, Grober H, Wintermark M, et al. Comparison of MRI techniques for detecting microadenomas in Cushing's disease. J Neurosurg 2018;128(4):1051–7.
17. McDonald RJ, McDonald JS, Kallmes DF, et al. Gadolinium deposition in human brain tissues after contrast-enhanced MR imaging in adult patients without intracranial abnormalities. Radiology 2017;285(2):546–54.

18. Bussi S, Coppo A, Botteron C, et al. Differences in gadolinium retention after repeated injections of macrocyclic MR contrast agents to rats. J Magn Reson Imaging 2018;47(3):746–52.
19. Nachtigall LB, Karavitaki N, Kiseljak-Vassiliades K, et al. Physicians' awareness of gadolinium retention and MRI timing practices in the longitudinal management of pituitary tumors: a "Pituitary Society" survey. Pituitary 2019;22(1):37–45.
20. Bonneville J-F. A plea for the T2W MR sequence for pituitary imaging. Pituitary 2019;22(2):195–7.
21. Ugga L, Cuocolo R, Solari D, et al. Prediction of high proliferative index in pituitary macroadenomas using MRI-based radiomics and machine learning. Neuroradiology 2019;61(12):1365–73.
22. Zeynalova A, Kocak B, Durmaz ES, et al. Preoperative evaluation of tumour consistency in pituitary macroadenomas: a machine learning-based histogram analysis on conventional T2-weighted MRI. Neuroradiology 2019;61(7):767–74.
23. Tjörnstrand A, Casar-Borota O, Heurling K, et al. Lower 68 Ga-DOTATOC uptake in nonfunctioning pituitary neuroendocrine tumours compared to normal pituitary gland-a proof-of-concept study. Clin Endocrinol (Oxf) 2019. https://doi.org/10.1111/cen.14144.
24. Zhao X, Xiao J, Xing B, et al. Comparison of (68)Ga DOTATATE to 18F-FDG uptake is useful in the differentiation of residual or recurrent pituitary adenoma from the remaining pituitary tissue after transsphenoidal adenomectomy. Clin Nucl Med 2014;39(7):605–8.
25. Wang H, Hou B, Lu L, et al. PET/MRI in the diagnosis of hormone-producing pituitary microadenoma: a prospective pilot study. J Nucl Med 2018;59(3):523–8.
26. Xiao J, Zhu Z, Zhong D, et al. Improvement in diagnosis of metastatic pituitary carcinoma by 68Ga DOTATATE PET/CT. Clin Nucl Med 2015;40(2):e129–31.
27. Garmes HM, Carvalheira JBC, Reis F, et al. Pituitary carcinoma: a case report and discussion of potential value of combined use of Ga-68 DOTATATE and F-18 FDG PET/CT scan to better choose therapy. Surg Neurol Int 2017;8:162.
28. Ferone D, Pivonello R, Lastoria S, et al. In vivo and in vitro effects of octreotide, quinagolide and cabergoline in four hyperprolactinaemic acromegalics: correlation with somatostatin and dopamine D2 receptor scintigraphy. Clin Endocrinol (Oxf) 2001;54(4):469–77. Available at: http://www.ncbi.nlm.nih.gov/pubmed/11318782.
29. Muhr C. Positron emission tomography in acromegaly and other pituitary adenoma patients. Neuroendocrinology 2006;83(3–4):205–10.
30. Bergström M, Muhr C, Lundberg PO, et al. PET as a tool in the clinical evaluation of pituitary adenomas. J Nucl Med 1991;32(4):610–5. Available at: http://www.ncbi.nlm.nih.gov/pubmed/2013801.
31. Jeong SY, Lee S-W, Lee HJ, et al. Incidental pituitary uptake on whole-body 18F-FDG PET/CT: a multicentre study. Eur J Nucl Med Mol Imaging 2010;37(12):2334–43.
32. Hyun SH, Choi JY, Lee K-H, et al. Incidental focal 18F-FDG uptake in the pituitary gland: clinical significance and differential diagnostic criteria. J Nucl Med 2011;52(4):547–50.
33. Maffei P, Marzola MC, Musto A, et al. A very rare case of nonfunctioning pituitary adenoma incidentally disclosed at 18F-FDG PET/CT. Clin Nucl Med 2012;37(5):e100–1.
34. Campeau RJ, David O, Dowling AM. Pituitary adenoma detected on FDG positron emission tomography in a patient with mucosa-associated lymphoid tissue lymphoma. Clin Nucl Med 2003;28(4):296–8.

35. Karapolat İ, Öncel G, Kumanlıoğlu K. Clinically occult pituitary adenoma can appear as a hypermetabolic lesion on whole body FDG PET imaging in a patient with lymphoma. Malecular Imaging Radionucl Ther 2013;22(1):18–20.

36. Gemmel F, Balink H, Collins J, et al. Occult prolactinoma diagnosed by FDG PET/CT. Clin Nucl Med 2010;35(4):269–70.

37. Joshi P, Lele V, Gandhi R. Incidental detection of clinically occult follicle stimulating hormone secreting pituitary adenoma on whole body 18-fluorodeoxyglucose positron emission tomography-computed tomography. Indian J Nucl Med 2011;26(1):34–5.

38. Koo CW, Bhargava P, Rajagopalan V, et al. Incidental detection of clinically occult pituitary adenoma on whole-body FDG PET imaging. Clin Nucl Med 2006; 31(1):42–3.

39. Maiza J-C, Zunic P, Revel C, et al. Acromegaly revealed by 18FDG-PET/CT in a plasmocytoma patient. Pituitary 2012;15(4):614–5.

40. Komori T, Martin WH, Graber AL, et al. Serendipitous detection of Cushing's disease by FDG positron emission tomography and a review of the literature. Clin Nucl Med 2002;27(3):176–8.

41. Seok H, Lee EJY, Choe EY, et al. Analysis of 18F-fluorodeoxyglucose positron emission tomography findings in patients with pituitary lesions. Korean J Intern Med 2013;28(1):81–8.

42. Alzahrani AS, Farhat R, Al-Arifi A, et al. The diagnostic value of fused positron emission tomography/computed tomography in the localization of adrenocorticotropin-secreting pituitary adenoma in Cushing's disease. Pituitary 2009;12(4):309–14.

43. Chittiboina P, Montgomery BK, Millo C, et al. High-resolution18F-fluorodeoxyglucose positron emission tomography and magnetic resonance imaging for pituitary adenoma detection in Cushing disease. J Neurosurg 2015;122(4):791–7.

44. Boyle J, Patronas NJ, Smirniotopoulos J, et al. CRH stimulation improves 18F-FDG-PET detection of pituitary adenomas in Cushing's disease. Endocrine 2019;65(1):155–65.

45. Xiangsong Z, Dianchao Y, Anwu T. Dynamic 13N-ammonia PET: a new imaging method to diagnose hypopituitarism. J Nucl Med 2005;46(1):44–7.

46. Wang Z, Mao Z, Zhang X, et al. Utility of 13N-ammonia PET/CT to detect pituitary tissue in patients with pituitary adenomas. Acad Radiol 2019;26(9):1222–8.

47. Haroon A, Zanoni L, Celli M, et al. Multicenter study evaluating extraprostatic uptake of 11C-choline, 18F-methylcholine, and 18F-ethylcholine in male patients: physiological distribution, statistical differences, imaging pearls, and normal variants. Nucl Med Commun 2015;36(11):1065–75. Available at: https://journals.lww.com/nuclearmedicinecomm/Fulltext/2015/11000/Multicenter_study_evaluating_extraprostatic_uptake.1.aspx.

48. Schillaci O, Calabria F, Tavolozza M, et al. 18F-choline PET/CT physiological distribution and pitfalls in image interpretation: experience in 80 patients with prostate cancer. Nucl Med Commun 2010;31(1):39–45.

49. Maffione AM, Mandoliti G, Pasini F, et al. Pituitary non-functioning adenoma disclosed at 18F-choline PET/CT to investigate a prostate cancer relapse. Clin Nucl Med 2016;41(10):e460–1.

50. Albano D, Bosio G, Bertagna F. Incidental pituitary adenoma detected by 18 F-FDG PET/CT and 18 F-choline PET/CT in the same patient. Rev Esp Med Nucl Imagen Mol 2018;37(4):250–2.

51. van der Hiel B, Stokkel MPM, Buikhuisen WA, et al. 18F-Choline PET/CT as a new tool for functional imaging of non-proliferating secreting neuroendocrine tumors. J Endocrinol Metab 2015;5(4):267–71.

52. Feng Z, He D, Mao Z, et al. Utility of 11C-methionine and 18F-FDG PET/CT in patients with functioning pituitary adenomas. Clin Nucl Med 2016;41(3):e130–4.

53. Tomura N, Saginoya T, Mizuno Y, et al. Accumulation of 11 C-methionine in the normal pituitary gland on 11 C-methionine PET. Acta Radiol 2017;58(3):362–6.

54. Ikeda H, Abe T, Watanabe K. Usefulness of composite methionine–positron emission tomography/3.0-Tesla magnetic resonance imaging to detect the localization and extent of early-stage Cushing adenoma. J Neurosurg 2010;112(4):750–5.

55. Rodriguez-Barcelo S, Gutierrez-Cardo A, Dominguez-Paez M, et al. Clinical usefulness of coregistered 11C-methionine positron emission tomography/3-T magnetic resonance imaging at the follow-up of acromegaly. World Neurosurg 2014; 82(3–4):468–73.

56. Koulouri O, Steuwe A, Gillett D, et al. A role for 11C-methionine PET imaging in ACTH-dependent Cushing's syndrome. Eur J Endocrinol 2015;173(4):M107–20.

57. Koulouri O, Hoole AC, English P, et al. Localisation of an occult thyrotropinoma with 11 C-methionine PET-CT before and after somatostatin analogue therapy. Lancet Diabetes Endocrinol 2016;4(12):1050.

58. Bashari W, Senanayake R, Koulouri O, et al. PET-guided repeat transsphenoidal surgery for previously deemed unresectable lateral disease in acromegaly. Neurosurg Focus 2020;48(6):E8.

59. Potorac I, Beckers A, Bonneville J-F. T2-weighted MRI signal intensity as a predictor of hormonal and tumoral responses to somatostatin receptor ligands in acromegaly: a perspective. Pituitary 2017;20(1):116–20.

60. Heck A, Emblem KE, Casar-Borota O, et al. Quantitative analyses of T2-weighted MRI as a potential marker for response to somatostatin analogs in newly diagnosed acromegaly. Endocrine 2016;52(2):333–43.

61. Varlamov EV, Hinojosa-Amaya JM, Fleseriu M. Magnetic resonance imaging in the management of prolactinomas; a review of the evidence. Pituitary 2020; 23(1):16–26.

62. Cazabat L, Dupuy M, Boulin A, et al. Silent, but not unseen: multimicrocystic aspect on T2-weighted MRI in silent corticotroph adenomas. Clin Endocrinol (Oxf) 2014;81(4):566–72.

63. Chernov MF, Kawamata T, Amano K, et al. Possible role of single-voxel 1H-MRS in differential diagnosis of suprasellar tumors. J Neurooncol 2009;91(2):191–8.

64. Pînzariu O, Georgescu B, Georgescu CE. Metabolomics—a promising approach to pituitary adenomas. Front Endocrinol (Lausanne) 2019;9:814.

65. Hainc N, Stippich C, Reinhardt J, et al. Golden-angle radial sparse parallel (GRASP) MRI in clinical routine detection of pituitary microadenomas: first experience and feasibility. Magn Reson Imaging 2019;60:38–43.

66. Manara R, Maffei P, Citton V, et al. Increased rate of intracranial saccular aneurysms in acromegaly: an MR angiography study and review of the literature. J Clin Endocrinol Metab 2011;96(5):1292–300.

67. Hakyemez B, Yildirim N, Erdoðan C, et al. Meningiomas with conventional MRI findings resembling intraaxial tumors: can perfusion-weighted MRI be helpful in differentiation? Neuroradiology 2006;48(10):695–702.

68. Bladowska J, Zimny A, Guziński M, et al. Usefulness of perfusion weighted magnetic resonance imaging with signal-intensity curves analysis in the differential diagnosis of sellar and parasellar tumors: preliminary report. Eur J Radiol 2013; 82(8):1292–8.

69. Rogg JM, Tung GA, Anderson G, et al. Pituitary apoplexy: early detection with diffusion-weighted MR imaging. AJNR Am J Neuroradiol 2002;23(7):1240–5. Available at: http://www.ncbi.nlm.nih.gov/pubmed/12169486. Accessed April 23, 2019.

70. Kunii N, Abe T, Kawamo M, et al. Rathke's cleft cysts: differentiation from other cystic lesions in the pituitary fossa by use of single-shot fast spin-echo diffusion-weighted MR imaging. Acta Neurochir (Wien) 2007;149(8):759–69.

71. de Rotte AAJ, Groenewegen A, Rutgers DR, et al. High resolution pituitary gland MRI at 7.0 Tesla: a clinical evaluation in Cushing's disease. Eur Radiol 2016;26(1):271–7.

72. Patel V, Liu CSJ, Shiroishi MS, et al. Ultra-high field magnetic resonance imaging for localization of corticotropin-secreting pituitary adenomas. Neuroradiology 2020.

73. Chatain GP, Patronas N, Smirniotopoulos JG, et al. Potential utility of FLAIR in MRI-negative Cushing's disease. J Neurosurg 2018;129(3):620–8.

74. Lang M, Habboub G, Moon D, et al. Comparison of constructive interference in steady-state and T1-weighted MRI sequence at detecting pituitary adenomas in Cushing's disease patients. J Neurol Surg B Skull Base 2018;79(06):593–8.

75. Yamamoto J, Kakeda S, Shimajiri S, et al. Tumor consistency of pituitary macroadenomas: predictive analysis on the basis of imaging features with contrast-enhanced 3D FIESTA at 3T. Am J Neuroradiol 2014;35(2):297–303.

76. Hughes JD, Fattahi N, Van Gompel J, et al. Magnetic resonance elastography detects tumoral consistency in pituitary macroadenomas. Pituitary 2016;19(3):286–92.

77. Pierallini A, Caramia F, Falcone C, et al. Pituitary macroadenomas: preoperative evaluation of consistency with diffusion-weighted MR imaging—initial experience. Radiology 2006;239(1):223–31.

78. Suzuki C, Maeda M, Hori K, et al. Apparent diffusion coefficient of pituitary macroadenoma evaluated with line-scan diffusion-weighted imaging. J Neuroradiol 2007;34(4):228–35.

79. Mahmoud OM, Tominaga A, Amatya VJ, et al. Role of PROPELLER diffusion-weighted imaging and apparent diffusion coefficient in the evaluation of pituitary adenomas. Eur J Radiol 2011;80(2):412–7.

80. Alimohamadi M, Sanjari R, Mortazavi A, et al. Predictive value of diffusion-weighted MRI for tumor consistency and resection rate of nonfunctional pituitary macroadenomas. Acta Neurochir (Wien) 2014;156(12):2245–52.

81. Yiping L, Ji X, Daoying G, et al. Prediction of the consistency of pituitary adenoma: a comparative study on diffusion-weighted imaging and pathological results. J Neuroradiol 2016;43(3):186–94.

82. Wang M, Liu H, Wei X, et al. Application of reduced-FOV diffusion-weighted imaging in evaluation of normal pituitary glands and pituitary macroadenomas. AJNR Am J Neuroradiol 2018;39(8):1499–504.

83. Sanei Taheri M, Kimia F, Mehrnahad M, et al. Accuracy of diffusion-weighted imaging-magnetic resonance in differentiating functional from non-functional pituitary macro-adenoma and classification of tumor consistency. Neuroradiol J 2019;32(2):74–85.

84. Ma Z, He W, Zhao Y, et al. Predictive value of PWI for blood supply and T1-spin echo MRI for consistency of pituitary adenoma. Neuroradiology 2016;58(1):51–7.

85. Linn J, Peters F, Lummel N, et al. Detailed imaging of the normal anatomy and pathologic conditions of the cavernous region at 3 Tesla using a contrast-enhanced MR angiography. Neuroradiology 2011;53(12):947–54.

86. Micko ASG, Wöhrer A, Wolfsberger S, et al. Invasion of the cavernous sinus space in pituitary adenomas: endoscopic verification and its correlation with an MRI-based classification. J Neurosurg 2015;122(4):803–11.
87. Watanabe K, Kakeda S, Yamamoto J, et al. Delineation of optic nerves and chiasm in close proximity to large suprasellar tumors with contrast-enhanced FIESTA MR imaging. Radiology 2012;264(3):852–8.
88. Suprasanna K, Vinay Kumar KM, Kumar A, et al. Comparison of pituitary stalk angle, inter-neural angle and optic tract angle in relation to optic chiasm location on 3-dimensional magnetic resonance imaging. J Clin Neurosci 2019;64:169–73.
89. Yu CS, Li KC, Xuan Y, et al. Diffusion tensor tractography in patients with cerebral tumors: a helpful technique for neurosurgical planning and postoperative assessment. Eur J Radiol 2005;56(2):197–204.
90. Salmela MB, Cauley KA, Nickerson JP, et al. Magnetic resonance diffusion tensor imaging (MRDTI) and tractography in children with septo-optic dysplasia. Pediatr Radiol 2010;40(5):708–13.
91. Anik I, Anik Y, Cabuk B, et al. Visual outcome of an endoscopic endonasal transsphenoidal approach in pituitary macroadenomas: quantitative assessment with diffusion tensor imaging early and long-term results. World Neurosurg 2018;112: e691–701.
92. Hu J, Yan J, Zheng X, et al. Magnetic resonance spectroscopy may serve as a presurgical predictor of somatostatin analog therapy response in patients with growth hormone-secreting pituitary macroadenomas. J Endocrinol Invest 2019; 42(4):443–51.
93. Hassan HA, Bessar MA, Herzallah IR, et al. Diagnostic value of early postoperative MRI and diffusion-weighted imaging following trans-sphenoidal resection of non-functioning pituitary macroadenomas. Clin Radiol 2018;73(6):535–41.

World Health Ozganization 2017 Classification of Pituitary Tumors

M. Beatriz S. Lopes, MD, PhD

KEYWORDS

- Pituitary gland • Pituitary adenoma • Pituitary neuroendocrine tumor
- Immunohistochemistry

KEY POINTS

- Pituitary neuroendocrine tumors are histologically classified according to adenohypophyseal cell lineage by assessment of specific pituitary hormones and transcription factors.
- Assessment of tumor proliferative potential by mitotic count and Ki-67 index is recommended in individual cases.
- Although most of the pituitary neuroendocrine tumors are benign neoplasm with a slow growing pattern, continuing efforts for detection of the small subset of aggressive tumors with new prognostic biomarkers are strongly recommended.

INTRODUCTION

The fourth edition of the World Health Organization (WHO) Classification of Tumors of the Pituitary Gland was released in 2017 (**Table 1**).[1] Several changes are recommended in the pathologic classification of tumors, in addition to description of new entities and redefinition of old entities. These changes include the following: (1) a novel approach for classifying pituitary neuroendocrine tumors according to adenohypophyseal cell lineages; (2) changes on the histologic grading of pituitary neuroendocrine tumors with the elimination of the term *atypical adenoma*; (3) changes in the classification of non-neuroendocrine pituitary tumors, including those tumors arising in the posterior pituitary; and (4) introduction of new entities.

In this review, the author focuses on the changes of tumors of the anterior pituitary gland, that is, pituitary neuroendocrine tumors. The reader is referred to the WHO Endocrine Tumors and Nervous System Tumors books for review of the non-neuroendocrine tumors and other tumors involving the pituitary gland.[1,2]

Department of Pathology, University of Virginia School of Medicine, 1215 Lee Street – Room 3060-HEP, Charlottesville, VA 22908-0214, USA
E-mail address: msl2e@virginia.edu

Endocrinol Metab Clin N Am 49 (2020) 375–386
https://doi.org/10.1016/j.ecl.2020.05.001
0889-8529/20/© 2020 Elsevier Inc. All rights reserved.

Table 1
2017 World Health Organization classification of pituitary adenomas

Adenoma Type	Morphologic Variants	Pituitary Hormones and Other Immunomarkers	Transcription Factors and Other Cofactors
Lactotroph adenomas	Sparsely granulated adenoma[a]	PRL	PIT-1, ERα
	Densely granulated adenoma	PRL	PIT-1, ERα
	Acidophilic stem cell adenoma	PRL, GH (focal and variable)	PIT-1, ERα
Somatotroph adenomas	Densely granulated adenoma[a]	GH ± PRL ± α-SU CK[b] perinuclear staining	PIT-1
	Sparsely granulated adenoma	GH ± PRL CK[b] highlights fibrous bodies	PIT-1
	Mammosomatotroph adenoma	GH + PRL (in same cells) ± α-SU	PIT-1, ERα
	Mixed somatotroph-lactotroph adenoma	GH + PRL (in different cells) ± α-SU	PIT-1, ERα
Thyrotroph adenomas		β-TSH, α-SU	PIT-1
Corticotroph Adenomas	Densely granulated adenoma[a]	ACTH	T-PIT
	Sparsely granulated adenoma	ACTH	T-PIT
	Crooke cell adenoma	ACTH CK[b] forming ringlike appearance	T-PIT
Gonadotroph adenoma		β-FSH, β-LH, α-SU (various combinations)	SF-1, GATA3, ERα
Null cell adenoma	Oncocytic variant	None or focal α-SU	None
Plurihormonal adenomas	Plurihormonal PIT-1 positive adenoma	GH, PRL, β-TSH ± α-SU	PIT-1
	Adenomas with unusual immunohistochemical combinations	Various combinations: ACTH/GH, ACTH/PRL	N/A

Abbreviation: ER-α, estrogen receptor alpha.
[a] Most common variant.
[b] CK = cytokeratin CAM5.2.
Reprinted from Osamura RY, Lopes MBS, Grossman A, et al. Introduction. In: Lloyd RV, Osamura RY, Klöppel G, Rosai J editors. WHO Classification of Tumours of Endocrine Organs. 4th Edition. Lyon, France: IARC Press; 2017:13-63; with permission.

GENERAL PRINCIPLES OF THE 2017 WHO CLASSIFICATION OF PITUITARY NEUROENDOCRINE TUMORS

Pituitary neuroendocrine tumors are classified in *pituitary adenomas* and *pituitary carcinomas*. Pituitary adenomas constitute most of the tumors arising in the pituitary gland and have been historically classified by their histopathological features, pituitary hormone content of the tumor cells as assessed by immunohistochemistry, and ultrastructural features of the tumor cells. A major change in the new WHO classification is the adaptation of a pituitary adenohypophyseal cell lineage as the main principle for classification of neuroendocrine tumors.

Several transcription factors and other differentiation driving factors have been described in the last decades as key players in the cellular differentiation of the adenohypophysis. These transcription factors are essential for differentiation and maturation of the neuroendocrine cells from the Rathke's pouch leading to 3 main cell lineages: the acidophilic, the gonadotroph, and the corticotroph lineages.[3,4] Three of these transcription factors are significant for clinicopathological practice due to their consistent expression in human pituitary tissues including PIT-1 (pituitary-specific POU-class homeodomain transcription factor) that leads differentiation of somatotrophs, lactotrophs, and thyrotrophs; SF-1 (steroidogenic factor 1) that regulates gonadotroph cell differentiation; and T-PIT (T-box family member TBX19) that drives the proopiomelanocortin lineage with differentiation of corticotrophs.[5-10] With this new paradigm, the 2017 WHO classification categorizes adenomas according to their pituitary cell lineage rather than a hormone-producing pituitary adenoma. Details of the different adenoma types and variants are described on **Table 1**.

The WHO recommends a stepwise method for the application of the new classification by means of immunohistochemistry for the main pituitary hormones and, when necessary, pituitary transcription factors and other factors. An initial panel of antibodies for pituitary hormones should be applied, including growth hormone (GH), prolactin (PRL), adrenocorticoptrohic hormone (ACTH), luteinizing hormone β (β-LH), follicle-stimulating hormone β (β-FSH), thyroid stimulating hormone β (β-TSH), and α-subunit of glycoproteins (α-SU). If a tumor is still not classifiable by the pituitary hormone expression according to a cell lineage, immunostaining for transcriptions factors—PIT-1, SF-1, and T-PIT—should be applied.

The use of pituitary transcription factor immunohistochemistry is critical in particular situations including the following: (1) when an adenoma exhibits focal/weak immunostaining for pituitary hormones (eg, SF-1 staining in an adenoma expressing only focal/weak α-SU); (2) performing the diagnosis of a null cell adenoma, now classified as an adenoma immunonegative for pituitary hormones and transcription factors; and (3) when the presence of a pituitary transcription factor is inherent to a tumor definition (eg, plurihormonal PIT-1-positive adenoma).

Additional immunohistochemical stains are helpful for the subclassification of adenomas in variants or subtypes. For instance, low-molecular-weight cytokeratin is very helpful in identifying corticotroph cell differentiation and Crooke's hyaline changes. In addition, cytokeratin highlights fibrous bodies in sparsely granulated somatotroph and acidophilic stem cell adenomas (see example on **Fig. 1**).[11] Immunostaining for estrogen receptor-α, a steroid receptor expressed in lactotroph and gonadotroph cells,[7] may be helpful in confirming lactotroph differentiation in mammosomatotroph adenomas, tumors that display somatotroph and lactotroph differentiation, and have a lesser cure rate than somatotroph adenomas (see example on **Fig. 2**).[7,12] GATA3 immunohistochemistry may be used as a surrogate for the expression of GATA2, a

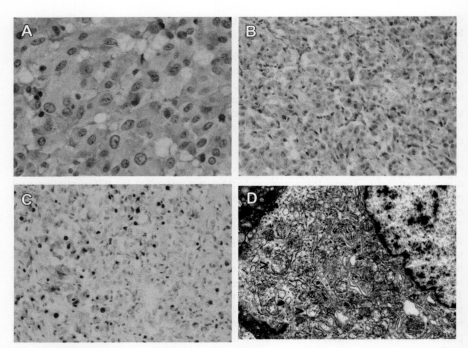

Fig. 1. *Acidophilic stem cell adenoma*—acidophilic stem cell adenoma (ASCA) is a rare sub-type of lactotroph adenoma accounting for the minority of clinically diagnosed prolactin-secreting adenomas.[51] Patients have varying degrees of hyperprolactinemia, but elevated growth hormone (GH) and insulin growth factor I (IGF-1) values may also be present.[24] Most of these tumors are rapidly growing macroadenomas with invasive features and behave more aggressively than any lactotroph adenoma with a lower surgical cure rate.[12,51] The tumors are characterized by cells with acidophilic cytoplasm with focal oncocytic changes (*A*). Immunostaining for PRL is variable with cells displaying both Golgi-pattern and more diffuse reactivity (*B*). Unlike lactotroph adenomas, ASCA display perinuclear, dotlike fibrous bodies confirmed by cytokeratin staining (*C*). A characteristic feature of ASCA is accumulation of mitochondria with sometimes dilated giant forms by ultrastructure (*D; arrowheads*).

transcription factor implicated in the development and function of thyrotrophs and gonadotrophs.[13]

With the combination of morphology and immunohistochemical markers, there is essentially minimal need for ultrastructural analysis for the classification of the adenomas.

REVIEW OF SPECIFIC PITUITARY NEUROENDOCRINE TUMORS
Gonadotroph Adenomas

Most gonadotroph adenomas are clinically nonfunctioning tumors with absence of hormone overproduction; clinically active gonadotroph adenomas are rare tumors. Despite the lack of clinical evidence of hormone hypersecretion, these adenomas express the gonadotropin hormones by immunohistochemistry in a variable and differential expression in addition to the transcription factor SF-1.[8,14]

The histologic features of gonadotroph adenomas are exemplified on **Fig. 3**. Immunohistochemistry demonstrates variable degrees and combinations of β-FSH, β-LH,

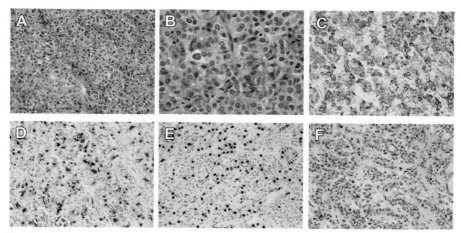

Fig. 2. *Mammosomatotroph adenoma*—mammosomatotroph adenoma (MSA) is quite similar to densely granulated somatotroph adenoma by H&E stain (*A*). The tumor cells are large, acidophilic, and with large central nucleus with prominent nucleoli (*B*). MSA displays immunoreactivity for GH (*C*) and PRL (*D*) in the same tumor cell. Lactotroph differentiation is confirmed by ER-α nuclear expression (*E*). MSA is strongly positive for PIT-1 (*F*).

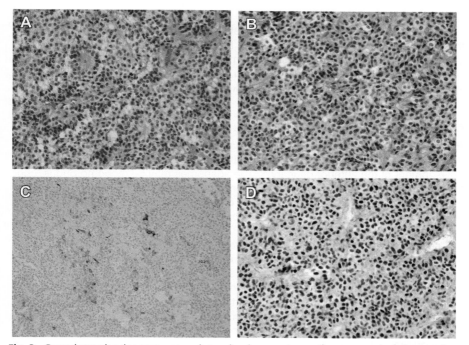

Fig. 3. *Gonadotroph adenoma*—gonadotroph adenoma is mostly composed of chromophobic cells arranged in several histologic arrangements including papillary formations, nests, and sinusoids (*A*, *B*). Immunostaining for the gonadotropins is variable; in this example, only focal and faint α-SU is present (*C*), but gonadotroph differentiation is confirmed by strong SF-1 immunoexpression (*D*).

and α-SU expression.[15] This uneven reactivity for the glycoprotein hormones has been of concern when distinguishing gonadotroph adenomas from null cell adenoma because the latter may display focal and weak α-subunit immunoreactivity.[16,17] Immunohistochemistry for SF-1 and/or GATA3 is an additional tool for characterization of gonadotroph adenomas, in particular in those cases in which glycoprotein hormones immunostaining is faint or uncertain.[13] In addition, several gonadotroph adenomas lack expression of hormones but express SF-1 only.[14]

Null Cell Adenomas

The introduction of new markers with more specific pituitary cell lineage differentiation has prompted a new definition of null cell adenomas by the 2017 WHO classification. They are now defined as tumors that do not exhibit expression for both pituitary hormones and pituitary transcription factors essential for cell lineage differentiation.[18] This new definition emphasizes the concept that "weakly immunoreactive" or "hormone-immunonegative" adenomas may display cell lineage differentiation by specific transcription factor and other cofactor expression.

The incidence of this newly defined null cell adenomas is unknown. In a large referral center-based series,[19] these adenomas represented 4.5% of surgical cases. Although only a few small series of cases using the new WHO classification guidelines have been reported, the clinical and laboratory features of the tumors are similar to gonadotroph adenomas[20,21]; most of them are macroadenomas with about half of the tumors showing cavernous sinus invasion at presentation.[21] Long-term follow-up of this newly defined group of adenomas is not yet available, and clinical behavior of these tumors has yet to be investigated.

Histologically, null cell adenomas are mostly chromophobic at light microscopy, and the tumor cells can be arranged in several histologic patterns and may demonstrate oncocytic changes.[18] The adenomas lack immunoreactivity for any pituitary hormone, but focal α-subunit reactivity may be seen.[14,18,19] By definition, the adenomas lack specific cytodifferentiation lineage with lack of expression of the transcription factors PIT-1, SF-1, and T-PIT.[18]

Plurihormonal and Double Adenomas

Plurihormonal adenomas are rare tumors that have unusual immunoreactivity for more than one type of pituitary hormone class that are unrelated by normal cytogenesis and development of the anterior pituitary.[22] The adenomas may be monomorphous, consisting of 1 cell type producing more than one hormone, or plurimorphous, composed of 2 (or more) distinct cells, each producing different hormones.[22] Rarely these tumors are functioning adenomas[23,24]; the majority are silent, clinically nonfunctioning adenomas.[22]

A newly defined entity is the *plurihormonal PIT-1 positive adenoma*.[22] This is a rare adenoma characterized by a monomorphous population of cells that express variable levels of GH, PRL, β-TSH, and α-SU.[22] This adenoma has been previously called silent adenoma subtype 3.[25–27] Most plurihormonal PIT-1-positive adenomas are clinically silent, although some patients may present with acromegaly, hyperprolactinemia, or hyperthyroidism.[25–27] Their recognition is of significance due to their intrinsic aggressive behavior with high degree of invasiveness, low rates of disease-free survival, and high tendency for recurrence.[25–27]

Double adenomas are composed of 2 distinct pituitary adenomas of different cell lineage.[22] Rare multiple (more than 2) distinct adenomas have also been described.[28] Although these rare cases of multiple adenomas may be clinically evident, cases are more commonly found incidentally at autopsies.[28]

Pituitary Carcinomas

Pituitary carcinomas are very rare, comprising less than 1% of all pituitary neoplasms.[29,30] Pituitary carcinomas are defined by demonstration of craniospinal dissemination and/or systemic metastases.[29,31] It is exceptionally rare for a pituitary carcinoma to present with synchronous metastasis. These tumors most commonly evolve from invasive, aggressive adenomas that recur over several years rather than presenting as *de novo* neoplasm. Most cases are endocrinologically functioning tumors; the most common are lactotroph tumors with hyperprolactinemia, followed by corticotroph tumors in the setting of Cushing disease.[29] Other subtypes of adenomas are less common and constitute about 20% of cases.[29]

No histologic features can distinguish a pituitary carcinoma from ordinary typical adenoma before metastasis; therefore, the diagnosis is based solely on the presence of metastasis. Standard morphologic features associated with malignancy including hypercellularity, nuclear and cellular pleomorphism, increased mitotic activity, and necrosis may be identified but are not necessarily present in the initial sellar tumor. Likewise, dural or bony invasion may be not necessarily present.[29] Ki-67 labeling indices are quite variable, with considerable overlap with ordinary pituitary adenomas, but some sellar primary tumors may show elevated Ki-67 labeling ($\geq$10%).[30]

PATHOLOGIC GRADING OF PITUITARY NEUROENDOCRINE TUMORS

A major change in the new WHO classification focused on the histologic grading of pituitary neuroendocrine tumors.[31] The current WHO classification grading scheme consists of pituitary adenomas and carcinomas. As discussed previously, no changes have been recommended for the diagnosis of *pituitary carcinomas*, and it is based on the presence of cerebrospinal and/or systemic metastasis.

Significantly, the new classification has abandoned the terminology *atypical adenoma* as defined by the 2004 WHO,[32] due to the lack of clinical evidence for a prognostic value of the diagnosis including lack of clinically aggressive behavior between typical and atypical adenomas.[33-37] The 2017 WHO classification did not introduce a new tumor grading system. Significance is given on evaluation of tumor proliferation (mitotic count and Ki-67 labeling index) and tumor invasion, both features that have been shown to correlate with a more aggressive tumor behavior.[33,37,38] However, no specific Ki-67 cut-off value is recommended. Moreover, it does not recommend p53 immunostaining on a regular basis due to the lack of evidence as a prognostic parameter.

In addition to the changes discussed earlier, important recommendation of the WHO in terms of "grading" is the recognition of special histologic variants that have shown a more aggressive clinical behavior. These variants of adenomas are considered "high-risk" pituitary adenomas. These tumors include the sparsely granulated somatotroph adenomas, the silent corticotroph adenoma (**Fig. 4**), the Crooke cell adenoma, the plurihormonal PIT-1 positive adenoma, and lactotroph adenomas in men.[31] Clinicians and surgeons should be alerted of these specific diagnoses.

As discussed earlier, most of the pituitary adenomas are benign, slow-growing tumors that show a very slow relapse rate over many years after surgical treatment. In a large series of nonfunctioning adenomas reported by Reddy and colleagues,[39] recurrence rates after complete surgical resection and lack of radiation therapy treatment was 6.9% after a mean follow-up of 9.1 years. Significantly, about 20% of recurrences in that series occurred after more than 10 years of follow-up.[39] Conversely, reports of complete tumor resection at first surgery indicates an overall success between 64.5%

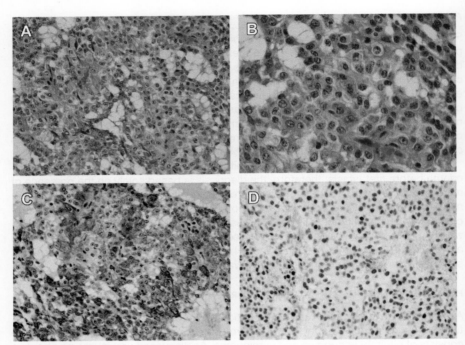

Fig. 4. *Corticotroph adenoma, clinically silent*—silent corticotroph adenoma may show features of a basophilic densely granulated adenoma with strong immunoreactivity for ACTH (silent corticotroph subtype 1) like this example (*A*) or may be more chromophobic and sparsely granulated adenomas with only focal immunoreactivity for ACTH (silent corticotroph subtype 2).[52] The cells may contain hyperchromatic nuclei with chromatin knobs, a feature seen mostly in functioning tumors (*B*). Immunostaining for ACTH (*C*) and T-PIT (*D*) is variable. Immunohistochemistry is variably for ACTH (*C*) and the transcription factor T-PIT (*D*).[14] Rarely, some silent adenomas lack ACTH immunoexpression but express the transcription factor T-PIT.[14]

and 69% in microscopic series and endoscopic series, respectively.[40] Therefore, a considerable percentage of patients with pituitary adenomas requires continued clinical surveillance and may need adjuvant treatment.

A small subset of pituitary adenomas may show a more aggressive clinical behavior that deviates from the benign behavior of a typical adenoma displaying early and multiple recurrences despite multimodal therapy including conventional treatment and radiation therapy.[41] The prevalence of these so-called *clinically aggressive pituitary adenomas* is unknown likely due to the variable definition of clinically aggressive adenomas in the literature.[37,41–43]

The identification of clinically aggressive adenomas in a prospective manner is complex. Prognostic predictors of tumor aggressive behavior are not well established and, despite numerous studies and advances in prognostic classification, no single pathologic marker has been shown to reliably predict pituitary adenoma behavior. Many studies have shown that several parameters including clinical and radiological features, tumor cell lineage subtype, tumor proliferation, and tumor invasiveness may need to be integrated for better prediction of "high-risk" pituitary adenomas.[37,38,44–46]

THE POST-WHO CLASSIFICATION

Since the release of the 2017 WHO classification, a few changes have been proposed by pituitary pathologists, endocrinologists, and neurosurgeons regarding classification and grading of pituitary tumors.[47] In particular, it has been proposed to change the nomenclature of pituitary adenomas to pituitary neuroendocrine tumors (PitNETs).[47] The rationale for these changes relies on the idea that "pituitary endocrine neoplasms exhibit a spectrum of behaviors that are not entirely benign and can cause significant morbidity, even when they are not metastatic."[47] Consequently, "the term 'adenoma', which defines a tumor as benign, does not seem appropriate to define aggressive and invasive pituitary tumors that cannot be resected and are refractory to therapy."[47] In addition, "this terminology would incorporate some of the basic principles of the pathology of neuroendocrine tumors of other anatomic locations and would reduce inconsistencies and contradictions among the various systems currently in use, allowing unification of classification concepts, despite organ-specific differences in classification criteria, tumor biology, and prognostic factors."[48]

Therefore, it has been proposed that pituitary neuroendocrine tumors be classified as NETs, that is, PitNETs rather than adenomas and carcinomas.[48] Although this nomenclature change has been a matter of controversy among members of Pathology and other specialties societies,[47,49,50] it is likely that future WHO Books will use the new classification system.[48]

SUMMARY

The 2017 WHO classification of tumors of the pituitary gland provides robust guidelines for the diagnosis of pituitary neuroendocrine tumors and other less common tumors involving the pituitary gland and sellar region. Pituitary adenomas are classified by specific cell lineage differentiation by using immunohistochemistry as the main ancillary diagnostic tool. Attempts for identification of potentially aggressive adenomas should be made on an individual basis using considerations of the adenoma subtype, proliferative potential, and tumor invasion assessment when available. In addition, the WHO emphasizes recognition of "high-risk" adenoma variants that have intrinsic substantial risk for recurrence and worse clinical behavior. Significantly, the WHO emphasizes the need for a more integrated diagnosis of pituitary neuroendocrine tumors with input of other disciplines in addition to pathology and discussion of the cases at multidisciplinary conferences.

DISCLOSURE

The author has nothing to disclose.

REFERENCES

1. Lloyd RV, Osamura RY, Klöppel G, et al, editors. WHO classification of tumours of endocrine organs. 4th edition. Lyon (France): IARC Press; 2017.
2. Louis DN, Hiroko O, Wiestler OD, et al, editors. WHO classification of tumours of the central nervous system. Revised 4th edition. Lyon (France): IARC Press; 2016.
3. Scully KM, Rosenfeld MG. Pituitary development: regulatory codes in mammalian organogenesis. Science 2002;295:2231–5.
4. Zhu X, Rosenfeld MG. Transcriptional control of precursor proliferation in the early phases of pituitary development. Curr Opin Genet Dev 2004;14:567–74.

5. Friend KE, Chiou YK, Laws ER Jr, et al. Pit-1 messenger ribonucleic acid is differentially expressed in human pituitary adenomas. J Clin Endocrinol Metab 1993; 77:1281–6.

6. Asa SL, Puy LA, Lew AM, et al. Cell type-specific expression of the pituitary transcription activator pit-1 in the human pituitary and pituitary adenomas. J Clin Endocrinol Metab 1993;77:1275–80.

7. Friend KE, Chiou YK, Lopes MB, et al. Estrogen receptor expression in human pituitary: correlation with immunohistochemistry in normal tissue, and immunohistochemistry and morphology in macroadenomas. J Clin Endocrinol Metab 1994; 78:1497–504.

8. Asa SL, Bamberger AM, Cao B, et al. The transcription activator steroidogenic factor-1 is preferentially expressed in the human pituitary gonadotroph. J Clin Endocrinol Metab 1996;81:2165–70.

9. Lloyd RV, Osamura RY. Transcription factors in normal and neoplastic pituitary tissues. Microsc Res Tech 1997;39:168–81.

10. Umeoka K, Sanno N, Osamura RY, et al. Expression of GATA-2 in human pituitary adenomas. Mod Pathol 2002;15:11–7.

11. Coons SW, Estrada SI, Gamez R, et al. Cytokeratin CK 7 and CK 20 expression in pituitary adenomas. Endocr Pathol 2005;16:201–10.

12. Kreutzer J, Vance ML, Lopes MB, et al. Surgical management of GH-secreting pituitary adenomas: an outcome study using modern remission criteria. J Clin Endocrinol Metab 2001;86:4072–7.

13. Mete O, Kefeli M, Çalışkan S, et al. GATA3 immunoreactivity expands the transcription factor profile of pituitary neuroendocrine tumors. Mod Pathol 2019;32: 484–9.

14. Nishioka H, Inoshita N, Mete O, et al. The complementary role of transcription factors in the accurate diagnosis of clinically nonfunctioning pituitary adenomas. Endocr Pathol 2015;26:349–55.

15. Yamada S, Osamura RY, Righi A, et al. Gonadotroph adenoma. In: Lloyd RV, Osamura RY, Klöppel G, et al, editors. Tumours of the pituitary gland. WHO classification of tumours of endocrine organs. 4th edition. Lyon (France): IARC Press; 2017. p. 34–6.

16. Sanno N, Teramoto A, Sugiyama M, et al. Application of catalyzed signal amplification in immunodetection of gonadotropin subunits in clinically nonfunctioning pituitary adenomas. Am J Clin Pathol 1996;106:16–21.

17. Yamada S, Sano T, Takahashi M, et al. Immunohistochemical heterogeneity within clinically nonfunctioning pituitary adenomas. Endocr Pathol 1995;6:217–21.

18. Nishioka H, Kontogeorgos G, Lloyd RV, et al. Null cell adenoma. In: Lloyd RV, Osamura RY, Klöppel G, et al, editors. Tumours of the pituitary gland. WHO classification of endocrine tumors. 4th edition. Lyon (France): IARC Press; 2017. p. 37–8.

19. Mete O, Cintosun A, Pressman I, et al. Epidemiology and biomarker profile of pituitary adenohypophysial tumors. Mod Pathol 2018;31:900–9.

20. Balogun JA, Monsalves E, Juraschka K, et al. Null cell adenomas of the pituitary gland: an institutional review of their clinical imaging and behavioral characteristics. Endocr Pathol 2015;26:63–70.

21. Almeida JP, Stephens CC, Eschbacher JM, et al. Clinical, pathologic, and imaging characteristics of pituitary null cell adenomas as defined according to the 2017 World Health Organization criteria: a case series from two pituitary centers. Pituitary 2019;22:514–9.

22. Kontogeorgos G, Kovacs K, Lloyd RV, et al. Plurihormonal and double adenomas. In: Lloyd RV, Osamura RY, Klöppel G, et al, editors. Tumours of the pituitary gland. WHO classification of endocrine tumors. 4th edition. Lyon (France): IARC Press; 2017. p. 39–40.

23. Mahler C, Verhelst J, Klaes R, et al. Cushing's disease and hyperprolactinemia due to a mixed ACTH- and prolactin-secreting pituitary macroadenoma. Pathol Res Pract 1991;187:598–602.

24. Rasul FT, Jaunmuktane Z, Khan AA, et al. Plurihormonal pituitary adenoma with concomitant adrenocorticotropic hormone (ACTH) and growth hormone (GH) secretion: a report of two cases and review of the literature. Acta Neurochir (Wien) 2014;156:141–6.

25. Horvath E, Kovacs K, Smyth HS, et al. Silent adenoma subtype 3 of the pituitary – immunohistochemical and ultrastructural classification: a review of 29 cases. Ultrastruct Pathol 2005;29:511–24.

26. Erickson D, Scheithauer B, Atkinson J, et al. Silent subtype 3 pituitary adenoma: a clinicopathologic analysis of the mayo clinic experience. Clin Endocrinol (Oxf) 2009;71:92–9.

27. Mete O, Gomez-Hernandez K, Kucharczyk W, et al. Silent subtype 3 pituitary adenomas are not always silent and represent poorly differentiated monomorphous plurihormonal pit-1 lineage adenomas. Mod Pathol 2016;29:131–42.

28. Kontogeorgos G, Kovacs K, Horvath E, et al. Multiple adenomas of the human pituitary. A retrospective autopsy study with clinical implications. J Neurosurg 1991; 74:243–7.

29. Roncaroli F, Kovacs K, Lloyd RV, et al. Pituitary carcinoma. In: Lloyd RV, Osamura RY, Klöppel G, et al, editors. Tumors of the pituitary gland. WHO classification of endocrine tumors. 4th edition. Lyon (France): IARC Press; 2017. p. 41–4.

30. Alshaikh OM, Asa SL, Mete O, et al. An institutional experience of tumor progression to pituitary carcinoma in a 15-year cohort of 1055 consecutive pituitary neuroendocrine tumors. Endocr Pathol 2019;30:118–27.

31. Osamura RY, Lopes MBS, Grossman A, et al. Introduction. In: Lloyd RV, Osamura RY, Klöppel G, et al, editors. WHO classification of tumours of endocrine organs. 4th edition. Lyon (France): IARC Press; 2017. p. 13.

32. Lloyd RV, Kovacs K, Young WFJr, et al. Pituitary tumors: Introduction. In: DeLellis RA, Lloyd RV, Heitz PU, et al, editors. World Health Organization classification of tumours: pathology and genetics of tumours of endocrine organs. 3rd edition. Lyon (France): IARC Press; 2004. p. 10–3.

33. Chiloiro S, Doglietto F, Trapasso B, et al. Typical and atypical pituitary adenomas: a single-center analysis of outcome and prognosis. Neuroendocrinology 2015; 101:143–50.

34. Del Basso De Caro M, Solari D, Pagliuca F, et al. Atypical pituitary adenomas: clinical characteristics and role of ki-67 and p53 in prognostic and therapeutic evaluation. A series of 50 patients. Neurosurg Rev 2017;40:105–14.

35. Yildirim AE, Divanlioglu D, Nacar OA, et al. Incidence, hormonal distribution and postoperative follow up of atypical pituitary adenomas. Turk Neurosurg 2013;23: 226–31.

36. Zada G, Woodmansee WW, Ramkissoon S, et al. Atypical pituitary adenomas: incidence, clinical characteristics, and implications. J Neurosurg 2011;114: 336–44.

37. Zaidi HA, Cote DJ, Dunn IF, et al. Predictors of aggressive clinical phenotype among immunohistochemically confirmed atypical adenomas. J Clin Neurosci 2016;34:246–51.
38. Trouillas J, Roy P, Sturm N, et al. A new prognostic clinicopathological classification of pituitary adenomas: a multicentric case-control study of 410 patients with 8 years post-operative follow-up. Acta Neuropathol 2013;126:123–35.
39. Reddy R, Cudlip S, Byrne JV, et al. Can we ever stop imaging in surgically treated and radiotherapy-naive patients with non-functioning pituitary adenoma? Eur J Endocrinol 2011;165:739–44.
40. Ammirati M, Wei L, Ciric I. Short-term outcome of endoscopic versus microscopic pituitary adenoma surgery: a systematic review and meta-analysis. J Neurol Neurosurg Psychiatry 2013;84:843–9.
41. Raverot G, Castinetti F, Jouanneau E, et al. Pituitary carcinomas and aggressive pituitary tumours: merits and pitfalls of temozolomide treatment. Clin Endocrinol (Oxf) 2012;76:769–75.
42. Chatzellis E, Alexandraki KI, Androulakis II, et al. Aggressive pituitary tumors. Neuroendocrinology 2015;101:87–104.
43. Di Ieva A, Rotondo F, Syro LV, et al. Aggressive pituitary adenomas–diagnosis and emerging treatments. Nat Rev Endocrinol 2014;10:423–35.
44. Asioli S, Righi A, Iommi M, et al. Validation of a clinicopathological score for the prediction of post-surgical evolution of pituitary adenoma: retrospective analysis on 566 patients from a tertiary care centre. Eur J Endocrinol 2019;180:127–34.
45. Raverot G, Burman P, McCormack A, et al, The European Society of Endocrinology. European Society of Endocrinology Clinical Practice Guidelines for the management of aggressive pituitary tumours and carcinomas. Eur J Endocrinol 2018;178:G1–24.
46. Raverot G, Dantony E, Beauvy J, et al. Risk of recurrence in pituitary neuroendocrine tumors: a prospective study using a five-tiered classification. J Clin Endocrinol Metab 2017;102:3368–74.
47. Asa SL, Casar-Borota O, Chanson P, et al, and attendees of 14th Meeting of the International Pituitary Pathology Club, Annecy, France, November 2016. From pituitary adenoma to pituitary neuroendocrine tumor (PitNET): an International Pituitary Pathology Club proposal. Endocr Relat Cancer 2017;24:C5–8.
48. Rindi G, Klimstra DS, Abedi-Ardekani B, et al. A common classification framework for neuroendocrine neoplasms: an International Agency for Research on Cancer (IARC) and World Health Organization (WHO) expert consensus proposal. Mod Pathol 2018;31:1770–86.
49. Villa C, Vasiljevic A, Jaffrain-Rea ML, et al. A standardised diagnostic approach to pituitary neuroendocrine tumours (PitNETs): a European Pituitary Pathology Group (EPPG) proposal. Virchows Arch 2019. https://doi.org/10.1007/s00428-019-02655-0 [Review].
50. Ho KKY, Fleseriu M, Wass J, et al. A tale of pituitary adenomas: to NET or not to NET: Pituitary Society position statement. Pituitary 2019;22:569–73.
51. Nosé V, Grossman A, Mete O. Lactotroph adenoma. In: Lloyd RV, Osamura RY, Klöppel G, et al, editors. WHO classification of tumours of endocrine organs. 4th edition. Lyon (France): IARC Press; 2017. p. 24–7.
52. Horvath E, Kovacs K, Killinger DW, et al. Silent corticotropic adenomas of the human pituitary gland: a histologic, immunocytologic and ultrastructural study. Am J Pathol 1980;98:617–38.

A Novel Etiology of Hypophysitis
Immune Checkpoint Inhibitors

Stuti Fernandes, MD[a], Elena V. Varlamov, MD[a,b,c],
Shirley McCartney, PhD[b], Maria Fleseriu, MD[a,b,c],*

KEYWORDS

- Hypophysitis • Adrenal insufficiency • Endocrine dysfunction
- Immune checkpoint inhibitors • Immunotherapy • T lymphocytes
- Cytotoxic T-lymphocyte-associated protein 4 • Programmed cell death

KEY POINTS

- Hypophysitis is more common with ipilimumab and combination immunotherapy; hypophysitis can develop soon after initiation and as late as 6 months after stopping immunotherapy.
- Headaches, anterior pituitary dysfunction, and mild pituitary enlargement are key features. Diabetes insipidus and vision changes are rare.
- Recovery of pituitary function is variable; adrenocorticotropic hormone deficiency usually persists.
- High-dose glucocorticoids do not improve outcomes in all cases and are recommended only for severe events: compressive symptoms and adrenal crisis.
- Screening for endocrine dysfunction should continue even after cessation of immunotherapy.

INTRODUCTION

Immune checkpoint inhibitor (ICPi) therapy used in cancer treatment exerts effect by blocking the actions of cytotoxic T-lymphocyte-associated protein 4 (CTLA-4) and programmed cell death protein 1 (PD-1).[1,2] These ICPi drugs have revolutionized oncology and improved survival in patients with advanced melanoma, non–small cell lung cancer, renal cell carcinoma, colorectal, and other cancers (**Table 1**).[1] ICPi

[a] Department of Medicine (Endocrinology, Diabetes and Metabolism), Oregon Health & Science University, 3181 Southwest Sam Jackson Park Road, Mail Code L607, Portland, OR 97239, USA; [b] Department of Neurological Surgery, Oregon Health & Science University, 3303 South Bond Avenue, Mail Code CH8N, Portland, OR 97239, USA; [c] Pituitary Center, Oregon Health & Science University, 3303 South Bond Avenue, Mail Code CH8N, Portland, OR 97239, USA
* Corresponding author. Department of Neurological Surgery, Oregon Health & Science University, 3303 South Bond Avenue, Mail Code CH8N, Portland, OR 97239.
E-mail address: fleseriu@ohsu.edu
Twitter: @MariaFleseriu (M.F.)

Endocrinol Metab Clin N Am 49 (2020) 387–399
https://doi.org/10.1016/j.ecl.2020.05.002
0889-8529/20/© 2020 Elsevier Inc. All rights reserved.

Table 1
Types of checkpoint inhibitors and incidence of hypophysitis

Immune Checkpoint Target	Drug Name	IgG Class[2]	Malignancy	Incidence of Hypophysitis (%)[ref]
CLTA-4	Ipilimumab	IgG1 (recombinant human)	Colorectal Melanoma Renal cell	1.8–17[1-15]
CLTA-4	Tremelimumab	IgG4 (fully human)	Colorectal Gastric and esophageal Melanoma Mesothelioma NSCLC	0–0.4[21,22]
PD-1	Nivolumab	IgG4 (fully human)	Colorectal HNSCC hepatocellular Hodgkin lymphoma Melanoma NSCLC Renal cell SCLC Urothelial	0–1[16,17]
	Pembrolizumab	IgG4 (recombinant human)	Cervical Colorectal Esophageal Endometrial Hodgkin Hepatocellular Gastric Melanoma Mediastinal large B-cell lymphoma Merkel cell NSCLC SCLC Renal cell Urothelial	1[18]
PD-L1	Atezolizumab	IgG1k (recombinant human)	Breast cancer (triple negative) NSCLC Urothelial	<0.1[19]
	Avelumab	IgG1 (fully human)	Merkel cell Renal cell Urothelial	<1
	Durvalumab	IgG1 (fully human)	Urothelial	<0.1[20]
Combination	Ipilimumab and nivolumab		Melanoma 11 Renal cell	8[23]

Abbreviations: HNSCC, head and neck squamous cell cancer; NSCLC, non-small cell lung cancer; SCLC, small cell lung cancer.
Data from Refs.[11-23]

drugs are used as monotherapy, in combination with other checkpoint inhibitors or along with chemotherapy agents.[2–4] However, ICPi therapy can trigger autoimmune adverse events affecting the skin, colon, lungs, and endocrine organs.[5] Endocrinopathies associated with ICPi therapy include hypophysitis, diabetes mellitus, primary adrenal insufficiency, and thyroid dysfunction. If not diagnosed and treated promptly these endocrinopathies can cause significant morbidity and mortality in already ailing patients. In this review article, we discuss the function of immune checkpoints, the action of ICPi drugs with a focus on pituitary adverse events, and provide evidence and recommendations for treatment of ICPi-induced hypophysitis.[2,3,5]

FUNCTION OF IMMUNE CHECKPOINTS

Immune checkpoints are molecules on the surface of T lymphocytes that play an important role in immune self-tolerance, prevention of autoimmunity, and regulation of the immune system response. CTLA-4 and PD-1 are two such molecules, which function to inhibit T-cell activity and are the targets of several medications used to treat cancers. CTLA-4 binds B7 ligands and prevents the early activation of naive and memory T cells, whereas PD-1 attenuates the function of T cells later in peripheral tissues through interaction with PD-L1 and PD-L2.[6–8]

CTLA-4 is a glycoprotein constitutively expressed on the surface of regulatory T cells but is mainly intracellular in conventional T cells. T-cell receptor activation in conventional T cells results in CTLA-4 movement to the cell surface. Once on the surface, CTLA-4 exerts an inhibitory function by binding to B7-1 and 2 (CD80 and CD86), on antigen-presenting cells (APCs), such as macrophages or dendritic cells. This blocks binding of CD28 (a stimulator of T-cell activity) to its ligand and results in endocytosis of B7 ligands, thus removing them from APCs. Binding also induces indoleamine 2,3-dioxygenase, which stimulates the production of regulatory cytokines, such as transforming growth factor-β, resulting in further inhibition of APCs or T cells.[2,8,9]

Like CTLA-4, PD-1 is a glycoprotein but is expressed on many different cells, including T cells, B cells, macrophages, and dendritic cells. PD-1 inhibits T-cell activation to a greater extent when compared with CTLA-4. PD-1 binding to ligands (PD-L1 or PD-L2) inhibits activation of phosphatidylinositol-4,5- bisphosphate 3-kinase, and Akt (PI3K/Akt pathway) by CD28, thus blocking glucose uptake. This results in T-cell exhaustion. PD-1 activation can also prevent induction of transcription factors and cell survival factor B-cell lymphoma-extra-large.[2,6,10] Tumor cells can evade immune destruction through overproduction of PD-1 and CTLA-4 on immune effector cells and PD-L1 on cancer cells (**Figs. 1** and **2**, see **Table 1**).[6,11–20]

PATHOGENESIS OF ENDOCRINE DYSFUNCTION CAUSED BY IMMUNE CHECKPOINT INHIBITORS

Checkpoint inhibitors result in an increase of effector T cells, which respond to self-antigens on tumor cells. However, this same mechanism, which makes these drugs effective against cancer cells, leads to autoimmunity. Autoimmunity occurs through self-antigen-mediated cytotoxicity and production of T-cell dependent self-antibodies. This causes tissue damage and release of self-antigens that prime more self-reactive T cells resulting in a positive feedback loop of autoimmunity. The degree of autoimmune effects may be correlated with tumor response to immunotherapy; in a retrospective study of patients with melanoma treated with anti-CTLA-4 therapy tumor regression strongly correlated with the development of grade 3 or 4 autoimmune toxicities.[21]

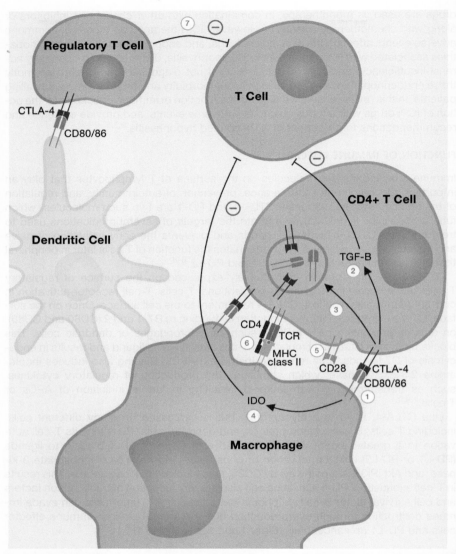

Fig. 1. Inhibitory actions of CTLA-4. (1) T cell binds to CD80/86 on an antigen-presenting cell (eg, a macrophage), which triggers inhibitory signaling. (2) Transforming growth factor-B (TGF-B) is released, which inhibits T-cell function. (3) CTLA-4 binding results in transendocytosis, thus removing CD80/86 from the surface of antigen-presenting cells and decreasing the availability of ligand. (4) Binding of CTLA-4 and CD80/86 results in induction of indoleamine 2,3 dioxygenase (IDO), which inhibits T-cell activity. (5) Binding of CD28 is out-competed by binding of CTLA-4, preventing activation of T cells. (6) Binding of major histocompatibility complex (MHC) class II and T-cell receptors on the CD4 cell enhances adhesion between the T cell and antigen-presenting cell. (7) Binding of CTLA-4 and CD80/86 on regulatory T cells results in inhibition of T cells. (©Meghan Toomayan.)

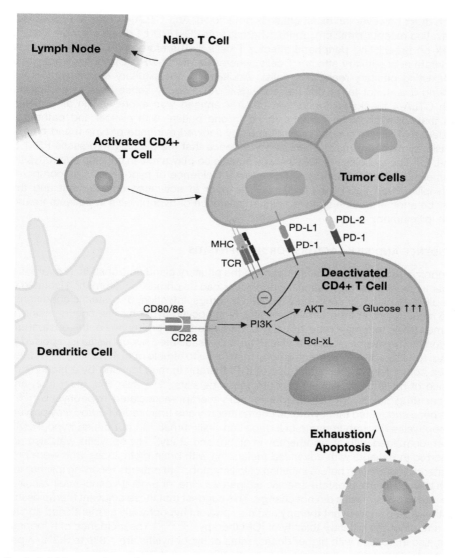

Fig. 2. Inhibitory actions of PD-1. Antigen-presenting cells (e.g. dendritic cells) activate the immune system by binding CD28. This results in activation of the PI3k pathway and increased glucose uptake for cell proliferation and effector function. Binding of PD-1 to PDL-1 inhibits this pathway leading to decreased glucose uptake and gluconeogenesis, ultimately causing cell death. Cell survival factor B-cell lymphoma–extra large (Bcl-xL) is also inhibited. (©Meghan Toomayan.)

Although other systems can be affected, some endocrine organs seem to be particularly at risk for adverse side effects of ICPi therapy; susceptibility may be caused by high vascularity of the pituitary, thyroid, and adrenal glands. Anti-CTLA-4 therapy is associated with hypophysitis more often than anti-PD-1/PD-L1 therapy.[3] This may be caused by a difference in the self-reactive effector T cells created in response to each drug; however, an exact cause is not known. Anti-CTLA-4 drugs are capable of activating recent thymic emigrants, whereas anti-PD-1/PD-L1 drugs are more likely to work on preexisting peripheral effector T cells.[22] Therefore anti-CTLA-4 drugs can generate new pituitary effector T cells, whereas anti-PD-1/PD-L1 enhance activity of preexisting pituitary reactive T cells.[3] Additionally, the pituitary expresses CTLA-4 making it a direct target for these drugs.[23] An autopsy series of patients (treated with CTLA-4 blockade) found that CTLA-4 antigen was expressed in all patients, but that the highest levels were found in one patient with clinical and pathologic evidence of severe hypophysitis. Pathology showed evidence of type II and type IV sensitivity mechanisms.[24] There is no evidence that the pituitary expresses PD-1 or PD-L1.[25] The IgG class of ICPi therapy could also play a role in causing hypophysitis. Tremelimumab (IgG4 subclass) has a lower incidence of hypophysitis as compared with ipilimumab (IgG1 subclass). IgG4 is poor at activating complement and this may be another reason as to the higher incidence of hypophysitis in patients treated with ipilimumab.[3]

INCIDENCE AND RISK FACTORS FOR HYPOPHYSITIS

Hypophysitis, defined as inflammation of the pituitary gland and/or stalk, is a rare disorder in the general population. Hypophysitis can be primary (inflammation isolated to the pituitary gland) or secondary (caused by drugs, infection, or systemic conditions). The most common form of hypophysitis, lymphocytic hypophysitis, occurs mainly in women (male to female ratio 1:6) and is associated with pregnancy or the postpartum period.[26] The overall incidence of ICPi therapy associated hypophysitis is reported to be up to 17%, with higher rates among men (male to female ratio 4:1).[12,14,24,27,28] Even when controlling for the higher use of ICPi therapy in men (caused by a higher incidence of melanoma), a male predominance persists.[12,14] Male sex, older age, and higher drug doses are risk factors for ICPi therapy–associated hypophysitis.[3,12] It has been suggested that cytotoxic chemotherapy and brain radiotherapy may prevent hypophysitis through immune cell depletion. Ipilimumab did not cause hypophysitis when combined with chemotherapy in all but one study.[5] Hypophysitis was also not reported in patients with advanced melanoma with brain metastases who were pretreated with radiation before initiation of ipilimumab.[29] In patients receiving ipilimumab with bevacizumab, prostate-specific antigen vaccine, or prostate cancer cell vaccine, the rate of hypophysitis did not change. This suggest that these adjuvant therapies (radiation is also an anjuvant therapy and may prevent hypophysitis as mentioned above) do not affect the pituitary toxicity of ICPi therapy.[3,18,30,31] The incidence of hypophysitis also increases with higher doses; rates of hypophysitis are 1.8% to 3.3% in patients on low-dose ipilimumab (<3 mg/kg)[21] versus 4.9% to 17% in patients on high-dose ipilimumab (>3 mg/kg).[32]

Anti-CTLA-4 therapies have a higher incidence of hypophysitis as compared with anti-PD-1/PD-L1 therapies. Furthermore, the combination of ICPi therapy (specifically ipilimumab and nivolumab) increases risk of hypophysitis.[33]

Screening for Hypophysitis

Patients should have a baseline biochemical evaluation before initiation of therapy. The ipilimumab package insert recommends clinical chemistries, adrenocorticotropic hormone (ACTH), and thyroid function testing before treatment and each dose escalation.[32] French Endocrine Society Guidelines recommend pretreatment evaluation with serum sodium, 8-AM cortisol, ACTH if morning cortisol less than 18 μg/dL, thyroid-stimulating hormone (TSH), free T4, and sex hormones (luteinizing hormone

[LH]/follicle-stimulating hormone [FSH]/testosterone in males; FSH/LH/estradiol in females with irregular periods; and FSH-only in postmenopausal females). These guidelines further recommend monitoring serum sodium, TSH, free T4, 8-AM cortisol, and testosterone (in males) at each treatment for the first 6 months, every other treatment for the following 6 months, and as needed later when clinical symptoms prompt evaluation.[34]

New onset of hyponatremia, malaise, and appetite loss should prompt an evaluation for adrenal insufficiency.[35] Additionally, patients and their families should be counseled about signs and symptoms of hypophysitis to improve detection between clinic visits.[2] Endocrine dysfunction has been reported even after discontinuation of ICPi therapy, most notably with nivolumab. Therefore, screening should continue even after cessation of immunotherapy, although the duration of surveillance is unclear.[35]

Clinical Presentation/MRI Findings

Hypophysitis develops usually early in the course of treatment, with median onset at 2 to 3 months; however, has been reported as early as 4 weeks after treatment initiation.[2] Late-onset ACTH deficiency has been reported 6 months after stopping the immunotherapy.[35] Symptoms are subtle and nonspecific, most commonly fatigue (59%–73%) and headache (32%–87%).[2] Other symptoms include hypotension, nausea, confusion, amenorrhea, and sexual dysfunction. In contrast to other forms of autoimmune hypophysitis, visual disturbances are uncommon, likely caused by an usually mild degree of pituitary enlargement.[36] Diabetes insipidus (DI) has only been reported in a few case reports and should prompt suspicion for pituitary metastases, which commonly cause DI.[2,28] Pituitary MRI may show enlargement of the pituitary, stalk thickening, and heterogeneous enhancement of the pituitary gland (**Fig. 3**). Rarely, optic chiasm compression is seen.[4,37] Pituitary MRI abnormalities often precede clinical manifestations of hypophysitis; in one

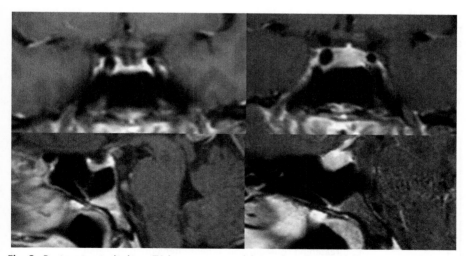

Fig. 3. Postcontrast pituitary T1 images, coronal (*upper*) and sagittal (*lower*). (*Left*) Normal MRI brain before initiation of checkpoint inhibitor therapy. (*Right*) MRI 6 weeks after starting nivolumab/ipilimumab (patient presented with new-onset headache, nausea, and vomiting). Pituitary is enlarged measuring 8 × 9 × 13 mm; heterogeneous enhancement postcontrast is noted.

study of patients treated with ipilimumab, MRI changes were observed at a median of 1 week before the development of biochemical deficiencies.[14] Therefore radiographic evidence of hypophysitis on surveillance MRIs should prompt close monitoring for development of pituitary dysfunction.[2] Frequently, however, there are no radiographic changes. A study of patients with CTLA-4 inhibitor–induced hypophysitis reported normal MRIs in 23% of cases. Thus, a normal-appearing pituitary does not rule out hypophysitis.[24]

When hypophysitis is suspected, laboratory work-up should be initiated with hormone measurements (cortisol, ACTH or cosyntropin stimulation test, TSH, free T4, FSH, LH, insulin-like growth factor [IGF]-1, prolactin, testosterone/estradiol, electrolytes, paired urine, and plasma osmolarity). Pituitary MRI is recommended if mass effect is suspected, if hormonal abnormalities are present, and to rule out pituitary metastases.[2,3,5,34] At diagnosis, corticotroph and thyrotroph dysfunction are most commonly observed.[2] Gonadotroph dysfunction is also frequently reported.[11,12] Deficiencies in IGF-1 and prolactin are rarer.[2] Reported frequencies of pituitary endocrine dysfunction at diagnosis of hypophysitis in patients receiving ipilimumab are varied: adrenal (50%–100%), thyroid (61%–100%), gonadal (38%–100%), IGF-1/GH (17%–43%), prolactin elevation (0%–11%), low prolactin (44%–92%), and DI (0%).[11–14] Grading of adrenal insufficiency/hypophysitis is shown in **Table 2**.[38]

Management

Initial recommendations were to discontinue ICPi therapy and initiate high-dose glucocorticoids (GC)[4]; however, this strategy has not been shown to improve outcomes. Retrospective studies showed that patients treated with high- versus low-dose steroids for ipilimumab-induced hypophysitis had no difference in frequency of or time to resolution of pituitary deficiencies or pituitary enlargement.[13,14,39] Additionally, it has been suggested that high-dose GC may decrease ICPi therapy effectiveness. A retrospective study of patients with melanoma and ipilimumab-induced hypophysitis showed that patients treated with high-dose as opposed to low-dose GC (replacement) had reduced survival and shorter time to treatment failure.[39] Therefore, in the absence of critical illness or compressive symptoms (intractable headaches or visual changes from optic chiasm compression) current recommendations are to treat pituitary deficiencies with replacement doses of GC and other hormones if not contraindicated. Severe hypophysitis with compressive symptoms should be, however, treated with high-dose GC (1 mg/kg/day of prednisone or equivalent).[2,3,5] High-dose GC may

Table 2	
Grades of adrenal insufficiency/hypophysitis	
Grade	**Symptoms**
1	Asymptomatic; clinical or diagnostic observations only; intervention not indicated
2	Moderate symptoms; medical intervention indicated
3	Severe symptoms; hospitalization indicated
4	Life-threatening consequences; urgent intervention indicated
5	Death

From Adverse Events/CTCAE. National Cancer Institute Web Site. https://evs.nci.nih.gov/ftp1/CTCAE/CTCAE_4.03/CTCAE_4.03_2010-06-14_QuickReference_5x7.pdf. Accessed September 22 2019; with permission.

also be indicated for other ICPi toxicities (dermatologic, rheumatologic, gastrointestinal/hepatic, or pneumonitis).

Adrenal Axis

A typical GC replacement regimen is 15 to 20 mg of hydrocortisone/day or equivalent. Patients presenting with adrenal crisis and/or severe hyponatremia should be treated with an initial stress dose GC (intravenous hydrocortisone preferred) and fluids with subsequent taper to physiologic replacement regimen.[40] Patients should be educated on sick day management and stress-dosing. Patients should also be advised to wear a medical alert bracelet and provided with an injectable high-dose GC kit for emergency use.[2]

Thyroid Axis

If central hypothyroidism is present, levothyroxine should be initiated. If there is concomitant adrenal insufficiency, GC replacement should precede thyroid hormone replacement. Because TSH is unreliable in central hypothyroidism, levothyroxine should be titrated to a goal of middle to upper half of the reference range for free T4.[2,40] In younger patients without cardiovascular disease it has been recommended to initiate treatment with half of replacement dose (0.8 μg/kg/day). This is to avoid overreplacement because ICPi-related hypothyroidism may be transient and patients treated with PD-1 might develop hyperthyroidism. For patients with known coronary artery disease it is recommended to start at lower doses. TSH and free T4 should be repeated in approximately 4 weeks. Triiodothyronine (L-T3), thyroid extract, or other formulations of thyroid hormone are not recommended because these can have variable amounts of active thyroid hormone and lead to fluctuations in thyroid levels. In contrast with other causes of central hypothyroidism, TSH monitoring is recommended because TSH elevation may signal recovery of pituitary thyrotrophs, development of primary hypothyroidism, or the recovery phase of nonthyroidal illness syndrome.[2]

Gonadal Axis

Replacement of sex steroids in men and women may be appropriate in select patients. Prostate cancer, breast cancer, and uterine cancer are contraindications to testosterone and estrogen replacement. Testosterone should be avoided in men desiring fertility in the near future. Sex hormone replacement is generally avoided in patients with high risk of clotting, cardiovascular disease, or stroke.[40]

Growth Hormone and Prolactin

Treatment of growth hormone deficiency with growth hormone replacement is contraindicated in the setting of active malignancy. Therefore, there is limited clinical utility in measuring IGF-1 and testing for growth hormone deficiency.

Prolactin is variable, it may be low; high prolactin is uncommon in ICPi-related hypophysitis and may be caused by other medications or stalk effect.[2]

Continuing Immune Checkpoint Inhibitor Therapy

Although initially recommendations included stopping ICPi therapy, development of hypophysitis does not necessitate permanent cessation because hormones can be replaced safely. A recent study investigated the reinitiation of anti-PD-1 or anti-PD-L1 in patients with grade 2 or higher immune adverse events (6.5% endocrine related) and found that 55% had a second adverse event. Of those with a recurrence, 43% had a recurrence of the same type of adverse event; however, no recurrences of endocrine

Table 3
Recovery of adrenal, thyroid, and gonadal axes in patient with checkpoint inhibitor–induced hypophysitis

	Authors	Adrenal	Thyroid	Gonadal
Proportion of patients who recovered (n)	Min et al,[14] 2015	0/22	14/22	7/15
	Albarel et al,[13] 2015	0/13	11/13	10/12
	Scott et al,[42] 2018	0/10	0/10	3/9
Median time to axis recovery (range) in all studies, wk (n)	Min et al,[14] 2015 Albarel et al,[13] 2015 Scott et al,[42] 2018	—	10.5 (1–44)	15 (2–92)

Data from Refs.[13,14,42]

adverse events were reported.[41] The European Society for Medical Oncology Guidelines recommend holding ICPi therapy in those with grade 2 or higher hypophysitis and states that in most cases ICPi therapy can be resumed but with no specific timeline given.[15] The prescribing information document for ipilimumab recommends reinitiation in patients with partial or complete resolution of adverse events (grade 0–1) and if receiving 7.5 mg of prednisone equivalent or less.[35] In one study of patients with ipilimumab-induced hypophysitis, discontinuation of the drug did not seem to affect the outcome of hypophysitis.[14]

PROGNOSIS

Pituitary enlargement is rare overall and resolves in most patients (83%–100%[12,14]), commonly resulting in diminished pituitary size or empty sella. Corticotroph deficiency is permanent in almost all patients, although recovery has been noted. There is variable recovery in gonadal and thyroid axes **(Table 3)**.[13,14,42]

SUMMARY

Clinicians should be aware of the side effects of immunotherapies. Checkpoint inhibitor–induced hypophysitis occurs early in the course of treatment and should be monitored with regular hormonal evaluation. Radiographic pituitary changes may not occur in all cases, but pituitary enlargement noted on routine surveillance brain imaging should prompt evaluation of the pituitary axes. In addition, awareness of clinical manifestations of adrenal and thyroid deficiency is essential, because these can be life threatening if not recognized and treated promptly. After recognition, treatment should be initiated promptly and ICPi therapy discontinued if the adverse reaction is severe; however, reinitiation of treatment is considered after resolution/improvement. Thyroid and gonadal axes can recover, but adrenal insufficiency is usually permanent, necessitating lifelong GC replacement therapy.

DISCLOSURE

The authors have nothing to disclose.

REFERENCES

1. Kyi C, Postow MA. Checkpoint blocking antibodies in cancer immunotherapy. FEBS Lett 2014;588(2):368–76.

2. Chang L-S, Barroso-Sousa R, Tolaney SM, et al. Endocrine toxicity of cancer immunotherapy targeting immune checkpoints. Endocr Rev 2019;40(1):17–65.

3. Joshi MN, Whitelaw BC, Palomar MTP, et al. Immune checkpoint inhibitor-related hypophysitis and endocrine dysfunction: clinical review. Clin Endocrinol 2016; 85(3):331–9.

4. González-Rodríguez E, Rodríguez-Abreu D. Immune checkpoint inhibitors: review and management of endocrine adverse events. Oncologist 2016;21(7):804.

5. Corsello SM, Barnabei A, Marchetti P, et al. Endocrine side effects induced by immune checkpoint inhibitors. J Clin Endocrinol Metab 2013;98(4):1361–75.

6. Lee JY, Lee HT, Shin W, et al. Structural basis of checkpoint blockade by monoclonal antibodies in cancer immunotherapy. Nat Commun 2016;7:13354.

7. Harding FA, McArthur JG, Gross JA, et al. CD28-mediated signalling costimulates murine T cells and prevents induction of anergy in T-cell clones. Nature 1992;356(6370):607–9.

8. Buchbinder EI, Desai A. CTLA-4 and PD-1 pathways: similarities, differences, and implications of their inhibition. Am J Clin Oncol 2016;39(1):98–106.

9. Walker LSK, Sansom DM. The emerging role of CTLA4 as a cell-extrinsic regulator of T cell responses. Nat Rev Immunol 2011;11(12):852–63.

10. Parry RV, Chemnitz JM, Frauwirth KA, et al. CTLA-4 and PD-1 receptors inhibit T-cell activation by distinct mechanisms. Mol Cell Biol 2005;25(21):9543–53.

11. Ryder M, Callahan M, Postow MA, et al. Endocrine-related adverse events following ipilimumab in patients with advanced melanoma: a comprehensive retrospective review from a single institution. Endocr Relat Cancer 2014;21(2): 371–81.

12. Faje AT, Sullivan R, Lawrence D, et al. Ipilimumab-induced hypophysitis: a detailed longitudinal analysis in a large cohort of patients with metastatic melanoma. J Clin Endocrinol Metab 2014;99(11):4078–85.

13. Albarel F, Gaudy C, Castinetti F, et al. Long-term follow-up of ipilimumab-induced hypophysitis, a common adverse event of the anti-CTLA-4 antibody in melanoma. Eur J Endocrinol 2015;172(2):195–204.

14. Min L, Hodi FS, Giobbie-Hurder A, et al. Systemic high-dose corticosteroid treatment does not improve the outcome of ipilimumab-related hypophysitis: a retrospective cohort study. Clin Cancer Res 2015;21(4):749–55.

15. Haanen J, Carbonnel F, Robert C, et al. Management of toxicities from immunotherapy: ESMO Clinical Practice Guidelines for diagnosis, treatment and follow-up. Ann Oncol 2017;28(suppl_4):iv119–42.

16. Ribas A, Puzanov I, Dummer R, et al. Pembrolizumab versus investigator-choice chemotherapy for ipilimumab-refractory melanoma (KEYNOTE-002): a randomised, controlled, phase 2 trial. Lancet Oncol 2015;16(8):908–18.

17. Topalian SL, Hodi FS, Brahmer JR, et al. Safety, activity, and immune correlates of anti-PD-1 antibody in cancer. N Engl J Med 2012;366(26):2443–54.

18. Robert C, Ribas A, Wolchok JD, et al. Anti-programmed-death-receptor-1 treatment with pembrolizumab in ipilimumab-refractory advanced melanoma: a randomised dose-comparison cohort of a phase 1 trial. Lancet 2014;384(9948): 1109–17.

19. Genetech. TECENTRIQ (atezolizumab) injection prescribing information 2019. Available at: https://www.gene.com/download/pdf/tecentriq_prescribing.pdf. Accessed September 22 2019.

20. Loibl S, Untch M, Burchardi N, et al. A randomised phase II study investigating durvalumab in addition to an anthracycline taxane-based neoadjuvant therapy

in early triple-negative breast cancer: clinical results and biomarker analysis of GeparNuevo study. Ann Oncol 2019;30(8):1279–88.

21. Attia P, Phan GQ, Maker AV, et al. Autoimmunity correlates with tumor regression in patients with metastatic melanoma treated with anti-cytotoxic T-lymphocyte antigen-4. J Clin Oncol 2005;23(25):6043–53.

22. Kvistborg P, Philips D, Kelderman S, et al. Anti-CTLA-4 therapy broadens the melanoma-reactive CD8 T cell response. Sci Transl Med 2014;6(254):254ra128.

23. Iwama S, De Remigis A, Callahan MK, et al. Pituitary expression of CTLA-4 mediates hypophysitis secondary to administration of CTLA-4 blocking antibody. Sci Transl Med 2014;6(230):230ra245.

24. Caturegli P, Di Dalmazi G, Lombardi M, et al. Hypophysitis secondary to cytotoxic T-lymphocyte–associated protein 4 blockade. Am J Pathol 2016;186(12): 3225–35.

25. Wang C, Thudium KB, Han M, et al. In vitro characterization of the anti-PD-1 antibody nivolumab, BMS-936558, and in vivo toxicology in non-human primates. Cancer Immunol Res 2014;2(9):846–56.

26. Caturegli P, Newschaffer C, Olivi A, et al. Autoimmune hypophysitis. Endocr Rev 2005;26(5):599–614.

27. Torino F, Barnabei A, De Vecchis L, et al. Hypophysitis induced by monoclonal antibodies to cytotoxic T lymphocyte antigen 4: challenges from a new cause of a rare disease. Oncologist 2012;17(4):525–35.

28. Dillard T, Yedinak CG, Alumkal J, et al. Anti-CTLA-4 antibody therapy associated autoimmune hypophysitis: serious immune related adverse events across a spectrum of cancer subtypes. Pituitary 2010;13(1):29–38.

29. Margolin K, Ernstoff MS, Hamid O, et al. Ipilimumab in patients with melanoma and brain metastases: an open-label, phase 2 trial. Lancet Oncol 2012;13(5): 459–65.

30. Madan RA, Mohebtash M, Arlen PM, et al. Ipilimumab and a poxviral vaccine targeting prostate-specific antigen in metastatic castration-resistant prostate cancer: a phase 1 dose-escalation trial. Lancet Oncol 2012;13(5):501–8.

31. van den Eertwegh AJ, Versluis J, van den Berg HP, et al. Combined immunotherapy with granulocyte-macrophage colony-stimulating factor-transduced allogeneic prostate cancer cells and ipilimumab in patients with metastatic castration-resistant prostate cancer: a phase 1 dose-escalation trial. Lancet Oncol 2012;13(5):509–17.

32. Maker AV, Yang JC, Sherry RM, et al. Intrapatient dose escalation of anti-CTLA-4 antibody in patients with metastatic melanoma. J Immunother 2006;29(4):455–63.

33. Barroso-Sousa R, Barry WT, Garrido-Castro AC, et al. Incidence of endocrine dysfunction following the use of different immune checkpoint inhibitor regimens. JAMA Oncol 2018;4(2):173.

34. Castinetti F, Albarel F, Archambeaud F, et al. French Endocrine Society Guidance on endocrine side-effects of immunotherapy. Endocr Relat Cancer 2018;26(2): G1–18.

35. Takeno A, Yamamoto M, Morita M, et al. Late-onset isolated adrenocorticotropic hormone deficiency caused by nivolumab: a case report. BMC Endocr Disord 2019;19(1):25.

36. Sznol M, Postow MA, Davies MJ, et al. Endocrine-related adverse events associated with immune checkpoint blockade and expert insights on their management. Cancer Treat Rev 2017;58:70–6.

37. Grob J, Hamid O, Wolchok J, et al. 9312 Antitumor responses to ipilimumab in advanced melanoma are not affected by systemic corticosteroids used to

manage immune-related adverse events (irAEs). Eur J Cancer Suppl 2009; 7(2):580.

38. National Cancer Institute. Available at: https://evs.nci.nih.gov/ftp1/CTCAE/ CTCAE_4.03/CTCAE_4.03_2010-06-14_QuickReference_5x7.pdf.   Accessed September 22 2019.

39. Faje AT, Lawrence D, Flaherty K, et al. High-dose glucocorticoids for the treatment of ipilimumab-induced hypophysitis is associated with reduced survival in patients with melanoma. Cancer 2018;124(18):3706–14.

40. Fleseriu M, Hashim IA, Karavitaki N, et al. Hormonal replacement in hypopituitarism in adults: an endocrine society clinical practice guideline. J Clin Endocrinol Metab 2016;101(11):3888–921.

41. Simonaggio A, Michot JM, Voisin AL, et al. Evaluation of readministration of immune checkpoint inhibitors after immune-related adverse events in patients with cancer. JAMA Oncol 2019;5(9):1310–7.

42. Scott ES, Long GV, Guminski A, et al. The spectrum, incidence, kinetics and management of endocrinopathies with immune checkpoint inhibitors for metastatic melanoma. Eur J Endocrinol 2018;178(2):173–80.

Advances in the Medical Treatment of Cushing Disease

Nicholas A. Tritos, MD, DSc*, Beverly M.K. Biller, MD

KEYWORDS

- Cushing disease • Ketoconazole • Metyrapone • Mitotane • Etomidate
- Cabergoline • Pasireotide • Mifepristone

KEY POINTS

- Medical therapy has an important, adjunctive role in the management of patients with Cushing disease.
- Available treatment options include steroidogenesis inhibitors, centrally acting agents, and glucocorticoid receptor antagonists.
- Several agents are currently in development and may eventually expand treatment options for Cushing disease.

INTRODUCTION

Cushing disease (CD) is caused by a corticotropin (ACTH)-secreting pituitary adenoma (or rarely carcinoma) and requires meticulous management to minimize excess morbidity and mortality associated with hypercortisolism.[1–4] Transsphenoidal pituitary surgery, performed by an experienced pituitary neurosurgeon, is the cornerstone of treatment of most patients with CD.[5–7] However, about 15% of patients with CD do not achieve remission after transsphenoidal pituitary surgery.[6,8] In addition, approximately 2% of patients recur annually after achieving surgical remission, leading to a cumulative recurrence rate that approaches 35% on long-term follow-up.[9]

Medical therapy is typically adjunctive in patients with CD.[5,10] It is generally administered to those who have recurred after surgery or patients who did not achieve remission postoperatively and are not considered repeat surgical candidates. In this group of patients, pituitary radiotherapy is frequently advised as definitive treatment, whereas medical therapy serves to control hypercortisolism until radiotherapy takes effect (after a period of months to years).[5,11] Less often, medical therapy is

Neuroendocrine Unit, Neuroendocrine and Pituitary Tumor Clinical Center, Massachusetts General Hospital, Harvard Medical School, 100 Blossom Street, Suite 140, Boston, MA 02114, USA
* Corresponding author.
E-mail address: NTRITOS@mgh.harvard.edu

Endocrinol Metab Clin N Am 49 (2020) 401–412
https://doi.org/10.1016/j.ecl.2020.05.003
0889-8529/20/© 2020 Elsevier Inc. All rights reserved.

endo.theclinics.com

recommended to optimize the status of patients preoperatively or administered to patients whose tumor location is uncertain despite extensive testing.[10,12]

Several medications are available to treat CD and others are in clinical development.[5,11] Currently available medical options are classified based on their site of action (**Fig. 1**). These include steroidogenesis inhibitors, centrally acting agents, and glucocorticoid receptor (GR) antagonists (**Table 1**).[5,13] The aims of the present article are to review medications that are used to manage patients with CD and highlight novel developments in the field. To compile the referenced literature, electronic searches were conducted using the keywords: Cushing's disease, hypercortisolism, medical therapy, ketoconazole, metyrapone, mitotane, etomidate, cabergoline, pasireotide, and mifepristone. Articles were included at the discretion of the authors.

STEROIDOGENESIS INHIBITORS

Steroidogenesis inhibitors act by inhibiting one or several enzymes involved in adrenal steroidogenesis, leading to a decrease in cortisol biosynthesis. They are effective in controlling hypercortisolism but all have the potential to cause adrenal insufficiency as an extension of their pharmacologic action. Regular and meticulous follow-up and monitoring is required to optimize clinical effectiveness while detecting and managing any toxicities associated with their use. Steroidogenesis inhibitors are titrated to achieve normal cortisol levels, generally 24-hour urinary free cortisol (UFC) or late night salivary cortisol. Alternatively, they are used as "block and replace" therapy, aiming at suppressing endogenous cortisol secretion and providing glucocorticoid replacement. The "block and replace" regimen option is particularly helpful in patients with

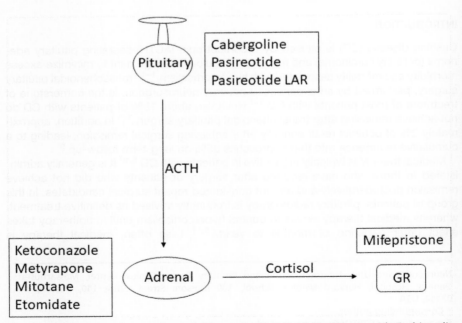

Fig. 1. Site of action of currently available medications used in patients with Cushing disease. Cabergoline, ketoconazole, metyrapone, mitotane, and etomidate are used off-label in this population in the United States. GR, glucocorticoid receptor; LAR, long-acting release.

Table 1
Medical therapies currently in use in Cushing disease

Drug Name	Usual Dose Range	Mechanism of Action	Effectiveness[a]	Adverse Effects
Ketoconazole	200–600 mg PO bid-tid	Steroidogenesis inhibitor	49% (24-h UFC)	Headache, nausea, dyspepsia, transaminitis, liver failure, pruritus
Metyrapone	250–1000 mg PO qid	Steroidogenesis inhibitor	55% (cortisol day curve); 43% (24-h UFC)	Nausea, dyspepsia, dizziness, hypertension, edema, hypokalemia, acne, hirsutism
Mitotane	0.5–3.0 g PO tid	Steroidogenesis inhibitor	72% (24-h UFC)	Gastrointestinal, metabolic, neurologic, ophthalmic, skin, genitourinary, and hematologic toxicities
Etomidate	0.03 mg/kg IV (bolus) followed by 0.1–0.3 mg/kg/h	Steroidogenesis inhibitor	Up to 100% (serum cortisol)	Sedation, vomiting, dystonia, myoclonus
Cabergoline	0.5–7.0 mg PO weekly	Dopamine receptor agonist (centrally acting)	25%–40% (24-h UFC)	Nausea, orthostatic dizziness, headache, psychiatric symptomatology
Pasireotide	0.3–0.9 mg SC bid	Somatostatin receptor agonist (centrally acting)	25% (24-h UFC)	Nausea, dyspepsia, diarrhea, cholelithiasis, diabetes mellitus/hyperglycemia, bradycardia
Pasireotide LAR	10–30 mg IM every 4 wk	Somatostatin receptor agonist (centrally acting)	40% (24-h UFC)	Same as pasireotide
Mifepristone	300–1200 mg PO daily	Glucocorticoid receptor antagonist	60% (improved glycemia); 38% (improved blood pressure); 87% (improved overall clinical status)	Headache, nausea, dizziness, joint aches, hypokalemia, endometrial thickening/metrorrhagia

All agents can result in hypoadrenalism as an extension of their pharmacologic effects. Only pasireotide, pasireotide LAR, and mifepristone are approved for use in patients with CD. Ketoconazole, metyrapone, mitotane, etomidate, and cabergoline are currently used off-label in the United States.

Abbreviations: bid, twice daily; IM, intramuscularly; IV, intravenously; LAR, long-acting release; PO, by mouth; qid, four times daily; SC, subcutaneously; tid, three times daily.

[a] Shown as the percentage of patients who achieved normalization (or improvement) of the corresponding end point within parentheses.

cyclic CD but caution is needed not to overreplace, resulting in iatrogenic (exogenous) hypercortisolism. Currently available steroidogenesis inhibitors include ketoconazole, metyrapone, mitotane, and etomidate. None of them are approved by the Food and Drug Administration (FDA) for use in CD. Of note, the European Medicines Agency (EMA) has licensed ketoconazole and metyrapone for use in patients with CD.

Ketoconazole is an imidazole derivative with antifungal activity, which also inhibits several enzymes involved in adrenal steroidogenesis.[14,15] The effectiveness of ketoconazole was recently reported in a retrospective, multicenter study of 200 patients with CD, who were treated with ketoconazole at a median dose of 600 mg daily.[16] In this study, 24-hour UFC normalization was reported in 49% of patients and a greater than or equal to 50% improvement in UFC was reported in 26% of study subjects. In addition, 40% to 50% of treated patients showed improvements in blood pressure, glycemia, and serum potassium levels during therapy.

In the same study, 20% of patients discontinued ketoconazole because of adverse events.[16] In addition to hypoadrenalism, adverse effects associated with ketoconazole therapy include dyspepsia, pruritus, hypogonadism (men), and liver inflammation. Mild transaminitis occurred in 13% of patients and was reversible on ketoconazole discontinuation. In addition, life-threatening hepatitis and hepatic failure have been reported after ketoconazole administration in approximately 1 out of 15,000 treated patients.[17] The FDA has mandated the insertion of a "black box" warning in the ketoconazole label to inform patients and physicians of the risk of serious hepatotoxicity associated with medication use and recommend regular monitoring of liver chemistries. Ketoconazole requires gastric acid for absorption; as a corollary, patients with hypochlorhydria (because of a medical condition or related to medications that decrease gastric acid secretion) may not absorb the medication well. In addition, ketoconazole has the potential for multiple drug-drug interactions, including those medications that are metabolized through the CYP3A pathway.

Metyrapone inhibits 11β-hydroxylase activity, leading to a decrease in cortisol synthesis.[18] In a retrospective, multicenter study of 195 patients with Cushing syndrome, including 115 patients with CD, metyrapone therapy led to normalization of serum cortisol levels (based on cortisol day curves) and 24-hour UFC in 55% and 43% of patients, respectively.[19] Metyrapone has been used to control hypercortisolism during pregnancy[20,21]; however, it is not specifically labeled for use during gestation. In addition to hypoadrenalism, adverse effects associated with metyrapone therapy include nausea, dyspepsia, hyperandrogenic effects (acne and hirsutism) in women as a result of accumulation of androgenic precursors, and mineralocorticoid effects (elevated blood pressure, edema, and hypokalemia) as a consequence of accumulation of precursors with mineralocorticoid activity.

Mitotane has structural similarities to an older insecticide (DDT) and has useful activity as a steroidogenesis inhibitor and an adrenolytic effect (especially with long-term use in higher doses). It is FDA-approved as treatment of adrenocortical carcinoma.[22,23] Its use in CD has been limited to few patients in the United States. In a retrospective study of 76 patients with CD, who were treated with mitotane (mean dose, 2.4 g/daily), 24-hour UFC normalization was reported in 72% of treated patients.[24] In addition, improvements in blood pressure and glycemia were reported. The salutary effects of mitotane were generally reversible on medication discontinuation in this study.[24]

Mitotane therapy has been associated with several adverse effects, including gastrointestinal toxicities, transaminitis, dyslipidemia, neutropenia, neurologic effects (dizziness, unsteadiness, dysarthria, tingling), skin rash, bladder, and ophthalmic toxic effects, among others. In the same study, 29% of patients treated with mitotane discontinued therapy because of adverse events.[24] In addition, mitotane is teratogenic and accumulates in adipose tissue, from which it is slowly cleared after drug discontinuation. As a consequence, it is advisable to defer pregnancy for 5 years after stopping this medication, which limits its use among premenopausal women.

Etomidate is generally used as an anesthetic and/or sedative in hospitalized patients. It inhibits primarily 11β-hydroxylase, leading to a rapid decrease in serum cortisol levels. Etomidate has been used in patients with life-threatening hypercortisolism, wherein it is helpful as a bridge to another intervention (generally surgery).[25] In a retrospective study of seven patients with severe Cushing (two of whom had CD), who were treated with etomidate, serum cortisol levels were reported to decrease rapidly into the target zone at a median interval of 38 hours in almost all patients (except one, who entered hospice care).[26] Etomidate therapy requires close monitoring in intensive care unit settings to detect and manage excessive sedation, which is dose-dependent.[25] Other possible adverse effects include nausea, vomiting, decrease in blood pressure, thrombophlebitis, kidney dysfunction, and myoclonus.

Several investigational steroidogenesis inhibitors are currently in development, including levoketoconazole, osilodrostat, ATR101, abiraterone acetate, ALD1613, and peptide antagonists of the melanocortin 2 receptor.

Levoketoconazole (2S,4R ketoconazole) is a ketoconazole enantiomer that possesses substantially higher potency as steroidogenesis inhibitor over the 2R,4S enantiomer in vitro.[27] A phase 3 study of levoketoconazole therapy in 94 patients with Cushing syndrome (including 80 subjects with CD) was recently published.[28] In this study, 38% of patients achieved normal 24-hour UFC after 6 months' therapy, including 30% who normalized 24-hour UFC without a dose increase. There were beneficial effects on body weight, symptoms and signs of CD, depression, quality of life, glycemia, and serum lipids.[28] Mild transaminitis (1–3 times greater than the upper limit of normal) was reported in 31% of patients; more severe transaminitis occurred in 10% of patients. There were no cases of hepatic failure. Transaminitis resolved in all patients after drug discontinuation without any sequelae.[28]

Osilodrostat is a potent inhibitor of 11β-hydroxylase and aldosterone synthase that showed promise as a steroidogenesis inhibitor in a phase 2 study of patients with CD.[29] The findings of a phase 3 study of osilodrostat in 137 patients with CD were recently reported.[30] This clinical trial included an 8-week randomized withdrawal phase, during which 86% of patients in the osilodrostat arm maintained normal 24-hour UFC versus 29% of patients on placebo, followed by open label osilodrostat therapy until the end of the study.[30] Beneficial effects on body weight, blood pressure, quality of life, and glycemia were also reported at the end of the study (48 weeks). Osilodrostat is generally well-tolerated. In addition to hypoadrenalism, which may occur as an extension to its pharmacologic effects, adverse effects include fatigue, headache, nausea, and arthralgias.[30] Hypokalemia, hyperandrogenism, and a small effect on QT prolongation have been reported, but serious arrhythmias have not been seen.

An inhibitor of acyl coenzyme A:cholesterol acyltransferase 1 (ACAT1), known as ATR101, has been studied in dogs and is currently being investigated in patients with CD.[31] Abiraterone acetate is another steroidogenesis inhibitor, blocking 17α-hydroxylase and 17,20 lyase. It is an approved therapy in men with metastatic prostate carcinoma.[32,33] There is a report of a patient with adrenocortical carcinoma who responded biochemically to this therapy.[34] A study of abiraterone acetate in adrenocortical carcinoma is in process. However, whether abiraterone acetate is efficacious in CD remains unknown. A monoclonal antibody (ALD1613) that neutralizes ACTH and peptide antagonists of the melanocortin 2 receptor, which mediates ACTH action, have been synthesized and are in early clinical development.[35,36]

CENTRALLY ACTING AGENTS

Centrally acting agents act on tumorous corticotrophs to decrease ACTH secretion. Currently used agents include cabergoline (prescribed off-label in CD), pasireotide, and pasireotide long-acting release (LAR), the latter two being approved by the FDA and the EMA for subgroups of patients with CD. The effectiveness of these agents is predicated by the presence of dopamine (D_2) receptors and somatostatin receptors (including SSTR2 and SSTR5) in most tumorous corticotrophs.[37,38]

Cabergoline is a selective D_2 receptor agonist that is licensed for use in patients with hyperprolactinemia.[39] The effectiveness of cabergoline in CD has been reported in several small studies (10–30 patients each), which were either retrospective or prospective.[40–44] In several of these studies, cabergoline therapy led to 24-hour UFC normalization in 25% to 40% of patients.[40–42,44] However, escape from the salutary effects of the medication was not infrequent. In yet another study of cabergoline therapy in CD, no patient achieved normal 24-hour UFC.[43] It should be noted that cabergoline doses used in these studies (1–7 mg/wk) were generally higher than the typical doses used in patients with hyperprolactinemia (0.5–2.0 mg/wk).

Cabergoline therapy is usually well-tolerated. However, adverse events may occur, including nausea, vomiting, and orthostatic dizziness.[39] Less often, headache, nasal congestion, constipation, digital vasospasm, vivid dreams or nightmares, anxiety, and depression have been reported. Cabergoline therapy can exacerbate psychosis and should be avoided in patients with psychosis. Impulsivity disorders have been recognized in several studies of patients with hyperprolactinemia treated with cabergoline.[45–49] In addition, cabergoline therapy (in higher doses) has been associated with cardiac valvulopathy in patients with Parkinson disease.[50,51] Most studies of patients with hyperprolactinemia on cabergoline therapy have been reassuring with regards to the occurrence of valvulopathy.[52] However, there are no such safety data in patients with CD on cabergoline therapy. It seems prudent to use the lowest possible effective cabergoline doses and periodically evaluate patients receiving higher than usual doses of cabergoline over several years with echocardiography.

Pasireotide and pasireotide LAR are somatostatin receptor agonists that activate multiple receptor isoforms (SSTR1, SSTR2, SSTR3, SSTR5).[38] Both agents have been shown to be effective in controlling hypercortisolism in CD. In a pivotal phase 3 study (162 patients) comparing two different, twice daily, subcutaneous doses of the drug, pasireotide therapy led to 24-hour UFC normalization in 25% of patients who were randomly allocated to the higher dose (900 μg twice daily).[53] There were improvements in blood pressure, lipids, body weight, and quality of life of study subjects. In addition, a decrease in tumor volume was reported among some patients with radiographically visible pituitary adenomas in the study.

Pasireotide shares many adverse effects with older somatostatin receptor agonists, including abdominal discomfort, bloating, diarrhea, cholelithiasis, and bradycardia. In addition, hypoadrenalism may occur as an extension of its pharmacologic action. However, hyperglycemia and diabetes mellitus have been more commonly reported among patients on pasireotide, occurring in 73% and 34% of study subjects, respectively.[53] Deterioration of glucose homeostasis on pasireotide therapy is a consequence of decreased insulinemia, which reflects direct inhibition of insulin secretion and suppression of incretin release from the gut.[54] Careful monitoring of glycemia is advisable. Patients who develop hyperglycemia or diabetes mellitus on pasireotide therapy may preferably be treated with metformin, incretin-based therapies, or insulin.

Pasireotide LAR, a long-acting formulation of pasireotide, was also shown to be efficacious in a pivotal phase 3 study of 150 patients, who were randomly allocated to either of two doses of the drug administered intramuscularly.[55] This therapy led to 24-hour UFC normalization in 40% of patients in the study. The safety profile of pasireotide LAR is essentially the same as that of pasireotide. Both agents are approved by the FDA and the EMA for use in patients with CD who have either failed surgery or are not surgical candidates.

Several centrally acting agents are in development, including gefitinib, r-roscovitine, isotretinoin, and silibinin. Recent studies have identified the presence of activating mutations of the ubiquitin-specific protease 8 (*USP8*) gene, which result in excessive deubiquitination of proteins normally targeted for proteasome degradation.[56] This leads to increased recycling of proteins, such as the epidermal growth factor receptor, to the plasma membrane, thus amplifying ACTH secretion.[57,58] An epidermal growth factor receptor tyrosine kinase inhibitor, gefitinib, is under study in patients with CD.[58] R-roscovitine is an inhibitor of cyclin-dependent kinase 2 and cyclin E, leading to decreased ACTH secretion and suppressed tumor growth in experimental studies.[59,60] R-roscovitine is also being investigated in patients with CD. Isotretinoin, an isomer of 13 *cis*-retinoic acid, was reported to control hypercortisolism in about 25% of patients with CD in small studies.[61,62] Silibinin acts by binding to heat shock protein 90 (HSP90), resulting in its dissociation from the GR.[63] In vitro and animal data suggest that silibinin therapy restores the negative feedback of cortisol on ACTH secretion and thus seems promising as a potential therapy in patients with CD.[63]

GLUCOCORTICOID RECEPTOR ANTAGONISTS

GR antagonists inhibit cortisol action by binding to its cognate receptor. Currently, mifepristone is the only agent in this class that is available for use; a second agent (relacorilant) is in clinical development.

Mifepristone was studied in a pivotal phase 3 study of 50 patients with Cushing syndrome, 43 of whom had CD.[64] Improvements in glycemia and blood pressure were reported in 60% of 29 and 38% of 21 patients, respectively, who had hyperglycemia or hypertension at baseline. The doses of glucose-lowering medications were decreased in several patients receiving mifepristone. In addition, 87% of study subjects had an improvement in overall clinical status.[64] Of note, ACTH and cortisol levels significantly increased greater than baseline in patients with CD on mifepristone therapy and may not be used to assess its clinical effectiveness.[65] As a corollary, the drug must be titrated based on clinical criteria alone. Mifepristone was approved by the FDA for use in patients with hyperglycemia with Cushing syndrome (including those with CD) who have failed surgery or are not surgical candidates.

Hypoadrenalism can develop in patients on mifepristone therapy as an extension of its pharmacologic action and must be diagnosed based on clinical grounds, because cortisol levels are not low in these patients.[64] If hypoadrenalism is suspected, mifepristone should be temporarily withdrawn until symptoms resolve. Patients with severe symptoms are rescued by administering dexamethasone in higher than replacement doses for several days.

Other adverse effects associated with mifepristone therapy include mineralocorticoid effects, such as hypokalemia, edema, and elevated blood pressure, which occur as a result of unopposed interaction of cortisol in high concentrations with the mineralocorticoid receptor.[64] Regular monitoring of serum potassium and administration of appropriate replacement therapy are clearly important in these patients, who may also benefit from spironolactone therapy. Endometrial thickening and metrorrhagia may occur as a result of progesterone receptor blockade but precancerous endometrial hyperplasia has not been observed.[64] Mifepristone terminates pregnancy and is contraindicated during gestation. Dyslipidemia and elevated thyroid-stimulating hormone levels have been also reported.[64] Regular surveillance of pituitary adenomas by periodic imaging is prudent. However, there are no concerning reports to suggest an increase in pituitary tumor size in patients on mifepristone therapy for the treatment duration studied thus far.[65] The drug has the potential to interact with other medications metabolized through several P-450 isoenzymes, including CYP3A4, thus necessitating review of all concurrent medications that patients use before initiating therapy.[66,67]

Relacorilant (CORT125134) is an investigational GR antagonist, which does not inhibit the progesterone receptor and is therefore unlikely to have adverse effects on the endometrium.[68] It is currently under investigation in patients with Cushing syndrome. A phase 2 study of 32 patients with Cushing syndrome (including those with CD) reported improvements in glycemia and blood pressure in response to relacorilant therapy.[69] Further investigation of relacorilant is under way.

SUMMARY

Medical therapy options for CD include steroidogenesis inhibitors, centrally acting agents, and GR antagonists. They are helpful in controlling hypercortisolism and are particularly used in patients who have either failed surgery or are not surgical candidates. All agents require careful monitoring to ensure that treatment targets are being met and evaluate for undue toxicity. Combination therapies, including several steroidogenesis inhibitors alone or in combination with centrally acting agents, have been studied in a small number of reports, but the exact role of this approach remains uncertain.[44,70–72] In recent years, there has been a flurry of interest in discovering and developing new drugs for CD, which may eventually lead to further expansion of available treatment options for this serious condition.

DISCLOSURE

N.A. Tritos has received institution-directed research support from Ipsen and Novartis. B.M.K. Biller has received institution-directed research support from Millendo, Novartis, and Strongbridge and occasional consulting honoraria from Novartis and Strongbridge.

REFERENCES

1. Cushing H. The basophil adenomas of the pituitary body and their clinical manifestations (pituitary basophilism). Bull Johns Hopkins Hosp 1932;50:137–95.
2. Cushing H. The basophil adenomas of the pituitary body. Ann R Coll Surg Engl 1969;44:180–1.
3. Clayton RN, Raskauskiene D, Reulen RC, et al. Mortality and morbidity in Cushing's disease over 50 years in Stoke-on-Trent, UK: audit and meta-analysis of literature. J Clin Endocrinol Metab 2011;96:632–42.
4. van Haalen FM, Broersen LH, Jorgensen JO, et al. Management of endocrine disease: mortality remains increased in Cushing's disease despite biochemical remission: a systematic review and meta-analysis. Eur J Endocrinol 2015;172: R143–9.
5. Nieman LK, Biller BM, Findling JW, et al. Treatment of Cushing's syndrome: an endocrine society clinical practice guideline. J Clin Endocrinol Metab 2015; 100:2807–31.

6. Swearingen B. Update on pituitary surgery. J Clin Endocrinol Metab 2012;97: 1073–81.

7. Tritos NA, Biller BM, Swearingen B. Management of Cushing disease. Nat Rev Endocrinol 2011;7:279–89.

8. Swearingen B, Barker FG 2nd, Zervas NT. The management of pituitary adenomas: the MGH experience. Clin Neurosurg 1999;45:48–56.

9. Roelfsema F, Biermasz NR, Pereira AM. Clinical factors involved in the recurrence of pituitary adenomas after surgical remission: a structured review and meta-analysis. Pituitary 2012;15:71–83.

10. Tritos NA, Biller BM. Cushing's disease. Handb Clin Neurol 2014;124:221–34.

11. Tritos NA, Biller BM. Medical management of Cushing's disease. J Neurooncol 2014;117:407–14.

12. Lacroix A, Feelders RA, Stratakis CA, et al. Cushing's syndrome. Lancet 2015; 386:913–27.

13. Fleseriu M, Petersenn S. Medical therapy for Cushing's disease: adrenal steroidogenesis inhibitors and glucocorticoid receptor blockers. Pituitary 2015;18: 245–52.

14. Sonino N, Boscaro M, Paoletta A, et al. Ketoconazole treatment in Cushing's syndrome: experience in 34 patients. Clin Endocrinol (Oxf) 1991;35:347–52.

15. Tabarin A, Navarranne A, Guerin J, et al. Use of ketoconazole in the treatment of Cushing's disease and ectopic ACTH syndrome. Clin Endocrinol (Oxf) 1991; 34:63–9.

16. Castinetti F, Guignat L, Giraud P, et al. Ketoconazole in Cushing's disease: is it worth a try? J Clin Endocrinol Metab 2014;99:1623–30.

17. McCance DR, Ritchie CM, Sheridan B, et al. Acute hypoadrenalism and hepato-toxicity after treatment with ketoconazole. Lancet 1987;1:573.

18. Verhelst JA, Trainer PJ, Howlett TA, et al. Short and long-term responses to metyrapone in the medical management of 91 patients with Cushing's syndrome. Clin Endocrinol (Oxf) 1991;35:169–78.

19. Daniel E, Aylwin S, Mustafa O, et al. Effectiveness of metyrapone in treating Cushing's syndrome: a retrospective multicenter study in 195 patients. J Clin Endocrinol Metab 2015;100(11):4146–54.

20. Gormley MJ, Hadden DR, Kennedy TL, et al. Cushing's syndrome in pregnancy: treatment with metyrapone. Clin Endocrinol (Oxf) 1982;16:283–93.

21. Lindsay JR, Jonklaas J, Oldfield EH, et al. Cushing's syndrome during pregnancy: personal experience and review of the literature. J Clin Endocrinol Metab 2005;90:3077–83.

22. Mauclere-Denost S, Leboulleux S, Borget I, et al. High-dose mitotane strategy in adrenocortical carcinoma: prospective analysis of plasma mitotane measurement during the first 3 months of follow-up. Eur J Endocrinol 2012;166:261–8.

23. Terzolo M, Angeli A, Fassnacht M, et al. Adjuvant mitotane treatment for adrenocortical carcinoma. N Engl J Med 2007;356:2372–80.

24. Baudry C, Coste J, Bou Khalil R, et al. Efficiency and tolerance of mitotane in Cushing's disease in 76 patients from a single center. Eur J Endocrinol 2012; 167:473–81.

25. Preda VA, Sen J, Karavitaki N, et al. Etomidate in the management of hypercorti-solaemia in Cushing's syndrome: a review. Eur J Endocrinol 2012;167:137–43.

26. Carroll TB, Peppard WJ, Herrmann DJ, et al. Continuous etomidate infusion for the management of severe Cushing syndrome: validation of a standard protocol. J Endocr Soc 2019;3:1–12.

27. Auchus RJ, Wu Y, Liu J. 2S, 4R-ketoconazole is the relevant enantiomer of keto-conazole for cortisol synthesis inhibition: steroidogenic P450 inhibition involves multiple mechanisms. Endocr Rev 2018;39.

28. Fleseriu M, Pivonello R, Elenkova A, et al. Efficacy and safety of levoketoconazole in the treatment of endogenous Cushing's syndrome (SONICS): a phase 3, multi-centre, open-label, single-arm trial. Lancet Diabetes Endocrinol 2019;7:855–65.

29. Bertagna X, Pivonello R, Fleseriu M, et al. LCI699, a potent 11beta-hydroxylase inhibitor, normalizes urinary cortisol in patients with Cushing's disease: results from a multicenter, proof-of-concept study. J Clin Endocrinol Metab 2014;99: 1375–83.

30. Biller BMK, Newell-Price J, Fleseriu M, et al. Osilodorstat treatment in Cushing's disease: results from a phase III, multicenter double-blind, randomized with-drawal study (LINC 3). J Endocr Soc 2019;3. OR16-2.

31. Langlois DK, Fritz MC, Schall WD, et al. ATR-101, a selective ACAT1 inhibitor, de-creases ACTH-stimulated cortisol concentrations in dogs with naturally occurring Cushing's syndrome. BMC Endocr Disord 2018;18:24.

32. Berruti A, Pia A, Terzolo M. Abiraterone and increased survival in metastatic pros-tate cancer. N Engl J Med 2011;365:766 [author reply: 7–8].

33. Gartrell BA, Saad F. Abiraterone in the management of castration-resistant pros-tate cancer prior to chemotherapy. Ther Adv Urol 2015;7:194–202.

34. Claps M, Lazzari B, Grisanti S, et al. Management of severe Cushing syndrome induced by adrenocortical carcinoma with abiraterone acetate: a case report. AACE Clin Case Rep 2016;2:e337–41.

35. Cuevas-Ramos D, Lim DST, Fleseriu M. Update on medical treatment for Cush-ing's disease. Clin Diabetes Endocrinol 2016;2:16.

36. Feldhaus AL, Anderson K, Dutzar B, et al. ALD1613, a novel long-acting mono-clonal antibody to control ACTH-driven pharmacology. Endocrinology 2017; 158:1–8.

37. Petrossians P, Thonnard AS, Beckers A. Medical treatment in Cushing's syn-drome: dopamine agonists and cabergoline. Neuroendocrinology 2010; 92(Suppl 1):116–9.

38. Boscaro M, Ludlam WH, Atkinson B, et al. Treatment of pituitary-dependent Cushing's disease with the multireceptor ligand somatostatin analog pasireotide (SOM230): a multicenter, phase II trial. J Clin Endocrinol Metab 2009;94:115–22.

39. Klibanski A. Clinical practice. Prolactinomas. N Engl J Med 2010;362:1219–26.

40. Pivonello R, De Martino MC, Cappabianca P, et al. The medical treatment of Cushing's disease: effectiveness of chronic treatment with the dopamine agonist cabergoline in patients unsuccessfully treated by surgery. J Clin Endocrinol Metab 2009;94:223–30.

41. Godbout A, Manavela M, Danilowicz K, et al. Cabergoline monotherapy in the long-term treatment of Cushing's disease. Eur J Endocrinol 2010;163:709–16.

42. Vilar L, Naves LA, Azevedo MF, et al. Effectiveness of cabergoline in monother-apy and combined with ketoconazole in the management of Cushing's disease. Pituitary 2010;13:123–9.

43. Burman P, Eden-Engstrom B, Ekman B, et al. Limited value of cabergoline in Cushing's disease: a prospective study of a 6-week treatment in 20 patients. Eur J Endocrinol 2016;174:17–24.

44. Barbot M, Albiger N, Ceccato F, et al. Combination therapy for Cushing's disease: effectiveness of two schedules of treatment: should we start with cabergoline or ketoconazole? Pituitary 2014;17:109–17.

45. Bancos I, Nannenga MR, Bostwick JM, et al. Impulse control disorders in patients with dopamine agonist-treated prolactinomas and nonfunctioning pituitary adenomas: a case-control study. Clin Endocrinol (Oxf) 2014;80:863–8.

46. Bancos I, Nippoldt TB, Erickson D. Hypersexuality in men with prolactinomas treated with dopamine agonists. Endocrine 2017;56:456–7.

47. Barake M, Evins AE, Stoeckel L, et al. Investigation of impulsivity in patients on dopamine agonist therapy for hyperprolactinemia: a pilot study. Pituitary 2014; 17:150–6.

48. Barake M, Klibanski A, Tritos NA. Management of endocrine disease. Impulse control disorders in patients with hyperpolactinemia treated with dopamine agonists: how much should we worry? Eur J Endocrinol 2018;179:R287–96.

49. De Sousa SMC, Baranoff J, Rushworth RL, et al. Impulse control disorders in dopamine agonist-treated hyperprolactinemia: prevalence and risk factors. J Clin Endocrinol Metab 2020;105(3):dgz076.

50. Zanettini R, Antonini A, Gatto G, et al. Valvular heart disease and the use of dopamine agonists for Parkinson's disease. N Engl J Med 2007;356:39–46.

51. Schade R, Andersohn F, Suissa S, et al. Dopamine agonists and the risk of cardiac-valve regurgitation. N Engl J Med 2007;356:29–38.

52. Valassi E, Klibanski A, Biller BM. Clinical review: potential cardiac valve effects of dopamine agonists in hyperprolactinemia. J Clin Endocrinol Metab 2010;95: 1025–33.

53. Colao A, Petersenn S, Newell-Price J, et al. A 12-month phase 3 study of pasireotide in Cushing's disease. N Engl J Med 2012;366:914–24.

54. Henry RR, Ciaraldi TP, Armstrong D, et al. Hyperglycemia associated with pasireotide: results from a mechanistic study in healthy volunteers. J Clin Endocrinol Metab 2013;98:3446–53.

55. Lacroix A, Gu F, Gallardo W, et al. Efficacy and safety of once-monthly pasireotide in Cushing's disease: a 12 month clinical trial. Lancet Diabetes Endocrinol 2017; 6(1):17–26.

56. Reincke M, Sbiera S, Hayakawa A, et al. Mutations in the deubiquitinase gene USP8 cause Cushing's disease. Nat Genet 2015;47:31–8.

57. Theodoropoulou M, Reincke M, Fassnacht M, et al. Decoding the genetic basis of Cushing's disease: USP8 in the spotlight. Eur J Endocrinol 2015;173:M73–83.

58. Fukuoka H, Cooper O, Ben-Shlomo A, et al. EGFR as a therapeutic target for human, canine, and mouse ACTH-secreting pituitary adenomas. J Clin Invest 2011; 121:4712–21.

59. Liu NA, Araki T, Cuevas-Ramos D, et al. Cyclin E-mediated human proopiomelanocortin regulation as a therapeutic target for Cushing disease. J Clin Endocrinol Metab 2015;100:2557–64.

60. Liu NA, Jiang H, Ben-Shlomo A, et al. Targeting zebrafish and murine pituitary corticotroph tumors with a cyclin-dependent kinase (CDK) inhibitor. Proc Natl Acad Sci U S A 2011;108:8414–9.

61. Pecori Giraldi F, Ambrogio AG, Andrioli M, et al. Potential role for retinoic acid in patients with Cushing's disease. J Clin Endocrinol Metab 2012;97:3577–83.

62. Vilar L, Albuquerque JL, Lyra R, et al. The role of isotretinoin therapy for Cushing's disease: results of a prospective study. Int J Endocrinol 2016;2016:8173182.

63. Riebold M, Kozany C, Freiburger L, et al. A C-terminal HSP90 inhibitor restores glucocorticoid sensitivity and relieves a mouse allograft model of Cushing disease. Nat Med 2015;21:276–80.

64. Fleseriu M, Biller BM, Findling JW, et al. Mifepristone, a glucocorticoid receptor antagonist, produces clinical and metabolic benefits in patients with Cushing's syndrome. J Clin Endocrinol Metab 2012;97:2039–49.
65. Fleseriu M, Findling JW, Koch CA, et al. Changes in plasma ACTH levels and corticotroph tumor size in patients with Cushing's disease during long-term treatment with the glucocorticoid receptor antagonist mifepristone. J Clin Endocrinol Metab 2014;99:3718–27.
66. Castinetti F, Fassnacht M, Johanssen S, et al. Merits and pitfalls of mifepristone in Cushing's syndrome. Eur J Endocrinol 2009;160:1003–10.
67. Fleseriu M, Molitch ME, Gross C, et al. A new therapeutic approach in the medical treatment of Cushing's syndrome: glucocorticoid receptor blockade with mifepristone. Endocr Pract 2013;19:313–26.
68. Hunt H, Donaldson K, Strem M, et al. Assessment of safety, tolerability, pharmacokinetics, and pharmacological effect of orally administered CORT125134: an adaptive, double-blind, randomized, placebo-controlled phase 1 clinical study. Clin Pharmacol Drug Dev 2018;7:408–21.
69. Moraitis A, Agrawal N, Bancos I, et al. Open label phase 2 study to assess safety and efficacy of relacorilant (CORT125134), a selective cortisol modulator, in the treatment of endogenous hypercortisolism. Endocr Pract 2018;24:300–1.
70. Kamenicky P, Droumaguet C, Salenave S, et al. Mitotane, metyrapone, and ketoconazole combination therapy as an alternative to rescue adrenalectomy for severe ACTH-dependent Cushing's syndrome. J Clin Endocrinol Metab 2011;96:2796–804.
71. Feelders RA, de Bruin C, Pereira AM, et al. Pasireotide alone or with cabergoline and ketoconazole in Cushing's disease. N Engl J Med 2010;362:1846–8.
72. Corcuff JB, Young J, Masquefa-Giraud P, et al. Rapid control of severe neoplastic hypercortisolism with metyrapone and ketoconazole. Eur J Endocrinol 2015;172:473–81.

Nelson's Syndrome
An Update

Athanasios Fountas, MD, MSc[a,b,c],
Niki Karavitaki, MD, MSc, PhD, FRCP[a,b,c],*

KEYWORDS

- Nelson's syndrome • Cushing's • Bilateral adrenalectomy
- Corticotroph tumor progression • Tumor growth

KEY POINTS

- Patients with Cushing's disease treated with bilateral adrenalectomy require long-term monitoring for the development of Nelson's syndrome.
- Corticotroph tumor growth is essential for Nelson's syndrome diagnosis; nonetheless, gradually increasing adrenocorticotropic hormone (ACTH) levels without demonstrable tumor enlargement needs to be included in the diagnostic algorithm.
- Data on factors predicting Nelson's syndrome development are conflicting; high ACTH during the first year after bilateral adrenalectomy is the one most consistently reported.
- Surgery followed or not by radiotherapy in cases of Nelson's syndrome is associated with higher tumor control rates compared with observation alone.
- A subset of patients with Nelson's syndrome demonstrates aggressive tumor behavior; predictive factors are unknown, management is individualized, and prognosis may be poor.

INTRODUCTION

Despite the advances in pituitary surgery, radiotherapy, and medical treatment of Cushing's disease (CD), bilateral adrenalectomy (BLA) still holds a place in the management of this condition, particularly in cases refractory to other therapeutic modalities, or as an emergency measure in patients with severe manifestations of hypercortisolemia. BLA offers immediate control of the cortisol excess but Nelson's syndrome (NS) is a potential complication with various adverse sequelae.[1–9]

[a] Institute of Metabolism and Systems Research, College of Medical and Dental Sciences, University of Birmingham, IBR Tower, Level 2, Birmingham, B15 2TT, UK; [b] Centre for Endocrinology, Diabetes and Metabolism, Birmingham Health Partners, Birmingham, B15 2TH, UK; [c] Department of Endocrinology, Queen Elizabeth Hospital, University Hospitals Birmingham NHS Foundation Trust, Birmingham, B15 2TH, UK
* Corresponding author. Institute of Metabolism and Systems Research, College of Medical and Dental Sciences, University of Birmingham, IBR Tower, Level 2, Birmingham, B15 2TT, UK.
E-mail address: n.karavitaki@bham.ac.uk

More than 60 years since the first description of the syndrome by Don Nelson and colleagues,[10] this condition still is surrounded by uncertainties in its diagnosis, management, and long-term outcomes. These are attributed mainly to the rarity of NS but also to the lack of sufficient quality data, as most of the studies have significant heterogeneity in their diagnostic criteria, monitoring/management approaches, and treatment endpoints.[2,4,7,8,11–13]

This review provides an update on NS, focusing on studies published after 1990, when the use of magnetic resonance imaging (MRI) was embedded in clinical practice, and areas requiring further research in this field are identified.

DEFINITION OF NELSON'S SYNDROME

Currently, there is no formal consensus on what defines NS, and the diagnostic criteria vary amongst available studies (**Table 1**). In most of the published literature, diagnosis of NS is based on 3 main axes: (1) radiographic evidence of corticotroph tumor growth (if tumor was evident on the pre-BLA imaging) or identification of tumor (if pre-BLA imaging was negative for tumor), (2) increased plasma adrenocorticotropic hormone (ACTH) levels, and (3) development of skin pigmentation.

Radiographic evidence of corticotroph tumor growth is the most frequently used criterion for NS diagnosis, either alone[4,13–16] or in combination with increased ACTH levels and/or pigmentation.[2,17–29] In the MRI era, early detection of marginal tumor growth (even before clinical manifestations become evident) is possible, giving ground to the concept of replacing the term *NS* with *corticotroph tumor progression*.[14] The definition of tumor growth varies significantly in the published studies. In the majority, no specific size or volume criteria have been described and simply radiographic evidence of corticotroph tumor growth or identification of new tumor (when previous pituitary imaging was negative) was sufficient for NS diagnosis.[2,15–17,19–21,23–26,28,29] In other studies, increase in tumor size of at least 2 mm in 1 dimension compared with previous imaging was a requirement,[4,14] whereas in another report, growth was accepted only if tumor volume exceeded 10% of its original one.[13] Further applied criteria include growth of adenoma that led to surgery or radiotherapy[12,30] or presence of a macroadenoma.[27]

Markedly elevated ACTH levels have been used as a sole diagnostic criterion of NS[31,32] or used together with imaging findings,[17] skin pigmentation,[33,34] or both.[19,20,22–25,27,28] However, the ACTH values differ between studies, and no specific cutoff has as yet been defined (see **Table 1**). Furthermore, the timing of the ACTH sampling rarely is reported or, when provided, varies considerably between the series (simply fasting ACTH[23,27] or at any time point[31,33] or in midafternoon[28]). Interestingly, despite the suppressive effect of glucocorticoid treatment on ACTH levels, the impact of timing of glucocorticoid administration on the ACTH values has been taken into account in only 3 studies; in Thompson and colleagues,[19] patients were refrained from steroid replacement for 24 hours, and in McCance and colleagues,[28] ACTH measurement was performed 6 to 8 hours after the last dose of hydrocortisone. Finally, ACTH levels greater than 200 pg/mL 120 minutes after the usual hydrocortisone morning dose, was considered diagnostic for NS by Jenkins and colleagues.[32]

Skin pigmentation has been used as a diagnostic criterion of NS in combination with corticotroph tumor growth and/or increased ACTH levels;[18–20,22–25,27–29,33,34] only 1 series has adopted it as the only criterion.[21] Nowadays, with the advances in the hormone assays and in neuroradiology techniques, diagnosis of NS can occur

Table 1
Diagnostic criteria and prevalence of Nelson's syndrome in studies published since 1990

Study	Period Covered	Diagnostic Criteria for Nelson's Syndrome	Number of Patients Diagnosed with Nelson's Syndrome (%)	Interval Between Bilateral Adrenalectomy and Nelson's Syndrome Diagnosis (Range)	Follow-up Since Bilateral Adrenalectomy (Range)
Cohen et al,[2] 2019	1974–2011	Imaging (expanding pituitary mass lesion after BLA in MRI or CT) and/or increased plasma ACTH levels (>500 pg/mL with rising levels on at least 3 consecutive occasions)	6/13 (46.2)	Mean 24 mo (8–47)	Mean 14 y (5–30) For those with NS, mean 13.1 y ± 7.2 y (5–20) For those without NS, mean 26.7 y ± 6.9 y (17–37)
Nagendra et al,[36] 2019	2005–2018	NR	6/14 (42.9)	Mean 32 mo	NR
Sarkis et al,[30] 2019	1990–2015	NS reported in patients who received surgery or radiotherapy for it	5/17 (29.4)	NR	NR
Graffeo et al,[4] 2017	1996–2015	Imaging (at least 2 mm of tumor growth in 1 dimension after BLA in comparison with previous MRI studies)	47/88 (53.4)	Mean 3 y ± 2 y (1–8)	For those with NS, mean 23 y ± 2 y (2–58) For those without NS, mean 8 y ± 1 y (1–42)
Espinosa-de-Los-Monteros et al,[17] 2017	1991–2014	Imaging (expanding pituitary mass compared to pre-BLA images) and increased plasma ACTH levels (>200 pg/mL in addition to a >30% increase on at least 3 consecutive occasions)	6/12 (50) (in 1 patient diagnosis was based only on imaging)	Median 2.5 y (IQR 2–8.5)	NR

(continued on next page)

Table 1
(continued)

Study	Period Covered	Diagnostic Criteria for Nelson's Syndrome	Number of Patients Diagnosed with Nelson's Syndrome (%)	Interval Between Bilateral Adrenalectomy and Nelson's Syndrome Diagnosis (Range)	Follow-up Since Bilateral Adrenalectomy (Range)
Prajapati et al,[37] 2015	1991–2013	NR	5/12 (41.7)	Median 32 mo (20–60)	Median 80.5 mo[a] (2–157)
Osswald et al,[12] 2014	1990–2013	Growth of a tumor leading to surgery or radiotherapy	7/29 (24.1)	Median 51 mo	Median 11 y[a] (0.8–51)
Mehta et al,[13] 2013	NR	Imaging (tumor growth when tumor exceeded 10% of its original volume in MRI)	1/20 (5)	NR	Median 5.4 y (0.6–12)
Tiyadatah et al,[38] 2012	2003–2011	NR	3/7 (42.9)	Median 1 y (4 mo–2 y)	Mean 32.6 mo[a] (6–73)
Xing et al,[18] 2008	1980–2005	Imaging (increase in pituitary adenoma size) and skin pigmentation	5/15 (33.3)	Mean 15.8 mo (1–24)	Mean 47 mo (9–120)
Prevedello et al,[39] 2008	1992–2005	NR	2/10 (20)	NR	NR
Thompson et al,[19] 2007	1994-unknown	Imaging (growing residual pituitary adenoma in MRI), increased plasma ACTH levels (>300 pg/mL) and skin pigmentation	3/35 (8.6)	NR	Mean 3.6 y (0.25–10)
Gil-Cárdenas et al,[20] 2007	1990–2005	Imaging (presence of a pituitary tumor in patients without preexisting pituitary enlargement or growth of a known pituitary tumor), increased plasma ACTH levels, and skin pigmentation	11/39 (28.2)	Mean 15 mo (2–33)	Mean 53 mo (12–188)

Assie et al,[14] 2007	1991–2002	Imaging (occurrence of pituitary tumor when no visible tumor on previous MRI studies or increase of at least 2 mm in 1 dimension of a preexisting tumor, associated with at least 1 of the following: (1) increase in stalk deviation, (2) increase in the upward convexity of the diaphragma sellae, and (3) increase in sellar floor asymmetry)	21/53 (39.6)	Median 2 y (1–7) Mean 2.19 y ± 1.78 y	Median 4.6 y (0.5–13.5)
Dalvi et al,[21] 2006	2001–2006	Imaging (recurrent pituitary tumor) or skin pigmentation	3/8 (37.5)	NR	Mean 24.16 mo[a] (4–61)
Hawn et al,[40] 2002	1994–2000	NR	1/10 (10)	3 y	Median 29 mo[a]
Wright-Pascoe et al,[41] 2001	1963–1983	NR	4/15 (26.7)	NR	NR
Vella et al,[42] 2001	1996–2000	NR	0/12 (0)	NR	Mean 2.7 y[a] (1.2–4.8)
Nagesser et al,[22] 2000	1953–1989	Full-blown NS: increased plasma ACTH levels, skin pigmentation, and expanding growth of pituitary adenoma causing visual field disturbances Beginning NS: increased plasma ACTH levels, skin pigmentation and nonexpanding pituitary microadenoma Hyperpigmentation syndrome: increased plasma ACTH levels, skin pigmentation and no radiographic evidence of pituitary adenoma	Full-blown NS: 4/44 (9.1) Beginning NS: 6/44 (13.6) Hyperpigmentation syndrome: 5/44 (11.4)	Full-blown NS, mean 15 y (7–24) Beginning NS, mean 16 y (10–23) Hyperpigmentation syndrome Mean 11 y (5–18)	Mean 19 y (1.0–39.8)

(continued on next page)

Table 1 (continued)					
Study	Period Covered	Diagnostic Criteria for Nelson's Syndrome	Number of Patients Diagnosed with Nelson's Syndrome (%)	Interval Between Bilateral Adrenalectomy and Nelson's Syndrome Diagnosis (Range)	Follow-up Since Bilateral Adrenalectomy (Range)
Invitti et al,[43] 1999	1979–1999	NR	8/23 (34.8)	Median: 23 mo (6–150) Mean 60 mo ± 25.4 mo	(2–15 y)
Pereira et al,[23] 1998	NR	Imaging (enlarging pituitary tumor in CT and/or MRI), increased fasting plasma ACTH levels, and skin pigmentation	14/30 (46.7)	Mean 4.6 y ± 2.9 y Median 4 y (11 mo–10 y)	Mean 8 y ± 6 y Median 6 y (2–21)
Feleke et al,[44] 1998	1985–1995	NR	3/5 (60)	NR	NR
Sonino et al,[24] 1996	1976–1996	Imaging (evidence of pituitary tumor), markedly elevated plasma ACTH levels, and skin pigmentation	29.8% ± 7.4% at 10-y follow-up	NR	Median 9 y (2–18)
Imai et al,[15] 1996	1957–1993	Imaging (evidence of pituitary tumor)	4/16 (25)	NR	Mean 24.6 y (14–35)
Chapuis et al,[45] 1996	1980–1995	NR	12/76 (15.8)	(2–10 y)	NR
Jenkins et al,[32] 1995	1946–1993	Plasma ACTH level >200 pg/mL 120 min after the usual morning dose of hydrocortisone replacement and skin pigmentation	11/38 (28.9) 11/34 (32.4) after exclusion of 4 patients with ACTH-dependent Cushing's of unknown etiology	Median 1 y (0.25–9.5)	Median 10 y[a] (0.5 mo–46 y)

Study	Time period	Diagnostic criteria	n/N (%)	Time to diagnosis	Follow-up
O'Riordain et al,[25] 1994	1980–1991	Imaging (evidence of pituitary tumor), increased plasma ACTH levels, and skin pigmentation	3/20 (15)	NR	Median 58 mo
Misra et al,[26] 1994	1984–1992	Neurologic or definite radiological evidence of pituitary tumor in radiograph or CT	2/18 (11.1)	NR	NR
Keming et al,[27] 1994	1962–1991	Imaging (evidence of pituitary tumor >1 cm), increased fasting plasma ACTH levels (>200 pmol/L) and skin pigmentation	8/48 (16.7)	Mean 6.6 y ± 4.3 y (1.5–13)	Median 9.5 y (1–30)
Favia et al,[46] 1994	1975–1991	NR	6/41 (14.6)	NR	Median 9 y (2–16)
Moreira et al,[16] 1993	NR	Imaging (evidence of pituitary tumor in CT)	3/7 (42.9)	Median 24 mo (14–26)	Median 33 mo (24–84)
McCance et al,[28] 1993	1972–1991	Imaging (evidence of pituitary tumor in CT), increased plasma ACTH levels, and skin pigmentation	9/26 (34.6)	NR	Median 5.25 y (0.6–19.1)
Grabner et al,[29] 1991	NR	Imaging (evidence of pituitary tumor) and skin pigmentation	10/109 (9.2)	Median 9.5 y (3–20)	Median 12.5 y (1–34)
Littley et al,[34] 1990	NR	Grossly elevated plasma ACTH levels and skin pigmentation	5/9 (55.6)	Median 68 mo (26–140)	Median 112 mo (80–171)

Abbreviations: CT, computed tomography; IQR, interquartile range; NR, not reported.
[a] The reported interval involves the whole group of patients with Cushing's disease and does not focus on those who had bilateral adrenalectomy.
Data from Refs.[2,4,12–30,32,34,36–46]

at an early stage, making pigmentation less common as a presenting manifestation of NS.

Taking into account these data but also the lack of studies establishing reliably diagnostic criteria for NS, the view of the authors is that diagnosis should rely on corticotroph tumor growth detected on pituitary MRI (evidence of tumor enlargement compared with pre-BLA imaging or, if previous pituitary imaging negative, new identification of tumor) and/or gradually increasing ACTH levels in a patient compliant on adequate glucocorticoid replacement. Specific cutoff values for ACTH have not been validated and a suggested approach includes an increase in plasma ACTH (taken at 8:00 AM, 20 hours after the last dose of glucocorticoid and before that morning's dose) of 100 pg/mL compared with a previous measurement (taken under the same conditions) or failure to suppress plasma ACTH to less than 200 pg/mL 2 hours after the morning glucocorticoid dose.[35]

EPIDEMIOLOGY

The prevalence of NS ranges between 0% and 60%[2,4,12–30,32,34,36–46] (see **Table 1**) and is influenced mainly by the diagnostic criteria, the length of follow-up, and possible referral bias of the reporting centers. In the study with rate of 0%, there is no information for the diagnostic approach and the length of the follow-up was short (mean: 2.7 years [range 1.2–4.8]).[42] Based on specific diagnostic criteria used, prevalence is between 5% and 53.4% for positive imaging[4,13–16]; the 5% rate was reported by Mehta and colleagues,[13] where definition of NS required greater than 10% increase of tumor volume compared with its original one, and, therefore, smaller growths were not included; in the remaining series, rates were greater than or equal to 25%.[4,14–16] Prevalence ranges between 32.4% and 55.6%[32,34] for increased ACTH levels combined or not with skin pigmentation and between 8.6% and 46.7% for radiological tumor growth, increased ACTH levels, and skin pigmentation.[19,20,22–25,27,28]

The interval between BLA and NS detection also varies between series (see **Table 1**) reflecting again the differences in the diagnostic strategy. When only positive imaging was required, NS was diagnosed at mean/median period of 2 to 3 years after BLA,[4,14,16] whereas when diagnosis was based on biochemical/clinical criteria, the median latency of NS onset was 1 to 5.7 years.[32,34] The mean interval between BLA and NS diagnosis also differs significantly in studies in which all criteria (radiographic, biochemical, and clinical) had to be met, ranging from 15 months to 16 years.[20,22,23,27]

PATHOGENESIS

Pathogenesis of NS remains unknown. Loss of the negative glucocorticoid feedback on the hypothalamus with subsequent increase in corticotropin-releasing hormone production leading to corticotroph neoplasia and NS has been proposed as one theory.[47] Although studies in rodents support this,[48,49] relevant evidence from human studies is still lacking. Furthermore, the fact the NS does not develop in all CD patients treated with BLA suggests that other factors also may be implicated. A second hypothesis suggests that NS represents the natural history of an aggressive corticotroph tumor. Despite the new insights, however, on the molecular pathogenesis of corticotroph tumors,[50] the mechanisms driving tumor progression and leading to NS remain poorly understood. Corticotroph tumor growth has been associated with reduced expression of E-cadherin (with Nelson's tumors demonstrating lowest expression compared with corticotroph microadenomas or macroadenomas); this molecule plays a role in cell-cell adhesion in epithelial tissues and its decreased expression has been correlated with increased invasiveness and metastatic potential for different types of tumors.[51] On the other hand, the prevalence of *USP8* mutations is similar between CD and Nelson's tumors, suggesting that *USP8* mutations do not drive corticotroph adenoma progression that leads to NS.[52]

PREDICTIVE FACTORS FOR DEVELOPMENT OF NELSON'S SYNDROME AFTER BILATERAL ADRENALECTOMY

Identification of factors predicting the development of NS has proved difficult, because several studies have provided conflicting results.

High ACTH levels in the first year after BLA is the most consistently found predictive factor in most,[2,14,16] but not all,[17] reports published after 1990. No definitive threshold value of ACTH has been, as yet, defined and, although Assie and colleagues[14] suggested that a greater than 100 pg/mL increase of ACTH levels in the first year after BLA is a predictor of corticotroph tumor growth, this finding has not been evaluated further.

Presence of a pituitary adenoma prior to BLA has also been proposed as a risk factor[24,32] but this has not been confirmed in other series.[14,20] Controversy also exists on the role of pituitary radiotherapy in preventing NS development (administered either as therapeutic intervention for the hypercortisolism [prior to BLA] or as prophylactic measure [at the time of BLA]). Although some studies have shown a protective effect,[20,22,32] this has not been confirmed in others.[23,24]

Young age at the time of BLA has been proposed as a risk factor by Kemink and colleagues,[27] but subsequent studies did not confirm this,[14,22,24] whereas short duration of CD also has been found to be predictive,[14] but not in all studies.[22,27] High urinary cortisol levels before BLA have been identified as a predictive factor in the study of Sonino and colleagues,[24] but not in the study of Pereira and colleagues,[23] whereas the presence of residual adrenal tissue after BLA has not been confirmed to be protective against the development of NS.[14,22] Finally, Nagesser and colleagues[22] suggested that insufficient glucocorticoid replacement therapy after BLA may be associated with NS development, but this factor has not been assessed in further studies.

MONITORING FOR DEVELOPMENT OF NELSON'S SYNDROME AFTER BILATERAL ADRENALECTOMY

Given the lack of widely accepted factors for the development of NS, all patients with CD treated with BLA require monitoring; this should be lifelong, because diagnosis of NS has been reported as late as 32 years after BLA.[1] Formal guidelines on an effective follow-up protocol are not available but this should include measurement of plasma ACTH levels and imaging surveillance.

Considering the impact of timing of ACTH measurements in relationship with the dose and type of glucocorticoid, blood sampling for ACTH needs to be performed at least 20 hours after the last administration of glucocorticoid and prior to the morning dose.[35,53] A second ACTH sample 2 hours after the morning glucocorticoid dose will help discriminate if ACTH responds or not to the negative feedback of steroids.[32,35,47] Increase of the morning plasma ACTH levels (20 hours off glucocorticoid) greater than 100 pg/mL compared with previous measurements and/or plasma ACTH greater than 200 pg/mL 2 hours after the morning glucocorticoid dose should be investigated further with a pituitary MRI.[35]

Biochemical surveillance is recommended at 6-monthly intervals for the first 3 years and annually thereafter. The frequency of the imaging monitoring varies amongst investigators[35,53,54] and a proposed approach includes high-resolution pituitary MRI 6 to

12 months after the BLA and then yearly. If plasma ACTH remains low after the initial 3 years of annual monitoring, the imaging interval can be extended to every other year.

MANAGEMENT OF NELSON'S SYNDROME

The long-term outcomes of patients with NS after primary management have been assessed poorly, especially in the modern era. Drawbacks of the limited published series include small number of patients, differences in the length of follow-up, and heterogeneity in the criteria defining successful treatment of NS (**Table 2**). Furthermore, in some studies, the inclusion in the analyses of tumors already showing regrowth after their primary management[3,5,7,55–59] and the lack of information on previous therapies[3,5,6,57–61] make the interpretation of their results difficult.

Surgery

Surgical removal of the Nelson's tumor has been associated with growth rates ranging between 0% and 50% during variable follow-up periods[1,2,7–9,11,62] (see **Table 2**). The series reporting 0% growth rate had only 4 patients monitored for a short interval (median 39 months).[10] In the largest study to date of patients with NS from 13 UK pituitary centers, the 10-year tumor progression-free survival was 80% for those treated by surgery.[1]

There is no consensus on the definition on NS remission after treatment and this has been delineated in only 4 studies.[7–9,11] The proposed criteria included (1) ACTH less than 200 pg/mL (<44 pmol/L) 2 hours after the morning glucocorticoid dose,[7] (2) ACTH less than 200 pmol/L (<909 pg/mL) after stopping glucocorticoid replacement therapy for at least 24 hours and tumor size less than 10 mm^3, (3) ACTH less than 70 pg/mL (<15.4 pmol/L) 2 hours after the morning glucocorticoid dose and no evidence of tumor growth,[9] and (4) ACTH less than 200 pg/mL (<44 pmol/L) after stopping glucocorticoid replacement therapy for 24 hours and no MRI evidence of tumor.[11] The reported remission rates were between 33% and 100%, but the small number of cases in each study (4–10 patients) challenges the validity of these rates. Nonetheless, small tumor size and no extrasellar extension have been associated with long-lasting remission.[8,11]

Radiotherapy

Radiotherapy is an alternative treatment of NS either alone or after pituitary surgery.

Adjuvant radiotherapy is used mainly in cases of incomplete tumor removal aiming to control its growth rate. Kelly and colleagues[7] reported tumor growth in 1 of 7 patients (14%) managed by surgery and radiotherapy during a 17-year median follow-up (range 9–20 years); however, this patient already had a recurrent tumor. Remission of NS (ACTH <200 pg/mL 2 hours after morning glucocorticoid dose) with no residual tumor was achieved in 4 (57%) patients; in the remaining 2, ACTH decreased and 1 had no residual tumor, whereas the second had stable residuum. In the UK Nelson's study, tumor growth probability was 19% at 10 years in those managed by surgery and radiotherapy.[1]

Pituitary irradiation as a primary treatment of NS has been used in patients not candidates for surgery, either due to tumor location or because of significant comorbidities. Tran and colleagues[63] reported normal ACTH levels in 50% (2/4) of patients treated with radiotherapy, with the remaining of them being on clinical remission (no clear definition for this was provided) during median follow-up of 3 years. In the series by Espinosa-de-Los-Monteros and colleagues,[17] primary treatment with radiotherapy in 4 patients followed-up for median period of 4.4 years resulted in tumor shrinkage in

Table 2
Primary treatment and outcomes of patients with Nelson's syndrome in studies published since 1990

Study	Period Covered	No of Patients	Treatment	Outcomes	Follow-up (Range)
Fountas et al,[1] 2019	1969–2018	68	10/68 surgery 18/68 surgery + radiotherapy (conventional in 16 patients and gamma knife in the other 2) 22/68 radiotherapy (conventional in 19 patients, gamma knife in 2 patients, and cyber knife in 1 patient) 16/68 observation 2/68 pasireotide	10-y tumor progression-free survival Surgery: 80% Surgery + radiotherapy: 81% Radiotherapy: 52% Observation: 51%	Median 13 y (1–45)
Cohen et al,[2] 2019	1974–2011	6	2/6 surgery 1/6 radiotherapy (gold implant) 1/6 radiosurgery (gamma knife) 1/6 observation 1/6 recently diagnosed–awaiting treatment decision	Surgery 1/2 in remission 1/2 further tumor growth and ACTH increase (despite treatment with octreotide, pasireotide, and cabergoline) Radiotherapy 1/1 in remission (gold implant) Radiosurgery 1/1 tumor stability (6 cycles of temozolomide and octreotide were also offered) Observation 1/1 further ACTH increase–no tumor in MRI	Median 7 y (4 mo–20 y)
Graffeo et al,[4] 2017	1956–2015	47	12/47 radiosurgery 2/47 surgery 33/47 observation	Radiosurgery 10/12 tumor control 2/12 further tumor growth No information for the remaining patients	Mean 23 y ± 2 y (2–58)

(continued on next page)

Table 2
(continued)

Study	Period Covered	No of Patients	Treatment	Outcomes	Follow-up (Range)
Espinosa-de-Los-Monteros et al,[17] 2017	1991–2014	6	4/6 radiotherapy 1/6 observation 1/6 no information available	Radiotherapy 2/4 decreased tumor size 2/4 stable tumor size Observation No information available	Median 4.4 y (0.5–7)
Zielinski et al,[11] 2015	2000–2005	10	10/10 surgery	5/10 in remission (defined as morning ACTH <200 pg/mL after stopping glucocorticoid for 24 h and no MRI evidence of tumor) 3/10 ACTH decrease and reduction of tumor size 2/10 further tumor growth	Mean 45.3 mo ± 17.8 mo (10–71)
Vik-Mo et al,[61] 2009	1989–2002	5[a]	5/5 radiosurgery (gamma knife)	1/5 normal ACTH and no residual tumor 1/5 ACTH decrease and no residual tumor 2/5 ACTH decrease and reduction of tumor size 1/5 stable ACTH and tumor size	Mean 9.4 y (2.9–13.5)
Xing et al,[62] 2002	1980–1999	23	23/23 surgery	19/23 normal or decreased ACTH and no residual tumor or stable residuum 4/23 further tumor growth	Mean 3.6 y (0.5–9)

Study	Years	N	Treatment	Outcomes	Follow-up
Kelly et al,[7] 2002	1978–1993	13	6/13 surgery 6/13 surgery + conventional radiotherapy 1/13 surgery + stereotactic multiple arc radiotherapy	Surgery 2/6 in remission (defined as ACTH <200 pg/mL 2 h after morning glucocorticoid dose) and no residual tumor 3/6 ACTH decrease and no residual tumor in 2 of them and stable residuum in the other 1 1/6 further tumor growth Surgery + radiotherapy 4/6 in remission and no residual tumor 2/6 ACTH decrease and no residual tumor in 1 patient and stable residuum in the other Surgery + stereotactic multiple arc radiotherapy 1/1 further tumor growth (already recurrent Nelson's)	Median 17 y (8–22)
Kemink et al,[8] 2001	1969–1998	15	6/15 surgery 1/15 conventional radiotherapy 8/15 observation	Surgery 2/6 in remission (defined as ACTH <200 pmol/L after stopping glucocorticoid for 24 h and tumor size <10 mm)—only 3 mo of follow-up 1/6 stable ACTH and tumor size 3/6 further tumor growth Radiotherapy 1/1 further tumor growth Observation 1/8 decreased ACTH and stable tumor volume (with quinagolide) 7/8 further tumor growth	Median 6 y (0.3–29)

(continued on next page)

Table 2
(continued)

Study	Period Covered	No of Patients	Treatment	Outcomes	Follow-up (Range)
Pereira et al,[23] 1998	NR	14	6/14 surgery 2/14 surgery + radiotherapy 2/14 radiosurgery 4/14 observation	Observation 4/4 stable tumor size (in 2 of them, follow-up was <1 y) Active treatment 1/10 in remission No available data regarding the remaining patients	Mean 9 y ± 5 y (3–20)
Ganz et al,[56] 1993	NR	3	3/3 radiosurgery (gamma knife)	2/3 improvement in ACTH and reduction in tumor size 1/3 stable ACTH and tumor size (already recurrent Nelson's)	NR
Tran et al,[63] 1991	1967–1985	5	4/5 conventional radiotherapy 1/5 surgery + conventional radiotherapy	Surgery + radiotherapy 1/1 normal ACTH Radiotherapy 2/4 normal ACTH 2/4 clinical remission (no further details are provided)	Median 3 y
Burke et al,[9] 1990	NR	4	4/4 surgery	4/4 in remission (defined as ACTH <70 pg/mL 2 h after the morning glucocorticoid dose and no evidence of tumor growth in follow-up)	Median 39 mo Mean 56 mo[b]

Abbreviation: NR, not reported.

[a] The total group consists of 10 patients, but 4 of them had already recurrent tumors and, for the fifth, it is unclear whether radiosurgery was performed as sole treatment of NS or as an adjuvant therapy after pituitary surgery.

[b] Follow-up for the total group of the study, which also included patients without NS.

Data from Refs.[1,2,4,7–9,11,17,23,56,61–63]

2 patients and stable size in the other 2 patients. The 10-year tumor progression-free survival for those treated solely with radiotherapy in the UK Nelson's study was 52%;[1] in this series, 4 of 22 patients from this group already had received a previous course of irradiation for their CD and the possibility that they had more aggressive tumors cannot be excluded.

Studies assessing the effects of stereotactic radiosurgery (SRS) in controlling Nelson's tumor growth have shown promising results (ranging between 60% and 100%).[3,5,6,56,58,59,61] However, these data need to be interpreted with caution as information on other therapeutic interventions prior to SRS is not provided.[3,5,6,58,59] In the 3 studies evaluating the efficacy of SRS as primary treatment of NS, no further tumor progression was reported in 83.4% (10/12) and in 100% (5/5 and 3/3) of the cases, respectively.[4,56,61] Selection bias and small sample size, however, challenge the practical significance of these data.

The effects of proton radiotherapy on NS have been reviewed in only 1 study;[60] normal ACTH levels were achieved in 75% (6/8) of the patients and tumor control in 100% (6/6) of them. Nonetheless, this study has limitations similar to those assessing SRS efficacy.

Observation

Imaging surveillance is considered mostly in patients with small tumors not causing mass effects to vital surrounding structures. In the UK Nelson's study, there was 51% tumor progression-free survival at 10 years in patients under surveillance, and in the majority of cases, active treatment (surgery, radiotherapy, medical therapy, or combination of these) subsequently was offered.[1] High tumor growth rates have also been reported by Kemink and colleagues,[8] with 87.5% (7/8) of the conservatively managed patients demonstrating further corticotroph tumor growth during median follow-up of 2.5 years. In 6 of these cases, surgery or radiotherapy was offered, whereas in the seventh, massive pituitary hemorrhage occurred 5 years after the diagnosis of NS. In contrast, in the study of Pereira and colleagues,[23] 4 patients were managed conservatively and in 2 of them (followed-up for 3 years and 4 years, respectively), no tumor growth was demonstrated; the other 2 were followed-up for less than 1 year.

Medical Therapy

Different types of pharmacotherapy have been used for the control of ACTH levels and/or the corticotroph tumor in patients with NS, including dopamine agonists, sodium valproate, octreotide and lanreotide, serotonin antagonists, and peroxisome proliferator-activated receptor γ agonists. Despite their beneficial effects in some cases, their efficacy has not been reproduced consistently.[35,47,64] It has been suggested, however, that pharmacotherapy could be an option when all other management approaches have failed.[54] Pasireotide has been recently investigated as a medical treatment in NS in a small case series where it resulted in reduction of ACTH levels, but with no significant change in the size of the tumor during a 28-week administration period.[65]

RECURRENT AND AGGRESSIVE NELSON'S SYNDROME

A small subset of patients demonstrates further corticotroph tumor growth after primary treatment of NS. Given the rarity of the condition, the identification of relevant predictive factors is challenging. In the UK Nelson's study, the highest risk was found in patients treated with pituitary surgery, radiotherapy, and BLA for their CD prior to NS diagnosis.[1] This group had received the most complex treatments for their CD, possibly reflecting an aggressive corticotroph tumor from the outset.[1]

Management of these patients is individualized and also tailored to previously offered treatments. Furthermore, the reported responses to treatment are variable and range from tumor stability (during variable monitoring intervals) to multiple growths and malignant transformation.[1,4,6–8] In the latter scenario, there is poor prognosis and increased mortality.[1–8,11,66] Temozolomide has been used for the treatment of such aggressive tumors with beneficial results in some[67,68] but not all published cases.[1,69]

SUMMARY AND FUTURE DIRECTIONS

More than 60 years since its first description, NS remains a fascinating but also enigmatic entity. A formal consensus on the diagnosis and management of this condition is still lacking. Patients with CD offered BLA require long-term monitoring for the development of NS. Corticotroph tumor growth is essential for diagnosis; nonetheless, gradually increasing ACTH levels without radiographic evidence of corticotroph tumor growth need to be included in the diagnostic algorithm. Surgery followed or not by radiotherapy is associated with higher tumor control rates compared with observation alone. The latter option can be offered to patients with small lesions, not causing mass effects to vital surrounding structures, but close follow-up is essential to detect further tumor progress and ensure appropriate treatment. The small subset of tumors demonstrating aggressive behavior is intriguing and may reflect an aggressive corticotroph tumor from the outset. Further studies focusing on all aspects of this condition are needed and, hopefully, will facilitate the development of tumor-targeted therapeutic agents.

DISCLOSURE

The authors have nothing to disclose. This work did not receive any specific grant from any funding agency in the public, commercial or not-for-profit sector.

REFERENCES

1. Fountas A, Lim ES, Drake WM, et al. Outcomes of patients with Nelson's syndrome after primary treatment: a multicenter study from 13 UK Pituitary centers. J Clin Endocrinol Metab 2019;105(5):1527–37.
2. Cohen AC, Goldney DC, Danilowicz K, et al. Long-term outcome after bilateral adrenalectomy in Cushing's disease with focus on Nelson's syndrome. Arch Endocrinol Metab 2019;63(5):470–7.
3. Caruso JP, Patibandla MR, Xu Z, et al. A long-term study of the treatment of nelson's syndrome with gamma knife radiosurgery. Neurosurgery 2018;83(3):430–6.
4. Graffeo CS, Perry A, Carlstrom LP, et al. Characterizing and predicting the Nelson's-Salassa syndrome. J Neurosurg 2017;127(6):1277–87.
5. Wilson PJ, Williams JR, Smee RI. Nelson's syndrome: single centre experience using the linear accelerator (LINAC) for stereotactic radiosurgery and fractionated stereotactic radiotherapy. J Clin Neurosci 2014;21(9):1520–4.
6. Pollock BE, Young WF Jr. Stereotactic radiosurgery for patients with ACTH-producing pituitary adenomas after prior adrenalectomy. Int J Radiat Oncol Biol Phys 2002;54(3):839–41.
7. Kelly PA, Samandouras G, Grossman AB, et al. Neurosurgical treatment of Nelson's syndrome. J Clin Endocrinol Metab 2002;87(12):5465–9.

8. Kemink SA, Grotenhuis JA, De Vries J, et al. Management of Nelson's syndrome: observations in fifteen patients. Clin Endocrinol (Oxf) 2001;54(1):45–52.

9. Burke CW, Adams CB, Esiri MM, et al. Transsphenoidal surgery for Cushing's disease: does what is removed determine the endocrine outcome? Clin Endocrinol (Oxf) 1990;33(4):525–37.

10. Nelson's DH, Meakin JW, Dealy JB Jr, et al. ACTH-producing tumor of the pituitary gland. N Engl J Med 1958;259(4):161–4.

11. Zielinski G, Witek P, Maksymowicz M. Outcomes in pituitary surgery in Nelson's syndrome–therapeutic pitfalls. Endokrynol Pol 2015;66(6):504–13.

12. Osswald A, Plomer E, Dimopoulou C, et al. Favorable long-term outcomes of bilateral adrenalectomy in Cushing's disease. Eur J Endocrinol 2014;171(2): 209–15.

13. Mehta GU, Sheehan JP, Vance ML. Effect of stereotactic radiosurgery before bilateral adrenalectomy for Cushing's disease on the incidence of Nelson's syndrome. J Neurosurg 2013;119(6):1493–7.

14. Assie G, Bahurel H, Coste J, et al. Corticotroph tumor progression after adrenalectomy in Cushing's Disease: A reappraisal of Nelson's Syndrome. J Clin Endocrinol Metab 2007;92(1):172–9.

15. Imai T, Funahashi H, Tanaka Y, et al. Adrenalectomy for treatment of Cushing's syndrome: results in 122 patients and long-term follow-up studies. World J Surg 1996;20(7):781–6 [discussion: 786–7].

16. Moreira AC, Castro M, Machado HR. Longitudinal evaluation of adrenocorticotrophin and beta-lipotrophin plasma levels following bilateral adrenalectomy in patients with Cushing's disease. Clin Endocrinol (Oxf) 1993;39(1):91–6.

17. Espinosa-de-Los-Monteros AL, Sosa-Eroza E, Espinosa E, et al. Long-term outcome of the different treatment alternatives for recurrent and persistent cushing disease. Endocr Pract 2017;23(7):759–67.

18. Xing B, Zhang N, Ren ZY, et al. [Effects of adrenalectomy on the treatment of Cushing's disease]. Zhonghua Wai Ke Za Zhi 2008;46(8):592–4.

19. Thompson SK, Hayman AV, Ludlam WH, et al. Improved quality of life after bilateral laparoscopic adrenalectomy for Cushing's disease: a 10-year experience. Ann Surg 2007;245(5):790–4.

20. Gil-Cárdenas A, Herrera MF, Diaz-Polanco A, et al. Nelson's syndrome after bilateral adrenalectomy for Cushing's disease. Surgery 2007;141(2):147–51 [discussion: 151–2].

21. Dalvi AN, Thapar PM, Vijay Kumar K, et al. Laparoscopic adrenalectomy: Gaining experience by graded approach. J Minim Access Surg 2006;2(2):59–66.

22. Nagesser SK, van Seters AP, Kievit J, et al. Long-term results of total adrenalectomy for Cushing's disease. World J Surg 2000;24(1):108–13.

23. Pereira MA, Halpern A, Salgado LR, et al. A study of patients with Nelson's syndrome. Clin Endocrinol (Oxf) 1998;49(4):533–9.

24. Sonino N, Zielezny M, Fava GA, et al. Risk factors and long-term outcome in pituitary-dependent Cushing's disease. J Clin Endocrinol Metab 1996;81(7): 2647–52.

25. O'Riordain DS, Farley DR, Young WF Jr, et al. Long-term outcome of bilateral adrenalectomy in patients with Cushing's syndrome. Surgery 1994;116(6): 1088–93 [discussion: 1093–4].

26. Misra D, Kapur MM, Gupta DK. Incidence of Nelson's syndrome and residual adrenocortical function in patients of Cushing's disease after bilateral adrenalectomy. J Assoc Physicians India 1994;42(4):304–5.

27. Kemink L, Pieters G, Hermus A, et al. Patient's age is a simple predictive factor for the development of Nelson's syndrome after total adrenalectomy for Cushing's disease. J Clin Endocrinol Metab 1994;79(3):887–9.

28. McCance DR, Russell CF, Kennedy TL, et al. Bilateral adrenalectomy: low mortality and morbidity in Cushing's disease. Clin Endocrinol (Oxf) 1993;39(3):315–21.

29. Grabner P, Hauer-Jensen M, Jervell J, et al. Long-term results of treatment of Cushing's disease by adrenalectomy. Eur J Surg 1991;157(8):461–4.

30. Sarkis P, Rabilloud M, Lifante JC, et al. Bilateral adrenalectomy in Cushing's disease: Altered long-term quality of life compared to other treatment options. Ann Endocrinol (Paris) 2019;80(1):32–7.

31. Smith PW, Turza KC, Carter CO, et al. Bilateral adrenalectomy for refractory Cushing's disease: a safe and definitive therapy. J Am Coll Surg 2009;208(6):1059–64.

32. Jenkins PJ, Trainer PJ, Plowman PN, et al. The long-term outcome after adrenalectomy and prophylactic pituitary radiotherapy in adrenocorticotropin-dependent Cushing's syndrome. J Clin Endocrinol Metab 1995;80(1):165–71.

33. Ding XF, Li HZ, Yan WG, et al. Role of adrenalectomy in recurrent Cushing's disease. Chin Med J (Engl) 2010;123(13):1658–62.

34. Littley MD, Shalet SM, Beardwell CG, et al. Long-term follow-up of low-dose external pituitary irradiation for Cushing's disease. Clin Endocrinol (Oxf) 1990; 33(4):445–55.

35. Munir A, Newell-Price J. Nelson's syndrome. Arq Bras Endocrinol Metabol 2007; 51(8):1392–6.

36. Nagendra L, Bhavani N, Pavithran PV, et al. Outcomes of bilateral adrenalectomy in cushing's syndrome. Indian J Endocrinol Metab 2019;23(2):193–7.

37. Prajapati OP, Verma AK, Mishra A, et al. Bilateral adrenalectomy for cushing's syndrome: pros and cons. Indian J Endocrinol Metab 2015;19(6):834–40.

38. Tiyadatah BN, Kalavampara SV, Sukumar S, et al. Bilateral simultaneous laparoscopic adrenalectomy in Cushing's syndrome: safe, effective, and curative. J Endourol 2012;26(2):157–63.

39. Prevedello DM, Pouratian N, Sherman J, et al. Management of Cushing's disease: outcome in patients with microadenoma detected on pituitary magnetic resonance imaging. J Neurosurg 2008;109(4):751–9.

40. Hawn MT, Cook D, Deveney C, et al. Quality of life after laparoscopic bilateral adrenalectomy for Cushing's disease. Surgery 2002;132(6):1064–8 [discussion: 1068–9].

41. Wright-Pascoe R, Charles CF, Richards R, et al. A clinico-pathological study of Cushing's syndrome at the University Hospital of the West Indies and a review of the literature. West Indian Med J 2001;50(1):55–61.

42. Vella A, Thompson GB, Grant CS, et al. Laparoscopic adrenalectomy for adrenocorticotropin-dependent Cushing's syndrome. J Clin Endocrinol Metab 2001;86(4):1596–9.

43. Invitti C, Pecori Giraldi F, de Martin M, et al. Diagnosis and management of Cushing's syndrome: results of an Italian multicentre study. Study Group of the Italian Society of Endocrinology on the Pathophysiology of the Hypothalamic-Pituitary-Adrenal Axis. J Clin Endocrinol Metab 1999;84(2):440–8.

44. Feleke Y, Abdulkadir J, Johnson O, et al. Cushing's syndrome: a ten year experience at Tikur Anbassa Hospital. Ethiop Med J 1998;36(1):19–26.

45. Chapuis Y, Pitre J, Conti F, et al. Role and operative risk of bilateral adrenalectomy in hypercortisolism. World J Surg 1996;20(7):775–9 [discussion: 779–80].

46. Favia G, Boscaro M, Lumachi F, et al. Role of bilateral adrenalectomy in Cushing's disease. World J Surg 1994;18(4):462–6.

47. Barber TM, Adams E, Wass JA. Nelson syndrome: definition and management. Handb Clin Neurol 2014;124:327–37.

48. Gertz BJ, Contreras LN, McComb DJ, et al. Chronic administration of corticotropin-releasing factor increases pituitary corticotroph number. Endocrinology 1987;120(1):381–8.

49. Wynn PC, Harwood JP, Catt KJ, et al. Regulation of corticotropin-releasing factor (CRF) receptors in the rat pituitary gland: effects of adrenalectomy on CRF receptors and corticotroph responses. Endocrinology 1985;116(4):1653–9.

50. Sbiera S, Deutschbein T, Weigand I, et al. The new molecular landscape of cushing's disease. Trends Endocrinol Metab 2015;26(10):573–83.

51. Evang JA, Berg JP, Casar-Borota O, et al. Reduced levels of E-cadherin correlate with progression of corticotroph pituitary tumours. Clin Endocrinol (Oxf) 2011; 75(6):811–8.

52. Perez-Rivas LG, Theodoropoulou M, Puar TH, et al. Somatic USP8 mutations are frequent events in corticotroph tumor progression causing Nelson's tumor. Eur J Endocrinol 2018;178(1):59–65.

53. Barber TM, Adams E, Ansorge O, et al. Nelson's syndrome. Eur J Endocrinol 2010;163(4):495–507.

54. Banasiak MJ, Malek AR. Nelson's syndrome: comprehensive review of pathophysiology, diagnosis, and management. Neurosurg Focus 2007;23(3):E13.

55. De Tommasi C, Vance ML, Okonkwo DO, et al. Surgical management of adrenocorticotropic hormone-secreting macroadenomas: outcome and challenges in patients with Cushing's disease or Nelson's syndrome. J Neurosurg 2005;103(5):825–30.

56. Ganz JC, Backlund EO, Thorsen FA. The effects of Gamma Knife surgery of pituitary adenomas on tumor growth and endocrinopathies. Stereotact Funct Neurosurg 1993;61(Suppl 1):30–7.

57. Levy RP, Fabrikant JI, Frankel KA, et al. Heavy-charged-particle radiosurgery of the pituitary gland: clinical results of 840 patients. Stereotact Funct Neurosurg 1991;57(1–2):22–35.

58. Marek J, Jezkova J, Hana V, et al. Gamma knife radiosurgery for Cushing's disease and Nelson's syndrome. Pituitary 2015;18(3):376–84.

59. Cordeiro D, Xu Z, Li CE, et al. Gamma Knife radiosurgery for the treatment of Nelson's syndrome: a multicenter, international study. J Neurosurg 2019;1–6. https://doi.org/10.3171/2019.4.JNS19273.

60. Wattson DA, Tanguturi SK, Spiegel DY, et al. Outcomes of proton therapy for patients with functional pituitary adenomas. Int J Radiat Oncol Biol Phys 2014;90(3):532–9.

61. Vik-Mo EO, Oksnes M, Pedersen PH, et al. Gamma knife stereotactic radiosurgery of Nelson's syndrome. Eur J Endocrinol 2009;160(2):143–8.

62. Xing B, Ren Z, Su C, et al. Microsurgical treatment of Nelson's syndrome. Chin Med J (Engl) 2002;115(8):1150–2.

63. Tran LM, Blount L, Horton D, et al. Radiation therapy of pituitary tumors: results in 95 cases. Am J Clin Oncol 1991;14(1):25–9.

64. Patel J, Eloy JA, Liu JK. Nelson's syndrome: a review of the clinical manifestations, pathophysiology, and treatment strategies. Neurosurg Focus 2015;38(2):E14.

65. Daniel E, Debono M, Caunt S, et al. A prospective longitudinal study of Pasireotide in Nelson's syndrome. Pituitary 2018;21(3):247–55.

66. Kasperlik-Zaluska AA, Bonicki W, Jeske W, et al. Nelson's syndrome – 46 years later: clinical experience with 37 patients. Zentralbl Neurochir 2006;67(1): 14–20.

67. Kurowska M, Nowakowski A, Zielinski G, et al. Temozolomide-induced shrinkage of invasive pituitary adenoma in patient with nelson's syndrome: a case report and review of the literature. Case Rep Endocrinol 2015;2015:623092.

68. Moyes VJ, Alusi G, Sabin HI, et al. Treatment of Nelson's syndrome with temozolomide. Eur J Endocrinol 2009;160(1):115–9.

69. Bruno OD, Juarez-Allen L, Christiansen SB, et al. Temozolomide therapy for aggressive pituitary tumors: results in a small series of patients from argentina. Int J Endocrinol 2015;2015:587893.

Update on the Genetics of Pituitary Tumors

Sayka Barry, PhD, Márta Korbonits, MD, PhD*

KEYWORDS

- Pituitary adenomas • Acromegaly • Prolactinoma • FIPA • AIP • MEN1
- Genetic testing

KEY POINTS

- Pituitary neuroendocrine tumors (PitNETs) are usually benign intracranial tumors that rarely metastasize. More than 95% of tumors are sporadic in origin, with around 5% harboring germline mutations causing syndromic or isolated pituitary adenomas.
- Over the last decades numerous genetic studies have led to the identification of the somatic (*GNAS*, *USP8*, *GPR101*) and germline mutations (*MEN1*, cyclin dependent kinase inhibitor genes, *AIP*, *DICER1*, *PRKAR1A*, *PRKACA*, *SDHx*, and *GPR101*) associated with pituitary tumors, which has advanced the understanding of pituitary tumorigenesis.
- We overview the genetics of pituitary tumors.
- Current challenges and implications of these genetic findings in clinical practice are discussed.

INTRODUCTION

The prevalence of symptomatic pituitary neuroendocrine tumors (PitNETs) is approximately 1 in 1000 in the general population. Most of these tumors occur sporadically and are not part of syndromic disorders. An estimated 5% of them are considered to have familial origin. There are a few well-defined genetic syndromes known to be associated with pituitary adenomas, including multiple endocrine neoplasia (MEN) type 1 and Carney complex (CNC), and nonsyndromic familial isolated pituitary adenomas (FIPA). PitNETs are slow-growing, usually benign tumors generally thought to be of monoclonal origin. However, they can cause considerable morbidity because of mass effects on surrounding tissues or altered hormonal secretion. Furthermore, tumors can invade into the surrounding structures leading to difficulties in complete surgical resection. Medical treatment is available with somatostatin analogues or dopamine agonist for some of the tumors, whereas for others surgery and radiotherapy are the only therapeutic options. Understanding the genetic background of

Centre for Endocrinology, William Harvey Research Institute, Barts and The London School of Medicine, Queen Mary University of London, Charterhouse Square, London EC1M 6BQ, UK
* Corresponding author.
E-mail address: m.korbonits@qmul.ac.uk

Endocrinol Metab Clin N Am 49 (2020) 433–452
https://doi.org/10.1016/j.ecl.2020.05.005
0889-8529/20/© 2020 Elsevier Inc. All rights reserved.

PitNETs can lead to early diagnosis associated with better outcomes and their molecular mechanisms should lead to novel targeted therapies even for sporadic tumors. We summarize here the genes and the syndromes associated with pituitary tumors.

GENETIC LANDSCAPE OF PITUITARY TUMORS - SOMATIC MUTATIONS

Despite numerous large-scale classical and recent studies, sporadic pituitary adenomas are characterized by recurrent somatic mutations only in two genes, *GNAS* and *USP8* (ubiquitin specific peptidase 8) (**Fig. 1**).[1–3] A unique form of somatic mutations, embryonic mutations leading to mosaicism, have been seen in *GNAS*, *GPR101*, and more recently in *MEN1*.

GNAS Mutations

The most frequently altered somatic heterozygous gain-of-function mutation of this gene is found in some 40% of somatotroph tumors.[4] *GNAS* encodes the *gsp* oncogene, the stimulatory G-protein subunit α (Gsα).[5–7] The mutations predominantly

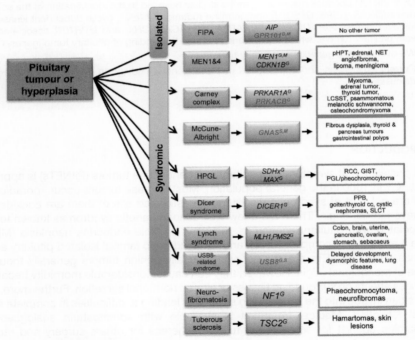

Fig. 1. Summary of familial pituitary adenomas, which is divided into two groups: an isolated group (FIPA), and a syndromic group, including MEN1, MEN4, Carney complex, McCune-Albright syndrome, HPGL, DICER1 syndrome, Lynch syndrome, USP8-related syndrome. Optic pathway gliomas in neurofibromatosis are typically associated with growth hormone excess. Neurofibromatosis and tuberous sclerosis cases with true pituitary adenomas probably represent coincidences. *Black* represents tumor suppressor gene; *red* represents oncogene. G, germline; GIST, gastrointestinal neuroendocrine tumor; HPGL, hereditary paraganglioma; LCCSCT, large-cell calcifying Sertoli cell tumors; M, mosaic; pHPT, primary hyperparathyroidism; PGL, paraganglioma; PPB, pleuropulmonary blastoma; RCC, renal cell cancer; S, somatic; SLCT, Sertoli-Leydig cell tumor.

occur in codon 201, whereas codon 227 mutations occur but are far less frequent. This mutation disrupts the GTPase activity of the Gsα, leading to constitutive activation of adenyl cyclase and increased cyclic adenosine monophosphate (cAMP) levels: cAMP binds the regulatory subunit of protein kinase A (PKA; coded by *PRKAR1A/1B* or *PRKAR2A/2B*) allowing the catalytic subunit (*PRKACA/B*) to increase levels of PKA, which subsequently activates cAMP response element binding protein (CREB). CREB activates the PIT1 (POU1F1) transcription factor, which stimulates growth hormone (GH) hypersecretion and increased somatotroph proliferation.[6,8–10] *GNAS* is an imprinted gene in the pituitary and mutations are always located on the maternal allele.[11] Several studies found that *gsp*-positive somatotroph tumors show a better response to somatostatin analogue treatment with distinct clinical features, including older age at diagnosis, smaller tumor size, less invasive nature, and a densely granulated pattern on histologic study.[1,12,13] *GNAS* mutations has been identified rarely in other tumor types, 1/21 and 1/14 in nonfunctioning pituitary adenomas (NFPAs)[14,15] and in one case of a corticotroph adenoma.[16] No other recurrent somatic mutations has been identified in somatotroph tumors.[1]

McCune-Albright Syndrome

If *GNAS* mutation occurs during embryonic development, the mosaic disease McCune-Albright syndrome (MAS) develops (see **Fig. 1**) with a variable phenotype, depending on what tissues are affected by the mutations. MAS is a systemic disorder characterized by polycystic fibrous dysplasia, precocious puberty, and café au lait spots. This is caused by gain-of-function mutations of the *GNAS* gene at an early post-zygotic stage leading to somatic mosaicism. *GNAS* is located on chromosome 20q13 encoding the cAMP pathway associated G protein Gsα, and represents the only recurrent mutation found in somatotroph adenomas.[10,17] The most common type of pituitary tumor related to MAS is a somatotroph adenoma (about 30%), with others showing pituitary hyperplasia.[18] The most frequent *GNAS* mutations in MAS are R201H or R201C. Mutations at these sites cause loss of the GTPase activity with consequent permanent activation of adenylate cyclase and constitutive activation of the cAMP-dependent PKA pathway. This results in increased cell proliferation in cAMP-responsive tissue, including the pituitary. The characteristics of patients depend on the affected tissues.[19–21]

USP8 Mutations

More recently identified recurrent somatic gain-of-function mutations are in the *USP8* gene in corticotropinomas (see **Fig. 1**).[22–24] This gene encodes a deubiquitinase that inhibits the lysosomal degradation of epidermal growth factor receptor (EGFR), thus leading to increased EGFR signaling and cell growth.[25] Mutations in *USP8* affect the 14-3-3 protein–binding domain that usually protects *USP8* from cleavage; mutations block the 14-3-3 binding site with the cleaved USP8 showing a higher deubiquitination activity resulting in more recycled EGFR and increased signaling through these receptors, then upregulating POMC expression. *USP8* mutation status, however, does not always correlate with EGFR expression.[26] A recent meta-analysis of 677 patients from 10 studies suggests that 32% of female and 24% of male patients with corticotrophinoma have a somatic *USP8* mutation.[27] Although data are variable, this meta-analysis found that average tumor size is 9 mm in *USP8*-mutated corticotroph tumors, with 42% of the microadenomas and 31% of the macroadenomas being mutated. Mutation-positive cases have a somewhat better chance of remaining in remission after surgery.[1,23,27–29] A heterozygous germline *USP8* mutation has also been reported recently[30] in a 16-year-old girl with recurrent Cushing disease including developmental delay, dysmorphic features, ichthyosiform hyperkeratosis, chronic lung and kidney disease, and cardiomyopathy.

GPR101 Mosaic Mutation

Germline *GPR101* duplication is typically seen in females as de novo mutations (see **Fig. 1**). To date, all male patients with X-linked acrogigantism (XLAG) without a family history have been found with a mosaic *GPR101* duplication,[31–33] whereas in the three familial kindreds described today, male offspring were identified with germline duplication.[34–36] No females have been described with mosaicism to date. There are no phenotypic differences between germline and mosaic cases.

MEN1 Mosaic Mutation

Patients with mosaic *MEN1* mutation and offspring with germline MEN1 have recently been described,[37,38] highlighting that mosaicism needs to be considered in patients with apparently sporadic de novo *MEN1* mutations.

GENETIC LANDSCAPE OF PITUITARY TUMORS - GERMLINE MUTATIONS

Patients with germline mutations associated with pituitary adenomas are divided into two groups: an isolated and a syndromic group (see **Fig. 1**).

Multiple Endocrine Neoplasia 1

MEN1 is an inherited autosomal-dominant syndrome associated with pituitary, parathyroid, and pancreatic tumors and facial angiofibromas, collagenomas, adrenal cortical adenomas, lipomata, meningiomas, and rarely pheochromocytomas.[39–41] Heterozygous inactivating mutations in *MEN1* have been found in 90% of cases, and show loss of heterozygosity in the tumors at 11q13.[42,43] Approximately 30% to 40% of patients with MEN1 develop pituitary tumors.[40,41] Prolactinomas are the most common clinically presenting pituitary tumors (~60% of clinically diagnosed *MEN1* pituitary adenomas), followed by NFPAs (15%–40%), somatotroph pituitary tumors (5%–10%), and, rarely, corticotroph or thyrotroph adenomas.[44–46] In patients with MEN1, pituitary tumors found to be larger and histologically more invasive,[40,44,45,47] although this has been disputed. The *MEN1* gene is located on the long arm of chromosome 11 and encodes for the tumor suppressor nuclear protein menin. It has numerous interacting partners involved in transcriptional regulation, genome stability, cell division, and proliferation.[40,48] More than 1500 germline mutations have been described to date,[48,49] most being truncating mutations caused by nonsense mutations and frameshifts because of deletions or insertions. Despite some controversial data,[50] no clear genotype–phenotype correlation has been established for pituitary tumors.[44,51]

Multiple Endocrine Neoplasia 4

MEN4 is an autosomal-dominant syndrome that results from germline heterozygous loss-of-function mutations in *CDKN1B* or other cyclin-dependent kinase inhibitor genes. Around 10% of patients with MEN1-like syndrome do not possess a mutation in *MEN1*, possibly caused by cryptic mutations in introns or promoters, or as phenocopies. However, some may show *CDKN1B* mutations, and thus represent a form of MEN, named as MEN4.[52] Pituitary tumors occur in 37% reported MEN4 cases.[53] Other tumors include parathyroid adenomas, adrenal tumors, renal angiomyolipomas, uterine fibroids, gastrinomas, neuroendocrine cervical carcinomas, bronchial carcinoids, papillary thyroid carcinomas, and gastric carcinomas. *CDKN1B* is located on chromosome 12q13 and encodes for p27, a cyclin-dependent kinase inhibitor involved in cell cycle regulation.[54] The *CDKN1B* mutations include frameshift, nonsense, missense, and 5'UTR mutations leading to reduced p27 expression.[52,55–64] Because of the rarity of MEN4, potential genotype–phenotype correlations remain to be confirmed.

Carney Complex

CNC is a rare autosomal-dominant syndrome characterized with skin pigmentation, cardiac myxomas, GH and prolactin-secreting pituitary adenomas, and Cushing syndrome from primary pigmented nodular adrenocortical disease.[65,66] Most often CNC is caused by germline mutations in the tumor suppressor *PRKAR1A* gene located on chromosome 17, encoding the type 1α regulatory subunit of PKA.[67] Inactivating mutations and large deletions of *PRKAR1A* lead to loss of function of the PKA 1α regulatory subunit, resulting in increased cAMP-dependent PKA activity.[68,69] Most common mutations are nonsense and frameshift mutations. A genotype-phenotype correlation has been observed in patients with CNC, with large deletions leading to more severe disease.[69,70] About 75% of patients with CNC demonstrate an abnormal GH axis; clinically evident acromegaly is not as common (10%–12%).[71,72] Childhood-onset GH excess leading to gigantism has rarely been reported.[71] Prolactinomas are rare,[72] whereas two cases of Cushing disease in association with CNC have been described.[73,74] A second locus on chromosome 2p16 has also been linked with CNC,[75] but no gene has been identified at this locus yet. Increased PKA activity is the result not just of loss of regulatory (i.e. inhibitory activity, loss-of-function PRKAR mutations), but also because of activation catalytic subunit mutations (*PRKACA* on chromosome 19 and *PRKACB* on chromosome 1). Somatic *PRKACA* point mutations are associated with cortisol-secreting adrenal adenomas,[76] whereas germline duplications and triplications can cause childhood or adult-onset bilateral micronodular or macronodular hyperplasias.[76,77] One of the germline duplication patients had skin lesions similar to CNC (pigmented inner canthus, pigmented spots on the vermilion border, and facial freckling), but no other CNC-related manifestations, whereas the other patients had no skin manifestation.[77] *PRKACB* duplication has been described in a patient with typical CNC.[78] Because adrenocortical adenomas and somatotroph adenomas are known to be reliant on the cAMP signaling pathway, the hotspot somatic L206R mutation affecting *PRKACA* and *PRKACB* was tested in sporadic somatotroph adenomas and other types of pituitary adenomas: no changes were identified in pituitary tumor tissue.[79]

Familial Isolated Pituitary Adenoma

FIPA is an autosomal-dominant disease defined by the presence of pituitary adenomas in two or more family members in the same family with no other syndromic features.[80] In 90% of FIPA families the gene resulting in genetic predisposition has not been identified to date.[81] However, heterozygote germline loss-of-function mutations have been identified in the aryl hydrocarbon receptor interacting protein (*AIP*) gene in 10% of FIPA families,[81] but because of incomplete penetrance, this gene has also been identified in apparently sporadic cases: 3.6% of unselected sporadic pituitary adenoma patients, and 10% to 20% of patients with pediatric pituitary adenoma. Most of the clinically presenting *AIP* mutation–positive cases present with somatotroph or somatolactotroph tumors, some 10% with lactotroph tumors, and rarely with clinically nonfunctioning adenomas, although on immunostaining these are usually positive for GH or prolactin.[82] There is a single TSHoma case,[83] whereas no corticotroph adenoma case has been described where the *AIP* variant is unequivocally pathogenic. *AIP* mutation–positive tumors have distinct clinical features that distinguish them from *AIP*-negative and sporadic tumors. In *AIP* mutation–positive patients, the disease occurs at a younger age (mean age of diagnosis, 18–24 years),[84] with the youngest case diagnosed at age 4 years.[85] We are unaware of an *AIP* mutation–positive case where the tumor was diagnosed older than the age of 30 years, if normal imaging and hormone levels were documented at 30 years.[81] Of the *AIP* mutation–positive cases, 44% have gigantism. Patients usually present with macroadenomas (~90%) and often with invasive tumors (>50%). Around 8% to 10% of all cases show pituitary apoplexy,[86] especially childhood pituitary apoplexy is a unique manifestation.[87] Decreased level of AIP protein in sporadic somatotrophinomas has been correlated with tumor invasiveness.[88] *AIP* mutation–positive tumors show increased numbers of immune infiltrates compared with the sporadic tumors.[89] Patients with *AIP* mutations need a multimodal therapeutic approach often more than a single operation. *AIP* mutation–positive tumors show relative resistance to treatment with somatostatin analogues[83,90] and an increased prevalence of *AIP* mutations has been found among patients with sporadic acromegaly who are resistant to somatostatin analogues.[91] Genetic screening of at-risk relatives can identify unaffected carriers who will benefit from clinical screening, which could result in early diagnosis in apparently asymptomatic subjects,[81,87] leading to early intervention, if necessary. Prospectively diagnosed mutation carriers should be managed according to the current guidelines. Prospectively diagnosed *AIP* mutation-positive patients compared with clinically presenting patients possess smaller lesions with less cavernous sinus invasion and less frequently require multimodal treatments. The spectrum for tumors identified during family screening prospectively is different from the clinically presenting cases: they show 45% GH excess; 12% are prolactinomas, usually microadenomas without invasion; and 41% are clinically nonfunctioning microadenomas.[81] The study by Marques and coworkers,[81] including a 12-year follow-up, highlighted the potential benefits of genetic and clinical screening.

AIP is located on chromosome 11q13.2, contains six exons, and encodes a 330 amino-acid protein. More than 100 *AIP* variants have been identified,[92] including deletions, insertions, segmental duplications, nonsense, missense, splice-site and promoter mutations, and large deletions of whole exons or the entire *AIP* gene. Mutations are present throughout the whole length of the gene and disrupt the protein. Seventy percent of known *AIP* variants result in a truncated protein.[87] Most of the missense mutations are typically clustered around the C-terminal part of the protein, thought to be crucial for its biologic function.[93] Clinical and functional data support its role as a tumor suppressor gene. Loss of heterozygosity is found in *AIP* mutation–positive tumors.[87,94,95]

The low penetrance of pituitary adenomas among *AIP* mutation carriers, together with their heterogeneous clinical phenotypes, suggests the involvement of other disease-modifying genes.[96,97]

Somatic mutations in *AIP* have not been found to date in sporadic pituitary adenomas.[98] Sporadic pituitary tumors with low AIP expression display increased invasiveness.[88,98–100] In other tumors, such as colorectal cancers, breast cancers, prostate tumors,[101] and endocrine tumors (thyroid lesions, adrenal lesions, carcinoids, parathyroid lesions, paragangliomas, pancreatic endocrine tumors, and adenocarcinoids), no somatic mutations of *AIP* have been found.[102,103]

AIP is a molecular cochaperone protein and as such interacts with a large number of partners, and probably plays a role in numerous vital pathways. Although heterozygous loss-of-function mutations are entirely compatible with life, and only approximately 20% of carriers develop a tumor, usually in one particular cell type (somatotrophs cells), its key role in physiology is suggested by the fact that homozygous knockout animal models (mouse, *Caenorhabditis elegans*, and *Drosophila*)[104–106] are lethal.

The first identified AIP partner was the nuclear xenobiotic receptor AhR (aryl hydrocarbon receptor). *AIP* regulates its subcellular localization and degradation. Other interacting partners including other nuclear receptors (AhR, GR, PPARα, ERα, and TRβ1), viral proteins (HBV-X and EBNA-3), G proteins (Gα13 and Gαq), chaperone proteins (Hsp90 and Hsp70), phosphodiesterases (PDE4A5, PDE2A3, and PDE3/SLFN12), mitochondrial proteins (TOMM20), cytoskeletal proteins (Actin, TUBB, and TUBB2A), and others (RET, survivin, TNNI3K, TIF-2, and p23) have been identified, which may indicate that *AIP* is involved in many and varied cellular pathways; however, the consequences of these interactions are not fully understood.[105,107–113]

It has been suggested, based on experimental findings, that *AIP* is involved in the cAMP-dependent PKA pathway, which plays a vital role in regulating GH expression and the proliferation of somatotroph cells.[114] *AIP* interacts with phosphodiesterase 4A4/5, which regulates the cAMP pathway,[108,115,116] and activation of the cAMP pathway is important in somatotroph tumorigenesis. *AIP* has also recently shown to interact with proteins involved in the organization of the cytoskeleton.[110]

Homozygous deletion of *AIP* is embryonically lethal because of cardiovascular developmental abnormalities and erythropoietic failure,[106] suggesting that *AIP* plays a crucial role in cardiac development and in maintaining erythropoiesis in mice. Heterozygote deletion of the *AIP* gene leads to the development of GH- and prolactin-secreting pituitary adenomas.[117] *Aip*-deficient mouse models generally recapitulate the human phenotype.[117,118] Another mouse model has been developed where *Aip* was deleted only in the somatotroph cells.[118] *Aip*-knockout mice were bigger than wild-type control animals at 12 weeks of age,[118] and GH and IGF-1 levels were significantly increased by 18 weeks of age. Macroscopic tumors were visible in 80% of knockout mice by the age of 20 weeks.

X-Linked Acrogigantism

XLAG has recently been described as a rare condition in patients with the early onset of GH excess. De novo germline or mosaic duplication of the *GRP101* gene, usually within a duplicated region (Xq23.6) on the X chromosome.[33,34,119] Although the originally identified Xq26.3 duplicated area involves four genes,[34] only the *GPR101* gene has been found to be upregulated at the mRNA level in pituitary tissue, and in one patient only this region was duplicated,[33] rendering the pathogenic role of this gene in the phenotype highly likely. The *GPR101* gene encodes a G-protein coupled receptor[119,120]; although previously an orphan receptor, more recently an endogenous ligand, the lipid molecule Resolvin D5, has been identified,[121] but the role of this ligand in GH regulation or XLAG pathogenesis is unclear. XLAG syndrome is characterized by excessive GH production and the early onset of accelerated growth, in most cases observed during the first 2 years of life, and in all patients before the age of 4 years,[119,122] often accompanied by signs of acromegaly (coarse facial features, sweating, headache) with the addition of increased appetite/food seeking behavior.[119] XLAG-related pituitary tumors show a typical sinusoidal and lobular architecture with frequent calcification and follicle-like structures.[33] Disease control is challenging because of resistance to therapy, often needing complete pituitary removal, or complex medical therapy with dopamine agonists, somatostatin analogues, GH receptor antagonists, and radiotherapy.[119,122,123]

The prevalence of XLAG is from 4.4% to 10% in gigantism cases.[119,124] Most cases are females.[33,34,119] These GH-secreting pituitary tumors are significantly more often macroadenomas with a suprasellar extension and cavernous sinus invasion. Pituitary hyperplasia is seen in around 25% cases. Hyperprolactinemia can occur in up to 85% of patients.[33] Two large studies of patients with gigantism identified altogether 31 cases with XLAG, either caused by a pituitary adenoma or pituitary hyperplasia.[33,125] Less than 40 cases have been reported to date.[126] In three families, mother-to-son transmission with full penetrance[127] has been observed as a rare cause of FIPA. GPR101 was overexpressed in the pituitary tumors of patients with XLAG, but is not expressed in sporadic somatotroph tumors or in the adult human pituitary gland.[34] The mechanisms underlying the pathogenesis of XLAG remain to be determined. No pathogenic GPR101 mutations or copy number variations were identified in patients with congenital isolated GH deficiency.[128]

DICER1 Syndrome

DICER1 is a rare autosomal-dominant disorder caused by germline heterozygous mutations in the DICER1 gene. Mutations in DICER1 lead to manifestation of variety of tumors, including pleuropulmonary blastoma, ovarian sex cord-stromal tumors (mostly Sertoli-Leydig cell tumors), cystic nephroma, nodular hyperplasia of the thyroid, differentiated thyroid cancer, pituitary blastoma, nasal chondromesenchymal hamartoma, ciliary body medulloepithelioma, renal sarcoma, genitourinary embryonal rhabdomyosarcoma, and pinealoblastoma.[129–131] Pituitary blastomas are a rare manifestation of DICER1 syndrome with a low penetrance (<1% of cases).[132] They develop in infancy (usually younger than the age of 2 years with adrenocorticotropic hormone–secreting pituitary blastoma) caused by mutations in the DICER1 gene. It is called a "blastoma" because the pituitary gland of these individuals appear akin to embryonic tissue.[132,133] DICER1 is located on chromosome 14q32.13: this is an RNA cleavage enzyme that cleaves precursor microRNA into mature miRNA; miRNAs are regulatory proteins that control the expression and/or degradation of specific RNA molecules.[134,135]

The tumors in patients with DICER1 mutation often show a germline loss-of-function mutation in one allele[136] and a second hit pathogenic somatic variant in another allele typically within the metal-binding sites of the catalytic RNase IIIa and IIIb domains of DICER1.[137,138] Mosaic RNase IIIa and IIIb domains mutations are associated with a severe phenotype, but no pituitary blastoma has been described in these patients to date.[139,140] Recently, the occurrence of a germline DICER1 mutation in a patient with microprolactinoma has been reported[141]; at this point this looks more as a coincidence rather than a causative relationship between the two diseases.

Pheochromocytoma/Paraganglioma with Pituitary Adenoma

The association of familial paragangliomas and pheochromocytomas and pituitary adenomas, called "the three P association," is a rare condition caused by germline SDHx mutations.[142] The prevalence of pituitary adenomas in SDHx is low, approximately 0.3%[143]; however, this may not be true representation, because SDHx mutation carriers are not routinely tested for pituitary tumors. Pituitary adenomas have been described in patients with mutations of all the succinate dehydrogenase (SDH) genes.[142,144–149] A unique feature of SDH-related pituitary adenomas is the intracytoplasmic vacuoles revealed by immunohistochemical analysis, which correspond to the presence of autophagic bodies.[144,145] SDH-related pituitary tumors are predominantly PRL- or GH-secreting or nonfunctioning adenomas, and are more likely to be resistant to standard therapy[150] and behave more aggressively, with a metastatic case also described.[29] The exact mechanisms of how loss of SDH function leads to tumorigenesis are not fully understood.

The SDH protein complex comprises multiple subunits (SDHA, SDHB, SDHC, and SDHD), and its associated assembly factor (SDHAF2). SDH, bound to the inner membrane of mitochondria, is a member of the Krebs cycle, and plays a role in oxidative phosphorylation. Mutations in any of the genes for the subunits can lead to impairment of the electron transfer chain, which leads to an accumulation of metabolites and the eventual accumulation of hypoxia-inducible factor-1a, which leads to vascular endothelial growth factor upregulation.[151] Hypoxia-inducible factor-1a is then responsible for causing resistance to apoptotic signals and enhances glycolysis in the tumor.[152] Furthermore, the association of pituitary adenomas and paragangliomas/pheochromocytomas appears also in other hereditary syndromes, such as ones related to mutations in the *MEN1*, *RET*, *VHL*, and *MAX* genes.[124,144]

OTHER GERMLINE VARIANTS LINKED WITH PITUITARY TUMORS

A heterozygous missense mutation in the *CDH23* gene has been identified in one FIPA kindred with two cases of acromegaly and two NFPA cases.[153] *CDH23* encodes for Cadherin-related 23, which is a member of the cadherin superfamily, involved in cell-to-cell adhesion. In 125 sporadic pituitary tumors 15 rare *CDH23* variants were identified and predicted to be potentially pathogenic.[153] Homozygous *CDH23* mutations are associated with deafness and Usher syndrome.[154] However, no functional data exist to explain how these mutations are involved in pituitary tumorigenesis, and no pituitary adenomas have ever been described in relation to Usher syndrome, so their pathogenicity for pituitary tumorigenesis remains unclear.

Germline *CABLES1* (CDK5 and ABL1 enzyme substrate 1) variants were found in four patients with sporadic corticotrophinomas (two young adults and two pediatric cases) in a cohort of 182 patients with Cushing disease[155]; however, no familial diseases were found. *CABLES1* is located on chromosome 18q11.2, and encodes a protein that is a negative regulator of cell cycle progression activated in corticotroph cells in response to glucocorticoids.[156] *CABLES1* protein expression is lost in around 50% of corticotrophinomas.[156,157] Further confirmatory studies are necessary to assess the occurrence of *CABLES1* mutations in patients with Cushing disease or other pituitary tumors.

Neurofibromatosis type 1 is a rare autosomal-dominant multisystem genetic disorder caused by inactivating mutation of *NF1* gene, manifest as benign and malignant tumors. This is associated with cutaneous neurofibromas, café au lait skin lesions, and intertriginous freckling.[158,159] Approximately 10% of patients with neurofibromatosis type 1 and optic gliomas present with features of clinical acromegaly with GH and IGF1 excess, but without a visible pituitary lesion.[160] *NF1* encodes neurofibromin; functions as a Ras-GTPase-activating protein; and deficiency of *NF1* leads to constitutive activation of Ras-dependent pathways, specifically Ras/Raf/MEK and Ras/PI3K/TSC/mTOR.[161] An NF1 patient with a GH-secreting adenoma has been reported with no loss-of-heterozygosity and the NF1 locus and a GNAS mutation, suggesting no role of NF1 in the pituitary tumorigenesis.[162] Future studies are needed to establish a link between NF1 mutations and pituitary tumors.

Tuberous sclerosis is an autosomal-dominant syndrome caused by genetic defects of *TSC1* or *TSC2* genes, which encode for hamartin and tuberin, respectively. TSC1/TSC2 mediate PI3K/Akt activation and lead to inhibition of the mTOR pathway.[161] Tuberous sclerosis is manifested by hamartomas, epilepsy, and mental retardation. To date, only four patients with possible mutated *TSC* and pituitary tumors have been found, two cases of adrenocorticotropic hormone, one GH, and one silent gonadotroph tumors.[163–166] Again, these cases could represent coincidences.

GENETIC SCREENING CHALLENGES AND RECOMMENDATIONS

The application of genetic screening guidelines for patients with PitNETs, similar to other genetic screening guidelines, such as breast and colon, is challenging. There are three questions to consider: (1) which patients with PitNET should be screened for one of the pituitary tumor predisposing genes, (2) what clinical screening should be done in carrier family members, and (3) the categorization of identified variants as pathogenic/likely pathogenic or benign/likely benign sequence alterations.

i. The frequency of germline mutations in sporadic pituitary adenoma cases is low, and therefore genetic screening for germline variants is not recommended for all patients. When there is a suggestion that a syndrome is present, then the appropriate gene or gene panel could be used for screening. A straightforward situation is a patient with MEN1 or MEN1-like clinical picture with a positive family history or presence of other manifestation of the syndrome. Because *MEN1* can be de novo mutation and pituitary adenoma may be the first manifestation of the disease, careful judgment is needed for testing in patients with a PitNET alone. In our opinion, aggressively growing childhood prolactinoma cases justify testing for *MEN1* mutations. CNC is often a clinical diagnosis based on the manifestations in the proband. There is 100% penetrance, usually by adult age: de novo mutations are well-described, even in a familial setting.[70] In exceptional *SDHx*-positive cases, the pituitary can also be the only manifestation.[145] Of the nonsyndromic diseases, GPR101 cases usually are recognized by clinical features (eg, patients with young-onset pituitary gigantism [<5 years of age]), and these cases should undergo genetic testing for *GPR101* duplications. Care should be taken to identify germline mutations using techniques recognizing even small duplications[33] or testing of pituitary or other tissues for mosaic mutations.[32] *AIP* screening is key for sporadic or familial young-onset GH excess, but because 10% of *AIP*-positive cases are prolactinomas, we also recommend testing for young-onset macroprolactinomas (although microprolactinoma has also been described with an *AIP* nonsense mutation).[81] Familial cases with older (>30 years) ages of onset are unlikely to be positive, but currently being still in the discovery phase of *AIP*-related research we recommend all FIPA cases to be screened, at least the youngest affected family members. One needs to be aware of phenocopies, well described in *AIP* families.[94,167] Genetic testing is moving toward panel testing, and currently several laboratories offer this option including most pituitary tumor–associated genes.

ii. Initial clinical screening of identified mutation-positive family members is important because already existing abnormalities are found at this stage, obviously depending on the particular disease and the age of the person. Further follow-up of apparently unaffected carrier family members is challenging. Although intensive clinical follow-up could identify disease at an early stage, it has the potential danger of precipitating screening-fatigue with the patient and family disengaging from screening, possibly by the time the risk of disease development becomes high. Lifelong surveillance has significant implications in terms of time, frequency, cost, incidental findings, and anxiety for the carriers. The discussion of comprehensive follow-up of carriers of syndromic disease genes is beyond the limits of this review. For the pituitary aspect of MEN1-like syndromes, screening is recommended from the age 5 years with yearly blood tests for pituitary-related hormones and 3-yearly MRIs. For the pituitary aspect of CNC, because the pituitary-related abnormality is primarily in the GH/PRL axis, following pituitary function and baseline pituitary MRI, yearly blood tests for GH, PRL, and IGF-1 with clinical follow-up if suggested. For SDHx mutation–positive patients the penetrance of pituitary disease is low; the routine body MRI screen can be extended to the pituitary fossa at first screening and then every 3 to 5 years. Because *DICER1* mutation–positive patients only develop pituitary abnormality younger than the age of 2 years, no further pituitary follow-up is needed. For *AIP* mutation carriers we suggest careful follow-up of growth and pubertal development from age 4 years through childhood and adolescence, with the first MRI around age 10 years unless needed earlier. Because development of disease after 30 years is unlikely, screening could be reduced or probably stopped after this age, although gathering data on this age group is still ongoing.[84] For *GPR101* because penetrance is 100%, carrier follow-up is not an issue. For *AIP* mutation–negative FIPA family members, because disease onset is usually middle age, penetrance is low, and carrier family members cannot be identified outside a clinical study, no particular follow-up has been suggested, although patient/family member education regarding possible symptoms is important.

iii. The categorization of identified variants is the most significant challenge for clinical geneticists. Numerous *in silico* prediction programs are now available and helpful online resources combine data from these (eg, www.varsome.com). Categorizing variants according to the American College of Medical Genetics and Genomics guidelines[168] to pathogenic, likely pathogenic, variant of uncertain significance, likely benign, and benign is used for decision making, but one needs to understand that these data may change and constant vigilance and readiness need to be present to change category, especially for the large group of variant of uncertain significance changes. To communicate this complex and often uncertain message to patients and their families is challenging.

SUMMARY

Pituitary adenomas are common intracranial neoplasms, with diverse phenotypes and associated syndromic features in some cases. Understanding the molecular pathogenesis of pituitary adenomas associated with germline, mosaic, or somatic mutations is vital for the development of novel therapeutic strategies.

ACKNOWLEDGMENTS

The authors are grateful for Prof Ashley Grossman for the careful review of this article.

DISCLOSURE

The authors have nothing to disclose.

REFERENCES

1. Neou M, Villa C, Armignacco R, et al. Pangenomic classification of pituitary neuroendocrine tumors. Cancer Cell 2020;37:123–34.e5.
2. Bi WL, Horowtiz P, Greenwald N, et al. Landscape of genomic alterations in pituitary adenomas. Clin Cancer Res 2016;23(7):1841–51.
3. Song ZJ, Reitman ZJ, Ma ZY, et al. The genome-wide mutational landscape of pituitary adenomas. Cell Res 2016;26:1255–9.
4. Landis CA, Masters SB, Spada A, et al. GTPase inhibiting mutations activate the alpha chain of Gs and stimulate adenylyl cyclase in human pituitary tumours. Nature 1989;340:692–6.
5. Aflorei ED, Korbonits M. Epidemiology and etiopathogenesis of pituitary adenomas. J Neuroncol 2014;117:379–94.

6. Spada A, Vallar L. G-protein oncogenes in acromegaly. Horm Res 1992; 38:90–3.

7. Gadelha MR, Trivellin G, Hernández-Ramírez LC, et al. Genetics of pituitary adenomas. Front Horm Res 2013;41:111–40.

8. Tada M, Kobayashi H, Moriuchi T. Molecular basis of pituitary oncogenesis. J Neurooncol 1999;45:83–96.

9. Lania A, Mantovani G, Spada A. Genetics of pituitary tumors: focus on G-protein mutations. Exp Biol Med 2003;228:1004–17.

10. Ronchi CL, Peverelli E, Herterich S, et al. Landscape of somatic mutations in sporadic GH-secreting pituitary adenomas. Eur J Endocrinol 2016;174:363–72.

11. Hayward BE, Barlier A, Korbonits M, et al. Imprinting of the G(s)alpha gene GNAS1 in the pathogenesis of acromegaly. J Clin Invest 2001;107:R31–6.

12. Zhou Y, Zhang X, Klibanski A. Genetic and epigenetic mutations of tumor suppressive genes in sporadic pituitary adenoma. Mol Cell Endocrinol 2014;386: 16–33.

13. Gadelha MR, Kasuki L, Korbonits M. Novel pathway for somatostatin analogs in patients with acromegaly. Trends Endocrinol Metab 2013;24:238–46.

14. Taboada GF, Tabet AL, Naves LA, et al. Prevalence of gsp oncogene in somatotropinomas and clinically non-functioning pituitary adenomas: our experience. Pituitary 2009;12:165–9.

15. Foltran RK, Amorim P, Duarte FH, et al. Study of major genetic factors involved in pituitary tumorigenesis and their impact on clinical and biological characteristics of sporadic somatotropinomas and non-functioning pituitary adenomas. Braz J Med Biol Res 2018;51:e7427.

16. Riminucci M, Collins MT, Lala R, et al. An R201H activating mutation of the GNAS1 (Gsalpha) gene in a corticotroph pituitary adenoma. Mol Pathol 2002; 55:58–60.

17. Valimaki N, Demir H, Pitkanen E, et al. Whole-genome sequencing of growth hormone (GH)-secreting pituitary adenomas. J Clin Endocrinol Metab 2015;100: 3918–27.

18. Salenave S, Boyce AM, Collins MT, et al. Acromegaly and McCune-Albright syndrome. J Clin Endocrinol Metab 2014;99:1955–69.

19. Chanson P, Salenave S, Orcel P. McCune-Albright syndrome in adulthood. Pediatr Endocrinol Rev 2007;4(Suppl 4):453–62.

20. Chanson P, Salenave S, Young J. Ovarian dysfunction by activating mutation of GS alpha: McCune-Albright syndrome as a model. Ann Endocrinol 2010;71: 210–3.

21. Boyce AM, Glover M, Kelly MH, et al. Optic neuropathy in McCune-Albright syndrome: effects of early diagnosis and treatment of growth hormone excess. J Clin Endocrinol Metab 2013;98:E126–34.

22. Reincke M, Sbiera S, Hayakawa A, et al. Mutations in the deubiquitinase gene USP8 cause Cushing's disease. Nat Genet 2015;47:31–8.

23. Ma ZY, Song ZJ, Chen JH, et al. Recurrent gain-of-function USP8 mutations in Cushing's disease. Cell Res 2015;25:306–17.

24. Perez-Rivas L, Theodoropoulou M, Ferraù F, et al. The ubiquitin-specific peptidase 8 (USP8) gene is frequently mutated in adenomas causing Cushing's disease. Exp Clin Endocrinol Diabetes 2015;122:OP2_01.

25. Normanno N, De Luca A, Bianco C, et al. Epidermal growth factor receptor (EGFR) signaling in cancer. Gene 2006;366:2–16.

26. Hayashi K, Inoshita N, Kawaguchi K, et al. The USP8 mutational status may predict drug susceptibility in corticotroph adenomas of Cushing's disease. Eur J Endocrinol 2016;174:213–26.

27. Wanichi IQ, de Paula Mariani BM, Frassetto FP, et al. Cushing's disease due to somatic USP8 mutations: a systematic review and meta-analysis. Pituitary 2019; 22:435–42.

28. Theodoropoulou M, Reincke M, Fassnacht M, et al. Decoding the genetic basis of Cushing's disease: USP8 in the spotlight. Eur J Endocrinol 2015;173:M73–83.

29. Tufton N, Roncaroli F, Hadjidemetriou I, et al. Pituitary carcinoma in a patient with an SDHB mutation. Endocr Pathol 2017;28:320–5.

30. Cohen M, Persky R, Stegemann R, et al. Germline USP8 mutation associated with pediatric Cushing disease and other clinical features: a new syndrome. J Clin Endocrinol Metab 2019;104:4676–82.

31. Daly AF, Yuan B, Fina F, et al. Somatic mosaicism underlies X-linked acrogigantism syndrome in sporadic male subjects. Endocr Relat Cancer 2016;23:221–33.

32. Rodd C, Millette M, Iacovazzo D, et al. Somatic GPR101 duplication causing X-linked acrogigantism (XLAG)-diagnosis and management. J Clin Endocrinol Metab 2016;101:1927–30.

33. Iacovazzo D, Caswell R, Bunce B, et al. Germline or somatic GPR101 duplication leads to X-linked acrogigantism: a clinico-pathological and genetic study. Acta Neuropathol Commun 2016;4:56.

34. Trivellin G, Daly AF, Faucz FR, et al. Gigantism and acromegaly due to Xq26 microduplications and GPR101 mutation. N Engl J Med 2014;371:2363–74.

35. Gordon RJ, Bell J, Chung WK, et al. Childhood acromegaly due to X-linked acrogigantism: long term follow-up. Pituitary 2016;19:560–4.

36. Wise-Oringer BK, Zanazzi GJ, Gordon RJ, et al. Familial X-linked acrogigantism: postnatal outcomes and tumor pathology in a prenatally diagnosed infant and his mother. J Clin Endocrinol Metab 2019;104:4667–75.

37. Beijers H, Stikkelbroeck NML, Mensenkamp AR, et al. Germline and somatic mosaicism in a family with multiple endocrine neoplasia type 1 (MEN1) syndrome. Eur J Endocrinol 2019;180:K15–9.

38. Mauchlen R, Carty D, Talla M, et al. Multiple endocrine neoplasia type 1 (MEN1) mosaicism caused by a c.124G>A variant in the MEN1 gene. Endocrine Abstracts 2019;65:CC4.

39. Thakker RV. Multiple endocrine neoplasia type 1 (MEN1). Best Pract Res Clin Endocrinol Metab 2010;24:355–70.

40. Thakker RV. Multiple endocrine neoplasia type 1 (MEN1) and type 4 (MEN4). Mol Cell Endocrinol 2014;386:2–15.

41. Schernthaner-Reiter MH, Trivellin G, Stratakis CA. MEN1, MEN4, and Carney complex: pathology and molecular genetics. Neuroendocrinology 2016;103: 18–31.

42. Chandrasekharappa SC, Guru SC, Manickam P, et al. Positional cloning of the gene for multiple endocrine neoplasia-type 1. Science 1997;276:404–7.

43. Lemmens I, Van de Ven WJ, Kas K, et al. Identification of the multiple endocrine neoplasia type 1 (MEN1) gene. The European Consortium on MEN1. Hum Mol Genet 1997;6:1177–83.

44. Verges B, Boureille F, Goudet P, et al. Pituitary disease in MEN type 1 (MEN1): data from the France-Belgium MEN1 multicenter study. J Clin Endocrinol Metab 2002;87:457–65.

45. Trouillas J, Labat-Moleur F, Sturm N, et al. Pituitary tumors and hyperplasia in multiple endocrine neoplasia type 1 syndrome (MEN1): a case-control study

in a series of 77 patients versus 2509 non-MEN1 patients. Am J Surg Pathol 2008;32:534–43.

46. de Laat JM, Dekkers OM, Pieterman CR, et al. Long-term natural course of pituitary tumors in patients with MEN1: results from the DutchMEN1 study group (DMSG). J Clin Endocrinol Metab 2015;100:3288–96.

47. Cuny T, Pertuit M, Sahnoun-Fathallah M, et al. Genetic analysis in young patients with sporadic pituitary macroadenomas: beside AIP don't forget MEN1 genetic analysis. Eur J Endocrinol 2013;168:533–41.

48. Lemos MC, Thakker RV. Multiple endocrine neoplasia type 1 (MEN1): analysis of 1336 mutations reported in the first decade following identification of the gene. Hum Mutat 2008;29:22–32.

49. Concolino P, Costella A, Capoluongo E. Multiple endocrine neoplasia type 1 (MEN1): an update of 208 new germline variants reported in the last nine years. Cancer Genet 2016;209:36–41.

50. Pieterman CRC, de Laat JM, Twisk JWR, et al. Long-term natural course of small nonfunctional pancreatic neuroendocrine tumors in MEN1-results from the Dutch MEN1 Study Group. J Clin Endocrinol Metab 2017;102:3795–805.

51. Kouvaraki MA, Lee JE, Shapiro SE, et al. Genotype-phenotype analysis in multiple endocrine neoplasia type 1. Arch Surg 2002;137:641–7.

52. Pellegata NS, Quintanilla-Martinez L, Siggelkow H, et al. Germ-line mutations in p27Kip1 cause a multiple endocrine neoplasia syndrome in rats and humans. Proc Natl Acad Sci U S A 2006;103:15558–63.

53. Alrezk R, Hannah-Shmouni F, Stratakis CA. MEN4 and CDKN1B mutations: the latest of the MEN syndromes. Endocrine Relat Cancer 2017;24:T195–208.

54. Chu IM, Hengst L, Slingerland JM. The Cdk inhibitor p27 in human cancer: prognostic potential and relevance to anticancer therapy. Nat Rev Cancer 2008;8: 253–67.

55. Georgitsi M, Raitila A, Karhu A, et al. Germline CDKN1B/p27Kip1 mutation in multiple endocrine neoplasia. J Clin Endocrinol Metab 2007;92:3321–5.

56. Agarwal SK, Mateo CM, Marx SJ. Rare germline mutations in cyclin-dependent kinase inhibitor genes in multiple endocrine neoplasia type 1 and related states. J Clin Endocrinol Metab 2009;94:1826–34.

57. Molatore S, Marinoni I, Lee M, et al. A novel germline CDKN1B mutation causing multiple endocrine tumors: clinical, genetic and functional characterization. Hum Mutat 2010;31:E1825–35.

58. Costa-Guda J, Marinoni I, Molatore S, et al. Somatic mutation and germline sequence abnormalities in CDKN1B, encoding p27Kip1, in sporadic parathyroid adenomas. J Clin Endocrinol Metab 2011;96:E701–6.

59. Belar O, De La Hoz C, Perez-Nanclares G, et al. Novel mutations in MEN1, CDKN1B and AIP genes in patients with multiple endocrine neoplasia type 1 syndrome in Spain. Clin Endocrinol 2012;76:719–24.

60. Tichomirowa MA, Lee M, Barlier A, et al. Cyclin dependent kinase inhibitor 1B (CDKN1B) gene variants in AIP mutation-negative familial isolated pituitary adenomas (FIPA) kindreds. Endocr Relat Cancer 2012;19:233–41.

61. Occhi G, Regazzo D, Trivellin G, et al. A novel mutation in the upstream open reading frame of the CDKN1B gene causes a MEN4 phenotype. PLoS Genet 2013;9:e1003350.

62. Tonelli F, Giudici F, Giusti F, et al. A heterozygous frameshift mutation in exon 1 of CDKN1B gene in a patient affected by MEN4 syndrome. Eur J Endocrinol 2014; 171:K7–17.

63. Elston MS, Meyer-Rochow GY, Dray M, et al. Early onset primary hyperparathyroidism associated with a novel germline mutation in CDKN1B. Case Rep Endocrinol 2015;2015:510985.

64. Sambugaro S, Di RM, Ambrosio MR, et al. Early onset acromegaly associated with a novel deletion in CDKN1B 5'UTR region. Endocrine 2015;49(1):58–64.

65. Carney JA, Gordon H, Carpenter PC, et al. The complex of myxomas, spotty pigmentation, and endocrine overactivity. Medicine (Baltimore) 1985;64:270–83.

66. Stratakis CA, Kirschner LS, Carney JA. Clinical and molecular features of the Carney complex: diagnostic criteria and recommendations for patient evaluation. J Clin Endocrinol Metab 2001;86:4041–6.

67. Kirschner LS, Carney JA, Pack SD, et al. Mutations of the gene encoding the protein kinase A type I-alpha regulatory subunit in patients with the Carney complex. Nat Genet 2000;26:89–92.

68. Casey M, Vaughan CJ, He J, et al. Mutations in the protein kinase A R1alpha regulatory subunit cause familial cardiac myxomas and Carney complex. J Clin Invest 2000;106:R31–8.

69. Salpea P, Horvath A, London E, et al. Deletions of the PRKAR1A locus at 17q24.2-q24.3 in Carney complex: genotype-phenotype correlations and implications for genetic testing. J Clin Endocrinol Metab 2014;99:E183–8.

70. Stelmachowska-Banas M, Zgliczynski W, Tutka P, et al. Fatal Carney complex in siblings due to de novo large gene deletion. J Clin Endocrinol Metab 2017;102:3924–7.

71. Caimari F, Korbonits M. Novel genetic causes of pituitary adenomas. Clin Cancer Res 2016;22:5030–42.

72. Correa R, Salpea P, Stratakis CA. Carney complex: an update. Eur J Endocrinol 2015;173:M85–97.

73. Kiefer FW, Winhofer Y, Iacovazzo D, et al. PRKAR1A mutation causing pituitary-dependent Cushing disease in a patient with Carney complex. Eur J Endocrinol 2017;177:K7–12.

74. Hernandez-Ramirez LC, Tatsi C, Lodish MB, et al. Corticotropinoma as a component of Carney complex. J Endocr Soc 2017;1:918–25.

75. Matyakhina L, Pack S, Kirschner LS, et al. Chromosome 2 (2p16) abnormalities in Carney complex tumours. J Med Genet 2003;40:268–77.

76. Beuschlein F, Fassnacht M, Assie G, et al. Constitutive activation of PKA catalytic subunit in adrenal Cushing's syndrome. N Engl J Med 2014;370:1019–28.

77. Lodish MB, Yuan B, Levy I, et al. Germline PRKACA amplification causes variable phenotypes that may depend on the extent of the genomic defect: molecular mechanisms and clinical presentations. Eur J Endocrinol 2015;172:803–11.

78. Forlino A, Vetro A, Garavelli L, et al. PRKACB and Carney complex. N Engl J Med 2014;370:1065–7.

79. Larkin SJ, Ferraù F, Karavitaki N, et al. Sequence analysis of the catalytic subunit of PKA in somatotroph adenomas. Eur J Endocrinol 2014;171:705–10.

80. Beckers A, Aaltonen LA, Daly AF, et al. Familial isolated pituitary adenomas (FIPA) and the pituitary adenoma predisposition due to mutations in the aryl hydrocarbon receptor interacting protein (AIP) gene. Endocr Rev 2013;34:239–77.

81. Marques P, Caimari F, Hernandez-Ramirez LC, et al. Significant benefits of AIP testing and clinical screening in familial isolated and young-onset pituitary tumors. J Clin Endocrinol Metab 2020;105(6):dgaa040.

82. Stiles CE, Korbonits M. Familial isolated pituitary adenoma. ENDOTEXT, Neuroendocrinology 2020. Chapter 11a11. Available at: http://www.endotext.org/neuroendo/neuroendo11a11/neuroendo11a11.htm. Accessed April 16, 2020.

83. Daly AF, Tichomirowa MA, Petrossians P, et al. Clinical characteristics and therapeutic responses in patients with germ-line AIP mutations and pituitary adenomas: an international collaborative study. J Clin Endocrinol Metab 2010;95: E373–83.

84. Korbonits M, Kumar AV. AIP-related familial isolated pituitary adenomas. In: Pagon RA, Bird TA, Dolan CR, et al, editors. GeneReviews. Seattle (WA): University of Washington; 2020. Available at: http://www.ncbi.nlm.nih.gov/books/NBK97965/. Accessed April 16, 2020.

85. Dutta P, Reddy KS, Rai A, et al. Surgery, octreotide, temozolomide, bevacizumab, radiotherapy, and pegvisomant treatment of an *AIP* mutation positive child. J Clin Endocrinol Metab 2019;104:3539–44.

86. Xekouki P, Mastroyiannis SA, Avgeropoulos D, et al. Familial pituitary apoplexy as the only presentation of a novel AIP mutation. Endocr Relat Cancer 2013;20: L11–4.

87. Hernandez-Ramirez LC, Gabrovska P, Denes J, et al. Landscape of familial isolated and young-onset pituitary adenomas: prospective diagnosis in AIP mutation carriers. J Clin Endocrinol Metab 2015;100:E1242–54.

88. Kasuki Jomori de PL, Vieira NL, Armondi Wildemberg LE, et al. Low aryl hydrocarbon receptor-interacting protein expression is a better marker of invasiveness in somatotropinomas than Ki-67 and p53. Neuroendocrinology 2011;94: 39–48.

89. Barry S, Carlsen E, Marques P, et al. Tumor microenvironment defines the invasive phenotype of AIP-mutation-positive pituitary tumors. Oncogene 2019;38: 5381–95.

90. Chahal HS, Trivellin G, Leontiou CA, et al. Somatostatin analogs modulate AIP in somatotroph adenomas: the role of the ZAC1 pathway. J Clin Endocrinol Metab 2012;97:E1411–20.

91. Oriola J, Lucas T, Halperin I, et al. Germline mutations of AIP gene in somatotropinomas resistant to somatostatin analogues. Eur J Endocrinol 2013;168:9–13.

92. Loughrey PB, Korbonits M. Genetics of pituitary tumours. In: Igaz P, Patocs A, editors. Genetics of endocrine diseases and syndromes. Cham, Switzerland: Springer; 2019. p. 171–211.

93. Ozfirat Z, Korbonits M. AIP gene and familial isolated pituitary adenomas. Mol Cell Endocrinol 2010;326:71–9.

94. Vierimaa O, Georgitsi M, Lehtonen R, et al. Pituitary adenoma predisposition caused by germline mutations in the AIP gene. Science 2006;312:1228–30.

95. Gadelha MR, Prezant TR, Une KN, et al. Loss of heterozygosity on chromosome 11q13 in two families with acromegaly/gigantism is independent of mutations of the multiple endocrine neoplasia type I gene. J Clin Endocrinol Metab 1999;84: 249–56.

96. Khoo SK, Pendek R, Nickolov R, et al. Genome-wide scan identifies novel modifier loci of acromegalic phenotypes for isolated familial somatotropinoma. Endocr Relat Cancer 2009;16:1057–63.

97. Lecoq AL, Bouligand J, Hage M, et al. Very low frequency of germline GPR101 genetic variation and no biallelic defects with AIP in a large cohort of patients with sporadic pituitary adenomas. Eur J Endocrinol 2016;174:523–30.

98. Leontiou CA, Gueorguiev M, van der Spuy J, et al. The role of the aryl hydrocarbon receptor-interacting protein gene in familial and sporadic pituitary adenomas. J Clin Endocrinol Metab 2008;93:2390–401.

99. Ibanez-Costa A, Korbonits M. AIP and the somatostatin system in pituitary tumours. J Endocrinol 2017;235:R101–16.

100. Jaffrain-Rea ML, Angelini M, Gargano D, et al. Expression of aryl hydrocarbon receptor (AHR) and AHR-interacting protein in pituitary adenomas: pathological and clinical implications. Endocr Relat Cancer 2009;16:1029–43.

101. Georgitsi M, Karhu A, Winqvist R, et al. Mutation analysis of aryl hydrocarbon receptor interacting protein (AIP) gene in colorectal, breast, and prostate cancers. Br J Cancer 2007;96:352–6.

102. Raitila A, Georgitsi M, Karhu A, et al. No evidence of somatic aryl hydrocarbon receptor interacting protein mutations in sporadic endocrine neoplasia. Endocr Relat Cancer 2007;14:901–6.

103. Tichomirowa MA, Barlier A, Daly AF, et al. High prevalence of AIP gene mutations following focused screening in young patients with sporadic pituitary macroadenomas. Eur J Endocrinol 2011;165:509–15.

104. Aflorei ED, Klapholz B, Chen C, et al. In vivo bioassay to test the pathogenicity of missense human AIP variants. J Med Genet 2018;55:522–9.

105. Chen B, Liu P, Hujber EJ, et al. AIP limits neurotransmitter release by inhibiting calcium bursts from the ryanodine receptor. Nat Commun 2017;8:1380.

106. Lin BC, Sullivan R, Lee Y, et al. Deletion of the aryl hydrocarbon receptor-associated protein 9 leads to cardiac malformation and embryonic lethality. J Biol Chem 2007;282:35924–32.

107. Cai W, Kramarova TV, Berg P, et al. The immunophilin-like protein XAP2 is a negative regulator of estrogen signaling through interaction with estrogen receptor alpha. PLoS One 2011;6:e25201.

108. Trivellin G, Korbonits M. AIP and its interacting partners. J Endocrinol 2011;210:137–55.

109. Tuominen I, Heliovaara E, Raitila A, et al. AIP inactivation leads to pituitary tumorigenesis through defective Galphai-cAMP signaling. Oncogene 2015;34:1174–84.

110. Hernandez-Ramirez LC, Morgan RML, Barry S, et al. Multi-chaperone function modulation and association with cytoskeletal proteins are key features of the function of AIP in the pituitary gland. Oncotarget 2018;9:9177–98.

111. Yano M, Terada K, Mori M. AIP is a mitochondrial import mediator that binds to both import receptor Tom20 and preproteins. J Cell Biol 2003;163:45–56.

112. Vargiolu M, Fusco D, Kurelac I, et al. The tyrosine kinase receptor RET interacts in vivo with aryl hydrocarbon receptor-interacting protein to alter survivin availability. J Clin Endocrinol Metab 2009;94:2571–8.

113. Kashuba EV, Gradin K, Isaguliants M, et al. Regulation of transactivation function of the aryl hydrocarbon receptor by the Epstein-Barr virus-encoded EBNA-3 protein. J Biol Chem 2006;281:1215–23.

114. Formosa R, Vassallo J. cAMP signalling in the normal and tumorigenic pituitary gland. Mol Cell Endocrinol 2014;392:37–50.

115. Bolger GB, Bizzi MF, Pinheiro SV, et al. cAMP-specific PDE4 phosphodiesterases and AIP in the pathogenesis of pituitary tumors. Endocr Relat Cancer 2016;23:419–31.

116. Igreja S, Chahal HS, King P, et al. Characterization of aryl hydrocarbon receptor interacting protein (AIP) mutations in familial isolated pituitary adenoma families. Hum Mutat 2010;31:950–60.

117. Raitila A, Lehtonen HJ, Arola J, et al. Mice with inactivation of aryl hydrocarbon receptor-interacting protein (Aip) display complete penetrance of pituitary adenomas with aberrant ARNT expression. Am J Pathol 2010;177:1969–76.

118. Gillam MP, Ku CR, Lee YJ, et al. Somatotroph-specific Aip-deficient mice display pretumorigenic alterations in cell-cycle signaling. J Endocr Soc 2017; 1:78–95.

119. Beckers A, Lodish MB, Trivellin G, et al. X-linked acrogigantism syndrome: clinical profile and therapeutic responses. Endocr Relat Cancer 2015;22:353–67.

120. Kamenicky P, Bouligand J, Chanson P. Gigantism, acromegaly, and GPR101 mutations. N Engl J Med 2015;372:1264.

121. Flak MB, Koenis DS, Sobrino A, et al. GPR101 mediates the pro-resolving actions of RvD5n-3 DPA in arthritis and infections. J Clin Invest 2020;130:359–73.

122. Iacovazzo D, Korbonits M. Gigantism: X-linked acrogigantism and GPR101 mutations. Growth Horm IGF Res 2016;30-31:64–9.

123. Daly AF, Lysy PA, Desfilles C, et al. GHRH excess and blockade in X-LAG syndrome. Endocr Relat Cancer 2016;23:161–70.

124. Pepe S, Korbonits M, Iacovazzo D. Germline and mosaic mutations causing pituitary tumours: genetic and molecular aspects. J Endocrinol 2019;240:R21–45.

125. Rostomyan L, Daly AF, Petrossians P, et al. Clinical and genetic characterization of pituitary gigantism: an international collaborative study in 208 patients. Endocr Relat Cancer 2015;22:745–57.

126. Vandeva S, Daly AF, Petrossians P, et al. Somatic and germline mutations in the pathogenesis of pituitary adenomas. Eur J Endocrinol 2019;181:R235–54.

127. Trivellin G, Hernandez-Ramirez LC, Swan J, et al. An orphan G-protein-coupled receptor causes human gigantism and/or acromegaly: molecular biology and clinical correlations. Best Pract Res Clin Endocrinol Metab 2018;32:125–40.

128. Castinetti F, Daly AF, Stratakis CA, et al. GPR101 mutations are not a frequent cause of congenital isolated growth hormone deficiency. Horm Metab Res 2016;48:389–93.

129. Doros L, Schultz KA, Stewart DR, et al. DICER1-Related disorders. In: Pagon RA, Bird TA, Dolan CR, et al, editors. GeneReviews. Seattle (WA): University of Washington; 2020. Available at: https://pubmed.ncbi.nlm.nih.gov/24761742/. Accessed April 30, 2020.

130. Schultz KAP, Williams GM, Kamihara J, et al. DICER1 and associated conditions: identification of at-risk individuals and recommended surveillance strategies. Clin Cancer Res 2018;24:2251–61.

131. Doros LA, Rossi CT, Yang J, et al. DICER1 mutations in childhood cystic nephroma and its relationship to DICER1-renal sarcoma. Mod Pathol 2014;27: 1267–80.

132. de Kock L, Sabbaghian N, Plourde F, et al. Pituitary blastoma: a pathognomonic feature of germ-line DICER1 mutations. Acta Neuropathol 2014;128:111–22.

133. Scheithauer BW, Kovacs K, Horvath E, et al. Pituitary blastoma. Acta Neuropathol 2008;116:657–66.

134. Choong CS, Priest JR, Foulkes WD. Exploring the endocrine manifestations of DICER1 mutations. Trends Mol Med 2012;18:503–5.

135. Krol J, Loedige I, Filipowicz W. The widespread regulation of microRNA biogenesis, function and decay. Nat Rev Genet 2010;11:597–610.

136. Rio FT, Bahubeshi A, Kanellopoulou C, et al. DICER1 mutations in familial multinodular goiter with and without ovarian Sertoli-Leydig cell tumors. JAMA 2011; 305:68–77.

137. Sahakitrungruang T, Srichomthong C, Pornkunwilai S, et al. Germline and somatic DICER1 mutations in a pituitary blastoma causing infantile-onset Cushing's disease. J Clin Endocrinol Metab 2014;99:E1487–92.

138. Schultz KAP, Rednam SP, Kamihara J, et al. PTEN, DICER1, FH, and their associated tumor susceptibility syndromes: clinical features, genetics, and surveillance recommendations in childhood. Clin Cancer Res 2017;23:e76–82.

139. Brenneman M, Field A, Yang J, et al. Temporal order of RNase IIIb and loss-of-function mutations during development determines phenotype in pleuropulmonary blastoma/DICER1 syndrome: a unique variant of the two-hit tumor suppression model. F1000Res 2015;4:214.

140. de Kock L, Wang YC, Revil T, et al. High-sensitivity sequencing reveals multi-organ somatic mosaicism causing DICER1 syndrome. J Med Genet 2016;53: 43–52.

141. Cotton E, Ray D. DICER1 mutation and pituitary prolactinoma. Endocrinol Diabetes Metab Case Rep 2018;2018. 18-0087.

142. Xekouki P, Szarek E, Bullova P, et al. Pituitary adenoma with paraganglioma/pheochromocytoma (3PAs) and succinate dehydrogenase defects in humans and mice. J Clin Endocrinol Metab 2015;100:E710–9.

143. Gill AJ, Toon CW, Clarkson A, et al. Succinate dehydrogenase deficiency is rare in pituitary adenomas. Am J Surg Pathol 2014;38:560–6.

144. Dénes J, Swords F, Rattenberry E, et al. Heterogeneous genetic background of the association of pheochromocytoma/paraganglioma and pituitary adenoma: results from a large patient cohort. J Clin Endocrinol Metab 2015;100:E531–41.

145. Maher M, Roncaroli F, Mendoza N, et al. A patient with a germline SDHB mutation presenting with an isolated pituitary macroprolactinoma. Endocrinol Diabetes Metab Case Rep 2018;2018:18–0078.

146. Tufton N, Shapiro L, Srirangalingam U, et al. Outcomes of annual surveillance imaging in an adult and paediatric cohort of succinate dehydrogenase B mutation carriers. Clin Endocrinol 2017;86:286–96.

147. Benn DE, Gimenez-Roqueplo AP, Reilly JR, et al. Clinical presentation and penetrance of pheochromocytoma/paraganglioma syndromes. J Clin Endocrinol Metab 2006;91:827–36.

148. Xekouki P, Pacak K, Almeida M, et al. Succinate dehydrogenase (SDH) D subunit (SDHD) inactivation in a growth-hormone-producing pituitary tumor: a new association for SDH? J Clin Endocrinol Metab 2012;97:E357–66.

149. Varsavsky M, Sebastian-Ochoa A, Torres VE. Coexistence of a pituitary macroadenoma and multicentric paraganglioma: a strange coincidence. Endocrinol Nutr 2012;60(3):154–6.

150. Guerrero-Perez F, Fajardo C, Torres Vela E, et al. 3P association (3PAs): pituitary adenoma and pheochromocytoma/paraganglioma. A heterogeneous clinical syndrome associated with different gene mutations. Eur J Intern Med 2019; 69:14–9.

151. Xekouki P, Stratakis CA. Succinate dehydrogenase (SDHx) mutations in pituitary tumors: could this be a new role for mitochondrial complex II and/or Krebs cycle defects? Endocr Relat Cancer 2012;19:C33–40.

152. Rutter J, Winge DR, Schiffman JD. Succinate dehydrogenase: assembly, regulation and role in human disease. Mitochondrion 2010;10:393–401.

153. Zhang Q, Peng C, Song J, et al. Germline mutations in CDH23, encoding cadherin-related 23, are associated with both familial and sporadic pituitary adenomas. Am J Hum Genet 2017;100:817–23.

154. Bolz H, von Brederlow B, Ramirez A, et al. Mutation of CDH23, encoding a new member of the cadherin gene family, causes Usher syndrome type 1D. Nat Genet 2001;27:108–12.

155. Hernandez-Ramirez LC, Gam R, Valdes N, et al. Loss-of-function mutations in the CABLES1 gene are a novel cause of Cushing's disease. Endocr Relat Cancer 2017;24:379–92.

156. Roussel-Gervais A, Couture C, Langlais D, et al. The Cables1 gene in glucocorticoid regulation of pituitary corticotrope growth and Cushing disease. J Clin Endocrinol Metab 2016;101:513–22.

157. Roussel-Gervais A, Bilodeau S, Vallette S, et al. Cooperation between cyclin E and p27(Kip1) in pituitary tumorigenesis. Mol Endocrinol 2010;24:1835–45.

158. Tadini G, Milani D, Menni F, et al. Is it time to change the neurofibromatosis 1 diagnostic criteria? Eur J Intern Med 2014;25:506–10.

159. Milani D, Pezzani L, Tadini G, et al. A multidisciplinary approach in neurofibromatosis 1. Lancet Neurol 2015;14:29–30.

160. Hannah-Shmouni F, Stratakis CA. Growth hormone excess in neurofibromatosis 1. Genet Med 2019;21:1254–5.

161. Rosner M, Hanneder M, Siegel N, et al. The mTOR pathway and its role in human genetic diseases. Mutat Res 2008;659:284–92.

162. Hozumi K, Fukuoka H, Odake Y, et al. Acromegaly caused by a somatotroph adenoma in patient with neurofibromatosis type 1. Endocr J 2019;66:853–7.

163. Tigas S, Carroll PV, Jones R, et al. Simultaneous Cushing's disease and tuberous sclerosis; a potential role for TSC in pituitary ontogeny. Clin Endocrinol 2005;63:694–5.

164. Nandagopal R, Vortmeyer A, Oldfield EH, et al. Cushing's syndrome due to a pituitary corticotropinoma in a child with tuberous sclerosis: an association or a coincidence? Clin Endocrinol 2007;67:639–41.

165. Dworakowska D, Grossman AB. Are neuroendocrine tumours a feature of tuberous sclerosis? A systematic review. Endocr Relat Cancer 2009;16:45–58.

166. Regazzo D, Gardiman MP, Theodoropoulou M, et al. Silent gonadotroph pituitary neuroendocrine tumor in a patient with tuberous sclerosis complex: evaluation of a possible molecular link. Endocrinol Diabetes Metab Case Rep 2018; 2018. 18-0086.

167. Williams F, Hunter S, Bradley L, et al. Clinical experience in the screening and management of a large kindred with familial isolated pituitary adenoma due to an aryl hydrocarbon receptor interacting protein (AIP) mutation. J Clin Endocrinol Metab 2014;99:1122–31.

168. Richards S, Aziz N, Bale S, et al, ACMG Laboratory Quality Assurance Committee. Standards and guidelines for the interpretation of sequence variants: a joint consensus recommendation of the American College of Medical Genetics and Genomics and the Association for Molecular Pathology. Genet Med 2015;17: 405–24.

The Role of Dopamine Agonists in Pituitary Adenomas

Erica A. Giraldi, MD[a], Adriana G. Ioachimescu, MD, PhD[a,b],*

KEYWORDS

- Dopamine agonist • Bromocriptine • Cabergoline • Prolactinoma • Acromegaly
- Cushing disease • Pituitary adenoma

KEY POINTS

- Dopamine agonists improve clinical manifestations, hyperprolactinemia, and tumor size in most patients with prolactinomas.
- A trial of cabergoline is reasonable for patients with biochemically mild acromegaly, whereas cabergoline/somatostatin receptor ligand combination is synergistic in up to 50% of patients.
- Large controlled studies are needed to identify patients with adrenocorticotropic hormone–negative and nonfunctional tumors who might benefit from cabergoline and the long-term outcomes of therapy.

INTRODUCTION

Dopamine inhibits prolactin secretion from lactotroph cells by modulation of prolactin gene expression, cellular proliferation, and neoplastic cell apoptosis.[1] Among the 5 types of dopamine receptors (DRs), D2R activation most potently inhibits prolactin secretion via decreasing cyclic AMP accumulation and cellular calcium levels.[1] Lactotroph, somatotroph, corticotroph, and nonfunctioning adenomas have variable expression of D2R receptors.[1–4]

Dopamine agonist (DA) therapy has been established for treatment of hyperprolactinemia and used off label in acromegaly, Cushing disease, and nonfunctioning pituitary adenomas (NFPAs). Several DAs were developed (**Box 1**). Bromocriptine and cabergoline are most commonly used, the latter with higher D2R selectivity/affinity and longer half-life.

The side effects include nausea, vomiting, postural hypotension, headache, dizziness,[5] and mood changes, including impulse control disorders,[6] typically resolved after medication discontinuation. In patients with Parkinson disease, high-dose

[a] Department of Medicine: Endocrinology and Metabolism, Emory University, Atlanta, GA 30322, USA; [b] Department of Neurosurgery, Emory University, Atlanta, GA, USA
* Corresponding author. 1365 B Clifton Road, Northeast, B6209, Atlanta, GA 30322.
E-mail address: aioachi@emory.edu

Endocrinol Metab Clin N Am 49 (2020) 453–474
https://doi.org/10.1016/j.ecl.2020.05.006
0889-8529/20/© 2020 Elsevier Inc. All rights reserved.

endo.theclinics.com

Box 1
Dopamine agonist therapy for prolactinomas

- Several DAs were developed, including bromocriptine, cabergoline, quinagolide, lisuride, pergolide, dihydroergocryptine, and mesulergine.

- Cabergoline and bromocriptine are most frequently used and yield prolactin normalization in 60% to 80% of patients.

- Direct comparison studies indicate superior biochemical and clinical effects for cabergoline.

- Tumor involution occurs in most patients treated with DAs, with more responders in cabergoline than bromocriptine studies.

- Withdrawal of DA therapy is associated with recurrent hyperprolactinemia in most patients.

- Patients with normoprolactinemia on a low-dose DA, and prior tumor shrinkage are more likely to maintain remission.

- Stopping DAs during pregnancy is safe in most patients, with neuro-ophthalmologic evaluation in case of large macroadenomas.

- During pregnancy, the risk of symptomatic enlargement in the absence of DAs is 16% for patients with macroadenomas without prior surgery or radiation and lower than 5% for the others.

---

cabergoline was associated with an increased risk of valvulopathy. This risk is usually not encountered at the smaller doses used for treatment of prolactinomas. Rarely, cerebrospinal fluid leak and pituitary apoplexy occur during DA therapy.[5]

DOPAMINE AGONISTS FOR PROLACTINOMAS

Prolactinomas represent 40% to 57% of pituitary adenomas[7,8] and predominantly affect women. Premenopausal women clinically present with amenorrhea, galactorrhea, or infertility, and radiographically mostly with microadenomas. Men present with headaches, vision changes, hypogonadism or gynecomastia, and higher prevalence of macroadenomas.

Indications and Overall Effects

DAs represent the first-line therapy in patients with prolactinomas, aiming for prolactin normalization, tumor control, and gonadal function restoration.[7]

The 2011 Endocrine Society guidelines recommended treatment of macroprolactinomas or symptomatic microprolactinomas.[7] In women with microprolactinomas and hypogonadism, either estrogen replacement or DAs can be used,[9] because tumor growth is unlikely.[10,11] In contrast, tumor-targeting therapy is recommended in macroprolactinomas.[9] Although 60% to 90% of men treated with DAs experience resolution of hypogonadism,[12,13] some require testosterone replacement, which was associated with tumor growth in some reports.[14,15]

A systematic review evaluated 3000 patients from 8 randomized and 178 non-randomized studies (39 bromocriptine, 26 cabergoline, and 15 quinagolide). Compared with no treatment, DAs reduced prolactin level (weighted mean difference −45; confidence interval [CI] −77 to −11) and the risk of persistent hyperprolactinemia (relative risk 0.90; CI 0.81–0.99).[16]

In the United States, cabergoline and bromocriptine are approved by the US Food and Drug Administration (FDA) for prolactinomas at maximal recommended dosages of 2 mg/wk and 15 mg/d respectively.

Bromocriptine

Bromocriptine was the first medical agent used for prolactinomas[17,18] at dosages of 2.5 to 15 mg/d.[19] A systematic review of 7 studies (1978–2011) indicated that most patients responded with normoprolactinemia (68%), tumor reduction (62%), resolution of visual defects (67%), galactorrhea (86%), amenorrhea (78%), sexual dysfunction (67%), and infertility (53%).[16]

In a 2013 retrospective study, all patients with invasive macroprolactinomas receiving bromocriptine (median 10 mg/d) experienced tumor shrinkage after a median of 30 months and 91.3% normoprolactinemia (69.6% within 6 months).[20]

Cabergoline

Cabergoline in dosages of 0.25 to 3 mg/wk is more effective in restoring normoprolactinemia than bromocriptine,[7,19] with occasional patients requiring dosages up to 11 mg/wk.[7]

A 2006 review of 14 prospective and 2 retrospective studies (1980 to early 2000) found normoprolactinemia in 81% to 96% and tumor shrinkage in 48% to 83% of patients.[19] A meta-analysis of 26 studies indicated normoprolactinemia in 50% to 100%, and tumor reduction in 47% to 97%.[16] In a retrospective study in 27 older men taking cabergoline, normoprolactinemia occurred in 85.7% and macroadenoma involution in 93%.[21]

Dopamine Agonist Choice

Most studies comparing cabergoline with bromocriptine addressed their biochemical outcomes and adverse effects.

In a multicentric trial of 459 women with hyperprolactinemic amenorrhea, patients received 1 of the 2 agents in a double-blinded fashion for 8 weeks, then nonblinded for 16 weeks. Prolactin normalized in 83% on cabergoline versus 59% on bromocriptine, and ovulation returned in 72% on cabergoline versus 52% on bromocriptine. Only 3% of patients discontinued cabergoline because of side effects versus 12% for bromocriptine.[22] A subsequent meta-analysis of 4 randomized trials (743 patients) directly comparing cabergoline with bromocriptine (including the aforementioned trial) reported higher likelihood of normoprolactinemia and lower risks of persistent amenorrhea and adverse effects for cabergoline.[23] In the 3000-patients systematic review, cabergoline was more likely to resolve hyperprolactinemia, amenorrhea, and galactorrhea than bromocriptine.[16]

Tumor size decreased by 50% to 75% in 65% to 100% of patients in bromocriptine studies,[24–26] and by 30% to 100% in 70% to 90% of patients in cabergoline studies.[7,27–29]

Few recent studies compared cabergoline with bromocriptine. In a meta-analysis of 24 patients with giant prolactinomas, mean tumor volume reduction (TVR) and proportion of responders were similar for bromocriptine and cabergoline. More patients achieved normoprolactinemia on cabergoline (60.4%) than on bromocriptine (35.3%).[30]

In summary, cabergoline seems superior to bromocriptine regarding clinical, biochemical, and radiographic effects. However, tumor shrinkage has not been evaluated by large direct comparison studies. In clinical practice, the DA choice also depends on drug availability and patient preference. The authors generally use cabergoline in patients with large or invasive tumors. Patients taking bromocriptine can be switched to cabergoline in cases of intolerance or less than satisfactory response.

Predictors of Response

Prediction of long-term biochemical and tumor reduction response in patients treated with DAs constitutes an important aspect, especially for patients with macroadenomas.

A prospective study of 110 patients with macroprolactinomas receiving cabergoline (maximal dosage 3.5 mg/wk) found that nadir prolactin levels during treatment were the most important predictor of tumor shrinkage, followed by the cabergoline dose, which inversely correlated with the radiological outcome.[29]

A retrospective study in 44 patients receiving cabergoline (maximal dosage 4.5 mg/wk) defined response as TVR greater than 50% alongside prolactin normalization. Patients with greater than 25% TVR and normoprolactinemia after 3 months were more likely to have long-term response.[31]

In a historical prospective study in 71 men with macroadenomas, the likelihood of normoprolactinemia was greater for lower prolactin levels and smaller adenomas at presentation. Also, lower prolactin levels and tumor shrinkage after 6 months of treatment were predictive of subsequent normoprolactinemia and tumor shrinkage, respectively. The maximal dosage of cabergoline used was 7 mg/wk, and patients achieving normoprolactinemia required smaller dosages compared with those who did not.[32]

In summary, baseline biochemical and radiological measurements, as well as response after 3 to 6 months, seem to play a role in predicting long-term outcomes of DA therapy. Responders seem to require smaller dosages, and further study is needed to identify patients who might benefit from increasing the dosage to greater than 2 mg/wk.

Dopamine Agonist Withdrawal

Per Endocrine Society guidelines, patients treated for more than 2 years can be considered for DA discontinuation if prolactin is normal and tumor no longer visible on imaging. This recommendation was based on 4 studies showing biochemical recurrence in 26% to 69% of patients after DA withdrawal.[28,33–35] Two were retrospective (89 and 46 patients),[33,35] 1 prospective (200 patients),[28] and 1 meta-analysis.[34] Since 2011, 2 other meta-analyses found 44% to 50% recurrence and better prognosis for patients with tumor shrinkage who used the lowest DA dosage before withdrawal (**Table 1**).[36,37]

In summary, close clinical and biochemical monitoring is important after a trial of DA withdrawal.

Role of Surgery

Surgery represented primary therapy for prolactinomas before the DA era. Surgery is currently recommended for resistance or intolerance to DAs, visual loss from tumor mass effect,[38] and absent tumor shrinkage in women with macroprolactinomas considering pregnancy.[7]

There are no head-to-head studies comparing the DA therapy with surgery. In a meta-analysis including 30 surgical studies (mean follow-up 4.9 years), biochemical remission was 68.8% and recurrence 18%.[39]

A meta-analysis evaluated 55 DA studies (3564 patients) and 25 surgical studies (1836 patients). In the DA studies, median treatment duration was 24 months with 12-month follow-up after withdrawal. In surgical studies, follow-up was 22 months postoperatively. Normoprolactinemia after DA withdrawal was maintained in 34% of cases (36% microprolactinomas, 28% macroprolactinomas) versus 67% postsurgery (83% microprolactinomas, 60% macroprolactinomas).[40]

Table 1
Meta-analysis studies of dopamine agonist therapy withdrawal

First Author, Year	DA Type (Number of Studies)	Patients (N)	Imaging Before DA	Maintained Remission After Withdrawal	Predictors of Durable Remission
Dekkers et al,[34] 2010	Cabergoline (4) Bromocriptine (12) Quinagolide (2) Dihydroergocryptine (1)	743	425 micro 263 macro 55 idiopathic hyperprolactinemia	21% micro 16% macro	Treatment >2 y
Hu et al,[36] 2015	Cabergoline (11)	637	467 micro 119 macro 32 unspecified	40% micro 25% macro	1. Lowest dose before withdrawal 2. Tumor shrinkage
Xia et al,[37] 2018	Cabergoline (10) Bromocriptine (11) Both (3)	1106	756 micro 306 macro 41 idiopathic 32 unspecified	36.6% overall	1. Lowest dose before withdrawal 2. Tumor shrinkage >50%

Abbreviations: macro, macroadenoma; micro, microadenoma.
Data from Refs.[34,36,37]

Recent studies in giant prolactinomas have shown that multimodality treatment including surgery, DA, and sometimes radiation achieved normoprolactinemia in 52% to 67%[41,42] and significant tumor shrinkage in 25% of patients.[42]

In summary, maintaining normoprolactinemia after successful surgery seems more likely than after cessation of DAs. The caveats are selection of patients undergoing surgery and surgical expertise. For patients with large tumors, surgery and medical treatment may be needed.

Pregnancy Implications

Correction of hyperprolactinemia restores ovulation in most patients. Two main concerns pertain to pregnancy: the safety profile of DA, and the risk of mass effect symptoms. The Endocrine Society guidelines recommend discontinuation of DAs in pregnancy, except women with tumors abutting the optic chiasm.[7] Neuroophthalmologic evaluation is essential in these cases.

A recent review analyzed 15 studies (764 patients) and found symptomatic tumor enlargement during pregnancy in 2.4% of microadenomas, 4.7% of macroadenomas with prior surgery or radiation, and 16.4% of macroadenomas without prior surgery or radiation.[43]

Bromocriptine has been shown to cross the placenta, whereas data are lacking for cabergoline.[43] In a study in 29 women (32 pregnancies) treated with DAs (81.2% bromocriptine, 18.8% cabergoline), patients were advised to discontinue the medication on confirmation of pregnancy. Of them, 8.7% discontinued before conception, 60.9% before the second month of pregnancy, 26.1% before the second trimester, and 4.3% afterward. Data were available for 22 births, of which 13.6% were premature. For 18 babies with known birth weights, these were low in 5.6% and very low in 5.6%. Of the 32 infants, 3.1% had clubfoot.[44] In a review of pregnancies with prior bromocriptine (6239) and cabergoline (1016) use, rates of spontaneous abortions, terminations, ectopic pregnancies, and malformations were similar to the general population.[43] In contrast, a French database of 57,408 women, of whom 0.3% had used DAs, found an association of DA exposure with preterm birth and early pregnancy loss, but not with birth defects.[45] In addition, a recent review summarized 15 patients taking cabergoline throughout most of their pregnancies: 13 had had no complications, 1 had severe preeclampsia and fetal death, and 1 had preterm labor at 36 weeks.[46]

In summary, women receiving DAs benefit from prepregnancy counseling. Unless the risk of symptomatic tumor enlargement seems significant, DAs should be discontinued once pregnancy is confirmed.

DOPAMINE AGONISTS FOR ACROMEGALY

The first line of treatment for acromegaly is surgery. Endocrine Society guidelines recommend medical therapy (somatostatin receptor ligands [SRLs], pegvisomant, or DAs) in patients with persistent or recurrent disease postoperatively.[47] SRLs and pegvisomant are FDA approved for acromegaly, whereas DAs are used off label. The mechanism of action entails DR expression in somatotroph adenomas, with DR2 being the predominant DR type.[48]

Bromocriptine Monotherapy

Studies using bromocriptine were published in the 1970s to 1990s. A 1994 review of 34 studies (616 patients) found that 10% of patients experienced growth hormone normalization and 10% to 20% tumor reduction.[49] In a more recent retrospective study in 133 patients, biochemical response was 18.8%.[50]

Cabergoline Monotherapy

A summary of cabergoline monotherapy is presented in **Table 2**.[50–55]

The 2014 Endocrine Society guidelines recommended a trial of DA monotherapy in patients with only modest increases of serum insulin-like growth factor 1 (IGF-1) levels and mild signs and symptoms of GH excess.[47] This recommendation was based on a meta-analysis and few prospective studies. The meta-analysis included 10 studies (150 patients) treated with cabergoline 0.3 to 7 mg/wk for an average of 10.8 months. Responders took cabergoline at a mean dosage of 2.5 ± 1.4 mg/wk for an average of 15 months. Normal IGF-1 level was achieved by 34% and GH level less than 2.5 ng/mL by 48% of patients.[56] In the largest prospective study from 1998, IGF-1 level less than 300 ng/mL was attained by 39%, GH less than 2 ng/mL by 46%, and tumor shrinkage greater than 50% by 24% of patients.[51] In later studies defining remission by IGF-1 normalization and GH thresholds of 0.5 to 2.5 ng/mL, cabergoline achieved IGF-1 control in 11% to 57% and GH control in 14% to 46% of patients.[50–52,54] Both IGF-1 and GH criteria were met in 14% to 36% of patients. Escape from cabergoline effect affected 37% of patients at 12 months[52] and 30 to 75% of patients at 16 to 18 months.[52,55] No tumor shrinkage was seen in 1 study at 6 months,[52] whereas another indicated that 24% of patients had greater than 50% tumor reduction during follow-up up to 40 months.[51]

Predictors of response were hyperprolactinemia, prolactin cosecretion,[51,55] and lower pretreatment IGF-1 levels.[51] In the meta-analysis, 50% of patients with baseline IGF-1 levels less than 150% more than the upper normal limit (UNL) achieved normal IGF-1 versus 30% with higher IGF-1 levels. Longer treatment duration and higher baseline prolactin levels were also predictors of response.

In summary, a trial of cabergoline monotherapy is reasonable in patients with mildly increased IGF-1 levels. Higher doses might be necessary compared with prolactinomas and escape can occur.

Cabergoline/Somatostatin Receptor Ligand Combination

The Endocrine Society guidelines suggest adding cabergoline or pegvisomant in patients with inadequate response to SRL postoperatively.[47]

In a meta-analysis of 5 studies with cabergoline/SRL combination (3 prospective, 2 retrospective, 77 patients), 70% of patients had prior surgery and 29% radiation. Patients were initially treated with SRLs, with subsequent cabergoline addition. Most patients achieved normal IGF-1 levels on cabergoline/SRL, with a 30% decrease from baseline for IGF-1 and 19% for GH. There was a 22% reduction in IGF-1 levels after cabergoline addition. Lower baseline IGF-1 level was predictive of response, whereas baseline prolactin level, length of treatment, and cabergoline dose were not. Similarly, GH reduction was related to baseline GH concentration and not to cabergoline dose or treatment duration.[56]

Since 2011, several studies including 10 to 82 patients reported effects of cabergoline (1–3.5 mg/wk) added onto SRL for 6 to 18 months. IGF-1 normalization occurred in 30% to 50% of patients, with 1 study showing GH less than 2.5 ng/mL in 46% of patients.[57] Two studies linked IGF-1 normalization to baseline IGF-1 levels (IGF-1 ≤ 2.2 more than UNL),[57,58] and 2 did not.[55,59] Three studies indicated lower pretreatment GH level as a predictor of response.[55,57,58]

In summary, cabergoline/SRL combination therapy seems synergistic in up to 50% of patients, and lower pretreatment IGF-1 and GH levels seem to predict the response.

Table 2
Studies evaluating cabergoline monotherapy in acromegaly

First Author, Year	Design	Patients	Duration (mo)	Regimen (mg/wk)	Prior Surgery or Radiation	Imaging	Definition of Response	Outcomes (% Responders)	Tolerance (N)
Abs et al,[51] 1998	Prospective	64	3–40	1–3.5	Surgery: 32 Radiation: 9	Macro: 25 Micro: 12 No lesion: 27	Good: <300 ng/mL for IGF-1 <2 ng/mL for GH Moderate: 300–450 ng/mL for IGF-I 2–5 ng/mL for GH Poor: >450 ng/mL for IGF-I >5 ng/mL for GH Tumor reduction >50%	Good: 39% IGF-1 46% GH Moderate: 28% IGF1 27% GH Poor: 33% IGF-1 27% GH Tumor reduction 24%	Nausea (2)
Freda et al,[52] 2004	Prospective	14	2–18	1–2	Surgery: 14	Macro: 12 Micro: 2	Normalized IGF-1 GH <0.5 ng/mL Tumor shrinkage (criteria NA)	At 24 wk: 57% IGF-1 14.3% GH Long-term: 21% IGF-1 No tumor shrinkage	Mood changes (2) Constipation (1) Headache (1) Hyperglycemia (1)
Higham et al,[53] 2012	Prospective	24	4.5	1–3.5	Surgery: 22	Macro: 15 Micro: 6 NA: 3	Normalized IGF-1	11%	Transaminitis (1)

Howlett et al,[54] 2013	Retrospective	355 treatment courses	NA	0.5–28	Surgery: number NA RT: number NA	NA	Normalized IGF-1 and GH ≤ 2 ng/mL	36%	NA
Vandeva et al,[50] 2015	Retrospective	70	Remission: 53.5 (7–119) Nonremission: 33.0 (5–144)	1–3	Surgery: 70 Radiation: 26	NA	Normalized IGF-1 and before 1999: GH<2.5 ng/mL 1999–2011: random GH <2.5 ng/mL or nadir GH <1 ng/mL 2011–2015: random GH <1 ng/mL or nadir GH <0.4 ng/mL	31.4%	NA
Kasuki et al,[55] 2018	Retrospective	28	14 (3–124)	1–3.5	Surgery: 23 Radiation: 3	Macro: 20 Micro/no lesion: 8	Normalized IGF1 and GH <1 ng/mL	Short term (3–6 mo): 21% Long term (>9 mo): 18%	Nausea/dizziness (1) Valvulopathy (0)

Abbreviations: IGF-1, insulin-like growth factor 1; NA, not available.
Data from Refs.[50–55]

Cabergoline and Pegvisomant Combination

A prospective study assessed 24 patients at 5 centers in an 18-week up-titration cabergoline phase, followed by adding pegvisomant (10 mg/d) until week 30, when cabergoline was stopped and pegvisomant was continued for 12 additional weeks. Most patients were taking cabergoline 3.5 mg/wk by week 12, and only 11% of patients achieved normal IGF-1 levels. After 12 weeks of combination therapy, 68% had normal IGF-1 levels. After cabergoline withdrawal, only 24% maintained normal IGF-1 on pegvisomant. The investigators concluded that cabergoline/pegvisomant combination was more effective than either treatment alone; however, the pegvisomant was not up-titrated.[53]

A retrospective cross-sectional study examined 14 patients resistant to SRL, of whom 13 had previously undergone surgery. They were switched to pegvisomant monotherapy (10–30 mg/d) for 40 ± 26 months. Cabergoline (1–3 mg/wk) was added for persistently increased IGF-1 level after greater than 6 months of pegvisomant monotherapy. Combination cabergoline/pegvisomant resulted in IGF-1 level normalization in 28% and IGF-1 improvement in 64% of patients. Predictors of response included baseline IGF-1 levels less than 160% of UNL, female gender, lower body weight, and higher prolactin levels. Baseline and follow-up echocardiograms in 12 cases were normal in 8 and unchanged in 4 patients.[60]

In summary, cabergoline/pegvisomant combination seems more effective than monotherapy and allows smaller drug doses. Prospective studies with larger sample sizes and standardized up-titration protocols are needed.

DOPAMINE AGONISTS FOR CUSHING DISEASE

The first-line treatment of Cushing disease (CD) is surgery, with remission rates of 65% to 90%; however, recurrence affects approximately 30% of patients. Management of persistent or recurrent hypercortisolism is challenging and entails pituitary reoperation, radiation, bilateral adrenalectomy, or medical treatment (steroidogenesis inhibitors, glucocorticoid receptor antagonists, and tumor-directed therapy).[61] The only approved tumor-targeting therapy is pasireotide, which normalizes the urine free cortisol (UFC) in a third and causes hyperglycemia in most patients.

A study in 16 corticotroph adenomas indicated that 68.7% were DR2 positive by in situ hybridization, although the correlation with immunohistochemistry was poor.[2] Another study in 20 corticotroph adenomas identified D2R in 75% of tumors by immunohistochemistry and 83% by reverse transcription polymerase chain reaction (PCR). DR2 expression correlated with the in vitro adrenocorticotropic hormone (ACTH) secretion inhibition in the cultured adenoma cells, and with the in vivo biochemical response to cabergoline.[3]

Bromocriptine Monotherapy

In the 1980s, 6 studies (49 patients) investigated bromocriptine therapy for 1 to 36 months in CD.[62] UFC decreased in 23% to 66%, and plasma ACTH level in 33% to 80% of patients.[62] One study showed no change in UFC or ACTH levels.[62]

Cabergoline Monotherapy

More recent studies investigated the biochemical response to cabergoline (**Table 3**).[3,63–70] Short-term (<7 months) analyses indicated UFC normalization in 35% to 39%, and partial UFC response in 10% to 40% of patients. Long-term (>12 months) UFC normalization occurred in 23% to 40% of patients.[63,64,70] One study did not find any changes in median UFC, salivary cortisol, or ACTH levels; however,

Table 3
Studies evaluating the role of cabergoline in Cushing disease

First Author, Year	Design	N	Duration (mo)	Regimen	Prior Surgery or Radiation	Imaging	Definition of Response	Outcomes (% Responders)	Tolerance (N)
Pivonello et al,[3] 2004	Prospective	10	3	CAB 1–3 mg/wk	Surgery	2 macro 13 micro 5 no lesion	UFC: • Full response: normalized • Partial response: ≥50% reduction • Resistant: <50% reduction	Full response: 40% Partial response: 20% Resistant: 40%	NA
Pivonello et al,[63] 2009	Prospective	20	3–24	CAB 1–7 mg/wk	Surgery	5 macro 12 micro 3 no lesion	UFC: • Full response: normalized • Partial response: ≥25% reduction • Resistant: <25% reduction Tumor shrinkage: >25% shrinkage	Short term (3 mo): • Full response: 35% • Partial response: 40% • Resistant: 25% Long term (24 mo): • Full response 40% Tumor shrinkage: 20%	Hypotension, asthenia (2) No valve issues by echo

(continued on next page)

Table 3
(continued)

First Author, Year	Design	N	Duration (mo)	Regimen	Prior Surgery or Radiation	Imaging	Definition of Response	Outcomes (% Responders)	Tolerance (N)
Godbout et al,[64] 2010	Retrospective	30	1–60	CAB 0.5–4 mg/wk	Surgery: 27 Radiation: 1	4 macro 21 micro 5 no lesion	UFC • Full response: normalized • Partial response: 100%–125% of ULN • Resistant: ≥125% of ULN	Short-term response (3–6 mo): • Full response: 36.6% • Partial response: 13.3% Resistant: 50.1% Long-term response: • 82% of short-term full responders • 0% of partial responders	No major AE No valve issues by echo (8)
Vilar et al,[65] 2010	Prospective	12	6 (CAB mono)	CAB 2–3 mg/wk CAB (2–3 mg/wk) + KET (200–400 mg/d)	Surgery	0 macro 6 micro 6 no lesion	UFC • Full response: normalized • Partial response: ≥25% reduction • Resistant: <25% reduction	CAB monotherapy (12 patients): • Full response: 3 (25%) • Partial response: 6 (50%) • Resistant: 3 (25%) CAB + KET (9 patients): • Full response: 6 (66.7%) • Partial response: 3 (33.3%)	No major AE No valve issues by echo

Study	Design	N		Treatment/Dose	Surgery/Radiation	Tumor	Criteria	Response	AE
Lila et al,[66] 2010	Prospective	18[a]	5–12	CAB 1–5 mg/wk	Surgery: 18 Radiation: 6	6 macro 3 micro 11 no lesion	Full response: MNSC <5 μg/dL or LDSC <1.8 μg/dL Partial response: >25% reduction in MNSC or >25% reduction of LDSC Resistant: none of the criteria met	Full response: 5 out of 18 (28%) Partial response: 2 out of 18 (11%) by MNSC, 3 out of 18 (16.7%) by LDSC Resistant: 8 (14.3%)	NA
Feelders et al,[67] 2010	Prospective	17	2.7	PAS (100–250 μg BID) PAS + CAB (2–6 mg/wk) PAS + CAB + KET (600 mg/d)	NA	NA	Full response: normalized UFC	Pasireotide: 29% Pasireotide + CAB: 24% Pasireotide + CAB + KET: 35%	NA
Barbot et al,[68] 2014	Prospective	14	6 (CAB mono)	CAB: 2–3 mg/wk KET: 600 mg/d	Surgery: 10	1 macro 6 micro 5 no lesion 2 indeterminate	Full response: UFC or MNSC normalization Partial response: >30% reduction of UFC Tumor shrinkage (10 patients had repeated MRI at end of treatment)	CAB: Full response 2 out of 6 (33%) Partial response 1 out of 6 (16.7%) KET: Full response 5 out of 8 (62.5%) Partial response 3 out of 8 (37.5%) CAB + KET: normalized UFC in 79% No tumor shrinkage	No major AE No valve issues by echo (8)

(continued on next page)

Table 3
(continued)

First Author, Year	Design	N	Duration (mo)	Regimen	Prior Surgery or Radiation	Imaging	Definition of Response	Outcomes (% Responders)	Tolerance (N)
Burman et al,[69] 2016	Prospective	20	1.5	CAB 2.5-5 mg/wk (fixed titration)	Surgery: 1	3 macro 13 micro 4 no lesion	Full response: >50% reduction UFC	No response	Visual hallucinations (1) Nausea/ constipation (1) Fatigue (1)
Ferriere et al,[70] 2017	Retrospective	53	7 (1-105) median	CAB 0.5-6 mg/wk	Surgery: 44	17 macro 23 micro 11 no lesion	UFC • Full response: normalized • Partial response: >50% reduction	Full response 40% Partial response 7% Resistant 53%	Grade 2 aortic insufficiency by echo (1); no baseline echocardiogram

Abbreviations: AE, adverse events; CAB, cabergoline; echo, echocardiogram; KET, ketoconazole; LDSC, low-dose dexamethasone suppression cortisol; MNSC, midnight salivary cortisol; mono, monotherapy; PAS, pasireotide; ULN, upper limit of normal.
[a] Twenty patients but 2 excluded because response attributed to radiotherapy.
Data from Refs.[3,63–70]

treatment course was only 6 weeks and patients did not have prior pituitary surgery.[69] Treatment escape was noted in 4 studies after 0.5 to 5 years in 18% to 43% of full responders and 25% to 100% of partial responders.[63,64,66,70]

Predictors of biochemical response included baseline hyperprolactinemia,[63] lower serum cortisol levels,[66] and lower UFC level.[68] However, the numbers of patients treated in each study were small, and findings were not substantiated across the literature. Prior radiation was associated with improved response in 1 study.[66]

Some studies showed improvement in hypertension,[63,66,67,70] hyperglycemia,[63,70] and obesity.[63,67,70]

Cabergoline/Ketoconazole Combination

Three studies, 2 prospective and 1 retrospective, reported UFC normalization in 56% to 79% of patients,[65,68,70] a higher response rate than with either therapy alone.[65,68] Dosages ranged from 1 to 3 mg/wk for cabergoline and 200 to 1200 mg/d for ketoconazole.

Cabergoline/Pasireotide/Ketoconazole Combination

In a prospective study with a progressive escalation protocol, patients initially received pasireotide alone, with UFC normalization in 29%. Cabergoline addition achieved control in 24% more patients. Ketoconazole addition achieved control in 35%, with 88% overall response.[67]

In summary, the data on bromocriptine are insufficient to support its use in CD. Cabergoline was associated with improved biochemical parameters of hypercortisolism in up to 40% of patients as monotherapy and up to 80% in combination with ketoconazole and pasireotide. Larger prospective studies are needed to confirm its efficacy and safety.

DOPAMINE AGONISTS FOR NONFUNCTIONING PITUITARY ADENOMAS

NFPAs are the second most common type of pituitary adenomas treated primarily by surgery. Complete tumor resection is achieved in 40% to 90% of cases. Strategies for management of the residual or recurrent tumor include observation, reoperation, and radiation. There is currently no consensus on pharmacologic therapy for NFPA. The lack of biochemical markers makes evaluation of medical treatment of NFPA difficult.

Studies examining the presence of the D2R in NFPAs yielded variable results. In a study of 20 NFPA and 5 normal pituitary samples, DR2 was expressed by PCR and immunohistochemistry in all.[71] A study of 198 adenomas found high D2R messenger RNA expression in 60% of samples, and much lower somatostatin receptor expression (<8%).[4] Studies investigating DR expression in patients treated with DAs did not indicate an association with clinical response.[71,72]

The early studies on clinical effect of DAs on NFPA used bromocriptine,[73–79] and most later studies cabergoline[3,71,72,80,81] **(Table 4)**. Three studies evaluated the effect of quinagolide.[82–84] The primary end points consisted of decrease in tumor size for most and progression-free survival for a few studies. Only 3 studies had control groups, and 1 was randomized.

Most bromocriptine studies did not show reduction in tumor size.[74,75,77] Notably, bromocriptine was used as primary therapy before surgery. One study showed a favorable effect of bromocriptine in dosages of 15 to 60 mg/d; however, most patients had mild increases of prolactin level and half had prior radiation.[73]

Quinagolide was used in 3 studies and largely showed no effect.[82–84]

Cabergoline studies included 13 to 79 patients, most having had prior surgery. Tumor shrinkage by greater than 25% was encountered in 28% to 67% of patients.[71]

Table 4
Studies evaluating the use of dopamine agonists in nonfunctional pituitary adenomas

First Author, Year	Design	Control Group	Treated Patients	Medical Treatment	Duration (mo)	Imaging (% Macro)	Prior Treatment	Tumor Changes (Number of Patients)
Wollesen et al,[73] 1982	Prospective	—	11	BCR 15–60 mg/d	2–33	100	Surgery 8 Radiation 6	>25% reduction: 6 18%–23% reduction: 3 12%–16% growth: 2
Barrow et al,[74] 1984	Prospective	—	4	BCR 7.5 mg/d	1.5	100	No	No change
Grossman et al,[75] 1985	Prospective	—	13	BCR 5–30 mg/d MES 2–4 mg/d PER 0.15 mg/d	3–36	100	Surgery 2	Reduction: 1[a] No change: 12
Zarate et al,[76] 1985	Prospective	—	7	BCR 15–22.5 mg/d	0.5–5.3	100	No	No change
Verde et al,[77] 1985	Prospective	—	20	BCR 7.5–20 mg/d	1–32	100	Surgery 8 Radiation 6	Reduction: 1 No change: 19
Bevan et al,[78] 1987	Prospective	—	7	BCR 7.5–40 mg/d	0.75–12	100	No	No change
Van Schaardenburg et al,[79] 1989	Prospective	—	25	BCR 5–22.5 mg/d	18 mean (1–73)	NA	Surgery 10 Radiation 8	Reduction: 4 No change: 20 Growth 1
Kwekkeboom et al,[82] 1992	Prospective	—	5	QUI 300 µg/d	12–18	100	No	Reduction: 1 Stable: 4
Ferone et al,[83] 1998	Prospective	—	6	QUI 600 µg/d	6–12	100	Surgery 6	>25% reduction: 2 No change: 4
Nobels et al,[84] 2000	Prospective	—	10	QUI 300 µg/d	57 median (36–93)	100	No	Short term (12 mo): >10% reduction: 3 No change: 3 Growth: 4 Long term (<92 mo): >10% reduction: 2 No change: 2 Growth: 6

Study	Design			Drug/dose	Duration	%	Surgery	Outcomes
Lohmann et al,[80] 2001	Prospective	—	13	CAB 1 mg/wk	12	100	Surgery 12	10%–20% reduction: 7 No change: 5 Growth: 1
Pivonello et al,[3] 2004	Prospective	—	9	CAB 3 mg/wk	12	100	Surgery: 9	>25% reduction: 5 4%–9% growth: 3 50% growth: 1
Garcia et al,[81] 2013	Prospective	—	19	CAB 2 mg/wk	6	100	Surgery: 11	>25% reduction: 6 10%–25% reduction: 3 No change: 6 Growth: 4
Vieira Neto et al,[71] 2015	Prospective	11	9	CAB 3 mg/wk	6	100	Surgery: 9	>25% reduction: 6 10%–25% reduction: 1 No change 2
Greenman et al,[85] 2016	Historical cohort	60	79 PT 55 RT 24	BCR 2.5–10 mg daily CAB 0.5–3.5 mg/wk	PT: 55 mean ± 39 RT: 40 mean ± 40	PT: 88 RT: 75 Control: 63.6	Surgery: 79	PT vs control: >2 mm diameter reduction: 21 vs 0 No change: 27 vs 28 Growth: 7 vs 32 RT vs control: >2 mm diameter reduction: 7 vs 0 No change: 7 vs 28 Growth: 10 vs 32
Batista et al,[72] 2019	Randomized clinical trial	57	59	CAB 3.5 mg/wk	22 mean ± 4.3	Study: 88 Control: 93	Surgery: 59	CAB vs control: ≥25% reduction: 17 vs 6 <25% reduction: 39 vs 42 ≥25% growth: 3 vs 9

Abbreviations: BCR, bromocriptine; MES, mesulergine; PER, pergolide; PT, preventive treatment group (patients with residual tumor detection on MRI); QUI, quinagolide; RT, remedial treatment group (patients with tumor growth detected on MRI).

a Attributed to infarction and not BCR.

Data from Refs.[3,71–85]

A historical cohort analysis examined 79 patients taking bromocriptine or cabergoline and 60 controls.[85] Patients treated with DAs had a higher 15-year progression-free survival rate than controls.

A randomized clinical trial included 59 patients receiving cabergoline 3.5 mg/wk for 2 years and 57 controls managed conservatively postsurgery.[72] In the DA-treatment group, tumor shrinkage occurred in 28.8% (vs 10.5% control), and tumor enlargement in 5% (vs 15.8% control). Progression-free survival rates were higher for the DA group than control. Serial echocardiographic evaluations did not find significant valvular changes.

In summary, there is no sufficient evidence to support bromocriptine or quinagolide treatment in NFPA. The results of the cabergoline studies are variable, with decreased size of the postoperative tumor residual in 28% to 67%. Larger prospective controlled studies are needed to establish its efficacy.

DISCLOSURE

The authors have nothing to disclose.

REFERENCES

1. Liu X, Tang C, Wen G, et al. The mechanism and pathways of dopamine and dopamine agonists in prolactinomas. Front Endocrinol (Lausanne) 2018;9:768.
2. Stefaneanu L, Kovacs K, Horvath E, et al. Dopamine D2 receptor gene expression in human adenohypophysial adenomas. Endocrine 2001;14(3):329–36.
3. Pivonello R, Ferone D, de Herder WW, et al. Dopamine receptor expression and function in corticotroph pituitary tumors. J Clin Endocrinol Metab 2004;89(5): 2452–62.
4. Gabalec F, Drastikova M, Cesak T, et al. Dopamine 2 and somatostatin 1-5 receptors coexpression in clinically non-functioning pituitary adenomas. Physiol Res 2015;64(3):369–77.
5. Ananthakrishnan S. The dark side to dopamine agonist therapy in prolactinoma management. Endocr Pract 2017. https://doi.org/10.4158/EP161709.CO.
6. Ioachimescu AG, Fleseriu M, Hoffman AR, et al. Psychological effects of dopamine agonist treatment in patients with hyperprolactinemia and prolactin-secreting adenomas. Eur J Endocrinol 2019;180(1):31–40.
7. Melmed S, Casanueva FF, Hoffman AR, et al. Diagnosis and treatment of hyperprolactinemia: an Endocrine Society clinical practice guideline. J Clin Endocrinol Metab 2011;96(2):273–88.
8. Rogers A, Karavitaki N, Wass JA. Diagnosis and management of prolactinomas and non-functioning pituitary adenomas. BMJ 2014;349:g5390.
9. Nassiri F, Cusimano MD, Scheithauer BW, et al. Prolactinomas: diagnosis and treatment. Expert Rev Endocrinol Metab 2012;7(2):233–41.
10. Weiss MH, Teal J, Gott P, et al. Natural history of microprolactinomas: six-year follow-up. Neurosurgery 1983;12(2):180–3.
11. Sisam DA, Sheehan JP, Sheeler LR. The natural history of untreated microprolactinomas. Fertil Steril 1987;48(1):67–71.
12. Auriemma RS, Galdiero M, Vitale P, et al. Effect of chronic cabergoline treatment and testosterone replacement on metabolism in male patients with prolactinomas. Neuroendocrinology 2015;101(1):66–81.
13. Colao A, Vitale G, Cappabianca P, et al. Outcome of cabergoline treatment in men with prolactinoma: effects of a 24-month treatment on prolactin levels, tumor

mass, recovery of pituitary function, and semen analysis. J Clin Endocrinol Metab 2004;89(4):1704–11.

14. Prior JC, Cox TA, Fairholm D, et al. Testosterone-related exacerbation of a prolactin-producing macroadenoma: possible role for estrogen. J Clin Endocrinol Metab 1987;64(2):391–4.

15. Sodi R, Fikri R, Diver M, et al. Testosterone replacement-induced hyperprolacti-naemia: case report and review of the literature. Ann Clin Biochem 2005;42(Pt 2):153–9.

16. Wang AT, Mullan RJ, Lane MA, et al. Treatment of hyperprolactinemia: a system-atic review and meta-analysis. Syst Rev 2012;1:33.

17. McGregor AM, Scanlon MF, Hall R, et al. Effects of bromocriptine on pituitary tumour size. Br Med J 1979;2(6192):700–3.

18. Thorner MO, Martin WH, Rogol AD, et al. Rapid regression of pituitary prolactino-mas during bromocriptine treatment. J Clin Endocrinol Metab 1980;51(3):438–45.

19. Gillam MP, Molitch ME, Lombardi G, et al. Advances in the treatment of prolacti-nomas. Endocr Rev 2006;27(5):485–534.

20. Cho KR, Jo KI, Shin HJ. Bromocriptine therapy for the treatment of invasive pro-lactinoma: the single institute experience. Brain Tumor Res Treat 2013;1(2):71–7.

21. Shimon I, Hirsch D, Tsvetov G, et al. Hyperprolactinemia diagnosis in elderly men: a cohort of 28 patients over 65 years. Endocrine 2019;65(3):656–61.

22. Webster J, Piscitelli G, Polli A, et al. A comparison of cabergoline and bromocrip-tine in the treatment of hyperprolactinemic amenorrhea. Cabergoline Compara-tive Study Group. N Engl J Med 1994;331(14):904–9.

23. dos Santos Nunes V, El Dib R, Boguszewski CL, et al. Cabergoline versus bromo-criptine in the treatment of hyperprolactinemia: a systematic review of random-ized controlled trials and meta-analysis. Pituitary 2011;14(3):259–65.

24. Molitch ME, Elton RL, Blackwell RE, et al. Bromocriptine as primary therapy for prolactin-secreting macroadenomas: results of a prospective multicenter study. J Clin Endocrinol Metab 1985;60(4):698–705.

25. van 't Verlaat JW, Croughs RJ. Withdrawal of bromocriptine after long-term ther-apy for macroprolactinomas; effect on plasma prolactin and tumour size. Clin En-docrinol (Oxf) 1991;34(3):175–8.

26. van 't Verlaat JW, Croughs RJ, Hendriks MJ, et al. Bromocriptine treatment of pro-lactin secreting macroadenomas: a radiological, ophthalmological and endocri-nological study. Acta Endocrinol (Copenh) 1986;112(4):487–93.

27. Biller BM, Molitch ME, Vance ML, et al. Treatment of prolactin-secreting macroa-denomas with the once-weekly dopamine agonist cabergoline. J Clin Endocrinol Metab 1996;81(6):2338–43.

28. Colao A, Di Sarno A, Cappabianca P, et al. Withdrawal of long-term cabergoline therapy for tumoral and nontumoral hyperprolactinemia. N Engl J Med 2003; 349(21):2023–33.

29. Colao A, Di Sarno A, Landi ML, et al. Macroprolactinoma shrinkage during caber-goline treatment is greater in naive patients than in patients pretreated with other dopamine agonists: a prospective study in 110 patients. J Clin Endocrinol Metab 2000;85(6):2247–52.

30. Huang HY, Lin SJ, Zhao WG, et al. Cabergoline versus bromocriptine for the treat-ment of giant prolactinomas: A quantitative and systematic review. Metab Brain Dis 2018;33(3):969–76.

31. Lee Y, Ku CR, Kim EH, et al. Early prediction of long-term response to cabergo-line in patients with macroprolactinomas. Endocrinol Metab (Seoul) 2014;29(3): 280–92.

32. Tirosh A, Benbassat C, Shimon I. Short-term decline in prolactin concentrations can predict future prolactin normalization, tumor shrinkage, and time to remission in men with macroprolactinomas. Endocr Pract 2015;21(11):1240–7.

33. Biswas M, Smith J, Jadon D, et al. Long-term remission following withdrawal of dopamine agonist therapy in subjects with microprolactinomas. Clin Endocrinol (Oxf) 2005;63(1):26–31.

34. Dekkers OM, Lagro J, Burman P, et al. Recurrence of hyperprolactinemia after withdrawal of dopamine agonists: systematic review and meta-analysis. J Clin Endocrinol Metab 2010;95(1):43–51.

35. Kharlip J, Salvatori R, Yenokyan G, et al. Recurrence of hyperprolactinemia after withdrawal of long-term cabergoline therapy. J Clin Endocrinol Metab 2009;94(7): 2428–36.

36. Hu J, Zheng X, Zhang W, et al. Current drug withdrawal strategy in prolactinoma patients treated with cabergoline: a systematic review and meta-analysis. Pituitary 2015;18(5):745–51.

37. Xia MY, Lou XH, Lin SJ, et al. Optimal timing of dopamine agonist withdrawal in patients with hyperprolactinemia: a systematic review and meta-analysis. Endocrine 2018;59(1):50–61.

38. Rutkowski MJ, Aghi MK. Medical versus surgical treatment of prolactinomas: an analysis of treatment outcomes. Expert Rev Endocrinol Metab 2018;13(1):25–33.

39. Roelfsema F, Biermasz NR, Pereira AM. Clinical factors involved in the recurrence of pituitary adenomas after surgical remission: a structured review and meta-analysis. Pituitary 2012;15(1):71–83.

40. Zamanipoor Najafabadi AH, Zandbergen IM, de Vries F, et al. Surgery as a viable alternative first-line treatment for prolactinoma patients. A systematic review and meta-analysis. J Clin Endocrinol Metab 2020;105(3):e32–41.

41. Hamidi O, Van Gompel J, Gruber L, et al. Management and outcomes of giant prolactinoma: a series of 71 patients. Endocr Pract 2019;25(4):340–52.

42. Iglesias P, Arcano K, Berrocal VR, et al. Giant prolactinoma in men: clinical features and therapeutic outcomes. Horm Metab Res 2018;50(11):791–6.

43. Molitch ME. Prolactin and pregnancy. In: Tritos NA, Klibanski A, editors. Prolactin disorders: from basic science to clinical management. Cham (Switzerland): Springer International Publishing; 2019. p. 161–74.

44. Araujo B, Belo S, Carvalho D. Pregnancy and tumor outcomes in women with prolactinoma. Exp Clin Endocrinol Diabetes 2017;125(10):642–8.

45. Hurault-Delarue C, Montastruc JL, Beau AB, et al. Pregnancy outcome in women exposed to dopamine agonists during pregnancy: a pharmacoepidemiology study in EFEMERIS database. Arch Gynecol Obstet 2014;290(2):263–70.

46. Glezer A, Bronstein MD. Prolactinomas, cabergoline, and pregnancy. Endocrine 2014;47(1):64–9.

47. Katznelson L, Laws ER Jr, Melmed S, et al. Acromegaly: an endocrine society clinical practice guideline. J Clin Endocrinol Metab 2014;99(11):3933–51.

48. Neto LV, Machado Ede O, Luque RM, et al. Expression analysis of dopamine receptor subtypes in normal human pituitaries, nonfunctioning pituitary adenomas and somatotropinomas, and the association between dopamine and somatostatin receptors with clinical response to octreotide-LAR in acromegaly. J Clin Endocrinol Metab 2009;94(6):1931–7.

49. Jaffe CA, Barkan AL. Acromegaly. Recognition and treatment. Drugs 1994;47(3): 425–45.

50. Vandeva S, Elenkova A, Natchev E, et al. Treatment outcome results from the Bulgarian Acromegaly Database: adjuvant dopamine agonist therapy is efficient

in less than one fifth of non-irradiated patients. Exp Clin Endocrinol Diabetes 2015;123(1):66–71.

51. Abs R, Verhelst J, Maiter D, et al. Cabergoline in the treatment of acromegaly: a study in 64 patients. J Clin Endocrinol Metab 1998;83(2):374–8.

52. Freda PU, Reyes CM, Nuruzzaman AT, et al. Cabergoline therapy of growth hormone & growth hormone/prolactin secreting pituitary tumors. Pituitary 2004;7(1): 21–30.

53. Higham CE, Atkinson AB, Aylwin S, et al. Effective combination treatment with cabergoline and low-dose pegvisomant in active acromegaly: a prospective clinical trial. J Clin Endocrinol Metab 2012;97(4):1187–93.

54. Howlett TA, Willis D, Walker G, et al. Control of growth hormone and IGF1 in patients with acromegaly in the UK: responses to medical treatment with somatostatin analogues and dopamine agonists. Clin Endocrinol (Oxf) 2013;79(5): 689–99.

55. Kasuki L, Dalmolin MD, Wildemberg LE, et al. Treatment escape reduces the effectiveness of cabergoline during long-term treatment of acromegaly in monotherapy or in association with first-generation somatostatin receptor ligands. Clin Endocrinol (Oxf) 2018;88(6):889–95.

56. Sandret L, Maison P, Chanson P. Place of cabergoline in acromegaly: a meta-analysis. J Clin Endocrinol Metab 2011;96(5):1327–35.

57. Vilar L, Azevedo MF, Naves LA, et al. Role of the addition of cabergoline to the management of acromegalic patients resistant to longterm treatment with octreotide LAR. Pituitary 2011;14(2):148–56.

58. Mattar P, Alves Martins MR, Abucham J. Short- and long-term efficacy of combined cabergoline and octreotide treatment in controlling igf-I levels in acromegaly. Neuroendocrinology 2010;92(2):120–7.

59. Suda K, Inoshita N, Iguchi G, et al. Efficacy of combined octreotide and cabergoline treatment in patients with acromegaly: a retrospective clinical study and review of the literature. Endocr J 2013;60(4):507–15.

60. Bernabeu I, Alvarez-Escola C, Paniagua AE, et al. Pegvisomant and cabergoline combination therapy in acromegaly. Pituitary 2013;16(1):101–8.

61. Langlois F, Chu J, Fleseriu M. Pituitary-directed therapies for cushing's disease. Front Endocrinol (Lausanne) 2018;9:164.

62. Cooper O, Greenman Y. Dopamine agonists for pituitary adenomas. Front Endocrinol (Lausanne) 2018;9:469.

63. Pivonello R, De Martino MC, Cappabianca P, et al. The medical treatment of Cushing's disease: effectiveness of chronic treatment with the dopamine agonist cabergoline in patients unsuccessfully treated by surgery. J Clin Endocrinol Metab 2009;94(1):223–30.

64. Godbout A, Manavela M, Danilowicz K, et al. Cabergoline monotherapy in the long-term treatment of Cushing's disease. Eur J Endocrinol 2010;163(5):709–16.

65. Vilar L, Naves LA, Azevedo MF, et al. Effectiveness of cabergoline in monotherapy and combined with ketoconazole in the management of Cushing's disease. Pituitary 2010;13(2):123–9.

66. Lila AR, Gopal RA, Acharya SV, et al. Efficacy of cabergoline in uncured (persistent or recurrent) Cushing disease after pituitary surgical treatment with or without radiotherapy. Endocr Pract 2010;16(6):968–76.

67. Feelders RA, de Bruin C, Pereira AM, et al. Pasireotide alone or with cabergoline and ketoconazole in Cushing's disease. N Engl J Med 2010;362(19):1846–8.

68. Barbot M, Albiger N, Ceccato F, et al. Combination therapy for Cushing's disease: effectiveness of two schedules of treatment: should we start with cabergoline or ketoconazole? Pituitary 2014;17(2):109–17.
69. Burman P, Eden-Engstrom B, Ekman B, et al. Limited value of cabergoline in Cushing's disease: a prospective study of a 6-week treatment in 20 patients. Eur J Endocrinol 2016;174(1):17–24.
70. Ferriere A, Cortet C, Chanson P, et al. Cabergoline for Cushing's disease: a large retrospective multicenter study. Eur J Endocrinol 2017;176(3):305–14.
71. Vieira Neto L, Wildemberg LE, Moraes AB, et al. Dopamine receptor subtype 2 expression profile in nonfunctioning pituitary adenomas and in vivo response to cabergoline therapy. Clin Endocrinol (Oxf) 2015;82(5):739–46.
72. Batista RL, Musolino NRC, Cescato VAS, et al. Cabergoline in the management of residual nonfunctioning pituitary adenoma: a single-center, open-label, 2-year randomized clinical trial. Am J Clin Oncol 2019;42(2):221–7.
73. Wollesen F, Andersen T, Karle A. Size reduction of extrasellar pituitary tumors during bromocriptine treatment. Ann Intern Med 1982;96(3):281–6.
74. Barrow DL, Tindall GT, Kovacs K, et al. Clinical and pathological effects of bromocriptine on prolactin-secreting and other pituitary tumors. J Neurosurg 1984; 60(1):1–7.
75. Grossman A, Ross R, Charlesworth M, et al. The effect of dopamine agonist therapy on large functionless pituitary tumours. Clin Endocrinol (Oxf) 1985;22(5): 679–86.
76. Zarate A, Moran C, Kleriga E, et al. Bromocriptine therapy as pre-operative adjunct of non-functional pituitary macroadenomas. Acta Endocrinol (Copenh) 1985;108(4):445–50.
77. Verde G, Oppizzi G, Chiodini PG, et al. Effect of chronic bromocriptine administration on tumor size in patients with "nonsecreting" pituitary adenomas. J Endocrinol Invest 1985;8(2):113–5.
78. Bevan JS, Adams CB, Burke CW, et al. Factors in the outcome of transsphenoidal surgery for prolactinoma and non-functioning pituitary tumour, including preoperative bromocriptine therapy. Clin Endocrinol (Oxf) 1987;26(5):541–56.
79. van Schaardenburg D, Roelfsema F, van Seters AP, et al. Bromocriptine therapy for non-functioning pituitary adenoma. Clin Endocrinol (Oxf) 1989;30(5):475–84.
80. Lohmann T, Trantakis C, Biesold M, et al. Minor tumour shrinkage in nonfunctioning pituitary adenomas by long-term treatment with the dopamine agonist cabergoline. Pituitary 2001;4(3):173–8.
81. Garcia EC, Naves LA, Silva AO, et al. Short-term treatment with cabergoline can lead to tumor shrinkage in patients with nonfunctioning pituitary adenomas. Pituitary 2013;16(2):189–94.
82. Kwekkeboom DJ, Lamberts SW. Long-term treatment with the dopamine agonist CV 205-502 of patients with a clinically non-functioning, gonadotroph, or alpha-subunit secreting pituitary adenoma. Clin Endocrinol (Oxf) 1992;36(2):171–6.
83. Ferone D, Lastoria S, Colao A, et al. Correlation of scintigraphic results using 123I-methoxybenzamide with hormone levels and tumor size response to quinagolide in patients with pituitary adenomas. J Clin Endocrinol Metab 1998;83(1): 248–52.
84. Nobels FR, de Herder WW, van den Brink WM, et al. Long-term treatment with the dopamine agonist quinagolide of patients with clinically non-functioning pituitary adenoma. Eur J Endocrinol 2000;143(5):615–21.
85. Greenman Y, Cooper O, Yaish I, et al. Treatment of clinically nonfunctioning pituitary adenomas with dopamine agonists. Eur J Endocrinol 2016;175(1):63–72.

Acromegaly
Update on Management and Long-Term Morbidities

Leandro Kasuki, MD, PhD[a,b,c], Ximene Antunes, MD, MSc[a],
Elisa Baranski Lamback, MD[a], Mônica R. Gadelha, MD, PhD[a,b,d],*

KEYWORDS

• Acromegaly • Somatotropinoma • Pituitary adenoma • Comorbidities • Treatment

KEY POINTS

• Surgery is first-line treatment for most patients but approximately 50% will need adjuvant medical treatment, with radiotherapy reserved for aggressive tumors resistant to surgical and medical treatment.

• Cardiovascular and cerebrovascular diseases, metabolic abnormalities, respiratory disease, and osteoarthropathy are common long-term comorbidities in patients with acromegaly.

• Growth hormone and insulinlike growth factor type I normalization improves cardiovascular, respiratory, and metabolic comorbidities in patients with acromegaly.

INTRODUCTION

Acromegaly is a systemic disease that is, the result of excessive growth hormone (GH) and insulin-like growth factor type I (IGF-I) and is associated with long-term comorbidities.[1] Acromegaly treatment and knowledge of its comorbidities have evolved significantly in the past decades and are addressed in this review.

UPDATE ON MANAGEMENT

Acromegaly treatment should be done in reference centers by a multidisciplinary team.[2] Goals of treatment are to normalize GH and IGF-I, to control tumor mass

[a] Endocrinology Division, Neuroendocrinology Research Center, Medical School and Hospital Universitário Clementino Fraga Filho – Universidade Federal do Rio de Janeiro, Rua Professor Rodolpho Paulo Rocco, 255, 9° andar – Setor 9, Ilha do Fundão, Rio de Janeiro 21941-913, Brazil; [b] Neuroendocrinology Division, Instituto Estadual do Cérebro Paulo Niemeyer, 156th Resende Street, Rio de Janeiro, RJ, Brazil; [c] Endocrinology Division, Hospital Federal de Bonsucesso, Rio de Janeiro, Brazil; [d] Neuropathology and Molecular Genetics Laboratory, Instituto Estadual do Cérebro Paulo Niemeyer, Rio de Janeiro, Brazil
* Corresponding author. Centro de Pesquisa em Neuroendocrinologia, Hospital Universitário Clementino Fraga Filho, Rua Professor Rodolpho Paulo Rocco, 255, 9° andar – Setor 9, Ilha do Fundão, Rio de Janeiro 21941-913, Brazil.
E-mail address: mgadelha@hucff.ufrj.br

Endocrinol Metab Clin N Am 49 (2020) 475–486
https://doi.org/10.1016/j.ecl.2020.05.007
0889-8529/20/© 2020 Elsevier Inc. All rights reserved.

and to preserve pituitary function, with consequent normalization of mortality rates.[3] Some instruments help in monitoring treatment and can also be used to assess disease status.[4,5]

There are currently 3 treatment modalities: surgery, medical treatment, and radiotherapy.[6]

Surgery

Surgery is the mainstay of treatment for most patients, with exception of those whose tumor is unresectable (almost all tumor inside the cavernous sinus), who refuse surgery, or have high surgical risk.[3] Transsphenoidal surgery is safe and leads to disease remission (defined as normal age-matched IGF-I and random GH <1.0 µg/L or nadir GH <0.4 on oral glucose tolerance test) in approximately 50% of cases when performed by experienced neurosurgeons.[3,7,8] Although endoscopic surgery may allow a better visualization of sellar region, until now there are no conclusive data showing superiority over microscopic approach, with main determinants of surgical cure being neurosurgeon experience and cavernous sinus invasion.[3,8,9]

Medical Treatment

First-generation somatostatin receptor ligands (SRLs), octreotide and lanreotide, are considered first-line medical therapy for patients not cured by surgery or for whom surgery cannot be considered.[3] They act mainly by interacting with somatostatin receptor subtype 2 (SST2).[10] Biochemical control is defined by random GH <1.0 µg/L and normal IGF-I for age and is observed in approximately 30% of patients.[11] Partial resistance may be characterized as GH and/or IGF-I reduction greater than 50%, without biochemical control.[8,9]

Three drugs are available for resistant patients and choice should be based on factors like tumor concern, glucose metabolism, patient preference, drug availability, tumor phenotype, presence of comorbidities, presence of headache, and GH and IGF-I.[12,13] The most recent guideline recommends that 3 aspects should be taken into account when choosing the next drug in patients with first-generation SRL-resistant acromegaly: GH and IGF-I, tumor remnant, and glucose status (**Fig. 1**).[6]

Cabergoline (CAB) is a dopamine agonist that binds to dopamine receptor type 2 (DR2) and can be used in monotherapy or in combination with SRL or pegvisomant (PEG).[14–17] More details regarding CAB treatment will be provided in a specific manuscript of this issue.

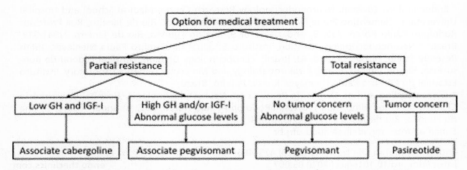

Fig. 1. Medical treatment algorithm for patients resistant to first-generation SRL.

Pasireotide is a second-generation SRL that differs from octreotide and lanreotide due to its higher affinity to SST3 and SST5.[18,19] Two large prospective randomized studies have shown that pasireotide has higher efficacy than first-generation SRL.[20,21]

The first study included 358 drug-naïve patients who were randomized to octreotide long-acting release (OCT-LAR) or pasireotide-LAR treatment.[20] Disease control was obtained in 19% of patients with OCT-LAR and 31% of patients with pasireotide-LAR ($P = .007$).[20]

The second study (PAOLA) included patients resistant to first-generation SRL treatment (n = 198) who were randomized to continue treatment with OCT-LAR (30 mg) or lanreotide autogel (120 mg) or to switch to pasireotide-LAR 40 or 60 mg.[21] After 24 weeks of treatment, disease control was obtained in 20% of patients with pasireotide-LAR 60 mg.[21] Also, tumor volume reduction was observed in 19% and 11% of patients in pasireotide-LAR 40 mg and 60 mg, respectively in comparison with only 2% in first-generation SRL group.[21]

Pasireotide presents a similar safety profile to first-generation SRL, with exception of glucose metabolism, in which a higher incidence and severity of hyperglycemia is observed in comparison with OCT-LAR (67% vs 30% in PAOLA study, respectively), being more common in those patients with abnormal fasting blood glucose previous to treatment.[20–22]

Pegvisomant is a GH receptor antagonist that binds to GH receptor without activating intracellular pathways.[23] Therefore, it does not act in the somatotropinoma but has the higher rates of IGF-I control in acromegaly.[6,24] Pegvisomant can be used as monotherapy or in combination therapy with SRL or CAB.[17,25–28] In the most recent publication of the largest drug database (Acrostudy), including 2090 patients, disease control was obtained in 73% after 10-year treatment period.[28]

Pegvisomant is generally well tolerated with most common side effects being local site injection reactions (pain, lipohypertrophy [3.1%]) and elevated liver enzymes (3% of patients).[28] Tumor size increase is observed in 6.8% of patients, indicating no effect of drug treatment on tumor size.[28] Opposed to SRLs, that have either neutral (first-generation SRL) or deleterious (pasireotide) effect on glucose metabolism, PEG has beneficial effects.[29–31]

Considering all options described previously, the near future of acromegaly treatment is a change to precision medicine, with biomarkers guiding the decision of the right drug to the right patient at the right moment.[32]

Radiotherapy

Radiotherapy is currently the third-line option, being indicated for those patients who present tumor growth despite surgical and medical therapy.[33]

Radiotherapy has a medium to long-term response. Tumor control ranges from 93% to 100% and biochemical control from 47% to 86% at 10 years after radiotherapy.[34,35] Main adverse effect is development of pituitary hormone deficiency, occurring in 44% to 80% of patients after 10 years.[36,37] Other adverse effects are cranial nerve deficit, brain necrosis, cerebrovascular accidents, and secondary brain tumors.[38,39] Rates of complications may be lower with more modern stereotaxic techniques, but follow-up of studies are not long enough to guarantee that frequencies are lower.[33,40]

UPDATE ON LONG-TERM MORBIDITIES
Cardiovascular and Cerebrovascular Disease

Cardiovascular disease is one of the commonest comorbidities in acromegaly.[1] Most GH effects on the heart are mediated by IGF-I.[1] It was previously considered the main cause of death, but recent series have shown that its severity has changed and that it is no longer the main cause of death.[1]

Left ventricular hypertrophy has been reported in up to 70% and 80% of patients based on cardiac MRI (CMRI) and echography studies, respectively.[1,41] Myocardial fibrosis is present in approximately 14% of patients seen on CMRI.[42] Moreover, diastolic dysfunction is described in up to 60% of patients based on echography studies, but is usually mild with no clinical repercussion.[1] Progression to systolic dysfunction is uncommon, being present in fewer than 3% of patients.[43,44]

Arterial hypertension (AH) is one of the most frequent complications and is present from the early stages of disease.[1,45] Its frequency varies from 17% to 23% using 24-hour ambulatory blood pressure monitoring (ABPM) and is overestimated if only clinical measurements are used (frequencies ranging from 32% to 42%).[1] Its pathophysiology has not been fully elucidated, but seems to result from extracellular fluid volume expansion secondary to sodium and water retention in kidney, peripheral vascular resistance increase and sleep apnea syndrome (SAS).[45,46]

In relation to valvular disease, its frequency seems to be increased.[1] Mild to moderate aortic regurgitation was described in 31% of patients with active acromegaly, 18% of patients with controlled acromegaly, and 7% in controls.[47] Mild mitral regurgitation was also increased (present in 26% of patients with active acromegaly and in 7% of controls).[47] Notably, progression of mitral regurgitation was associated with excess GH and IGF-I in a prospective study with 2 years of follow-up.[48]

Other cardiovascular abnormalities do not seem to be increased in patients with acromegaly. Clinically significant or sustained arrhythmias were not shown in patients with active disease with 24-hour Holter monitoring.[49] Coronary heart disease also does not seem to be increased in patients with acromegaly compared with controls, as shown by assessing coronary artery calcium content and observing similar Framingham scores in both groups.[42,50] Myocardial infarction rates are similar in patients with acromegaly compared with the healthy population.[51,52]

In addition, cerebrovascular disease seems to be increased secondary to AH and not acromegaly per se.[51] In a recent study, stroke in patients with acromegaly was similar to the healthy population.[51] However, higher prevalence of AH was observed in patients who suffered stroke compared with controls.[51] The scenario changes in patients submitted to radiotherapy as stroke incidence increases.[53]

An echography and measurement of blood pressure at diagnosis are recommended for all patients with acromegaly based on current guidelines.[1] In patients with AH, 24-hour ABPM might be advisable. In patients with abnormal cardiac rhythm detected at clinical examination, an electrocardiogram should be considered.[1]

Respiratory Disease

Acromegaly is associated with SAS and respiratory insufficiency.[54] Anatomic changes in craniofacial region and upper respiratory tract result from GH/IGF-I excess and are associated with SAS.[54,55] Frequency of SAS is increased in patients with acromegaly (14%–26%) compared with the general population (5%–10%), but is likely underestimated because of low polysomnography screening.[1] In active acromegaly, it has been described in more than 70% of patients.[56] Acromegaly treatment may improve SAS, but biochemical control does not predict complete reversal.[57,58] Prospective studies suggest that 40% of patients with controlled acromegaly have persistent SAS.[1,57]

Assessment of SAS in all patients with acromegaly at diagnosis is recommended, the gold standard for this is polysomnography.[1]

Bone

GH and IGF-I have important roles in bone metabolism, regulating both bone formation and reabsorption.[59] In acromegaly, GH and IGF-I excess increase bone turnover,
leading to skeleton fragility and vertebral fractures (VFs).[60,61] Prevalence of radiological VFs has been reported in up to 60% of patients with acromegaly, much higher than
that in the general population (14%).[59,62] It occurs regardless bone mineral density
(BMD), especially in the thoracic spine and happened early after diagnosis.[63,64] Coex-
isting conditions also contribute to higher risk of VFs (**Box 1**).[59,65]

BMD measurement by dual-energy x-ray absorptiometry is the cornerstone method
currently used to evaluate skeleton fragility in general population. However, in acromegaly, its interpretation has several problems due to specific changes in bone micro-
architecture caused by acromegaly and lack of diagnosis validation in this
population.[59] Furthermore, some studies show increased risk of fractures independent of BMD.[62,66]

Long disease duration and biochemically active disease are also additional factors
that impair bone health in acromegaly.[59] Risk of VFs remains high even when
biochemical control is achieved.[59] Progression of VFs was observed in up to 25%
of patients over 2 to 3 years, even though biochemical control was obtained.[63,64]

There are no data on the effects of anti-osteoporosis drugs in acromegaly, and no
specific therapeutic recommendations for these patients. Current guidelines recommend screening patients for osteoporosis risk factors and imaging studies for all patients regardless of disease status.[3,67] It is recommended to perform radiographic or
vertebral fracture assessment at diagnosis and to repeat imaging every 2 to 3 years
depending on osteoporosis risk factors, kyphosis, and presence of symptoms.[67]

Arthropathy

Acromegaly arthropathy (AA) is a common condition observed in 50% to 70% of patients,[68] which represents twice the frequency in the general population.[43] Shoulder,
knee, and hip are the most frequent affected joints, and pain is the most prominent
symptom.[68,69]

Treatment of acromegaly provides partial reversion of structural alterations like
cartilage hypertrophy and joint thickening.[1] Normalization of joint thickening in shoulder and knee was described in 60% and 90%, respectively, of patients treated for
1 year with SRL.[70]

Currently recommendations for management of AA are similar to primary Osteoar-
thitis (OA), including analgesia and improving mobility.

Metabolic disorders

Glucose

Abnormalities in glucose metabolism are a consequence of insulin resistance (IR),
resulting in hyperglycemia, despite an increased insulin secretion being also a

---

Box 1
Conditions associated with high risk of vertebral fracture in acromegaly

- Diabetes mellitus
- Hypovitaminosis D
- Hyperparathyroidism (in patients with multiple endocrine neoplasia type 1)
- Hypogonadism
- Overreplacement of glucocorticoids

---

consequence of GH excess.[71] GH and IGF-I have different actions on glucose metabolism, which are described in **Fig. 2.**[1] Prevalence of diabetes mellitus (DM) varies in the literature.[71] In large multicenter series, this rate was approximately 30%.[72,73]

Several factors have been associated with abnormalities in glucose metabolism, such as older age, positive family history of DM, higher GH and IGF-I, and disease duration.[72] Severity of DM varies into patients as a result of genetic predisposition, but most patients have mild disease and usually achieve glucose control with diet alone or in combination with metformin.[71] Effects of acromegaly treatment on glucose metabolism vary in different modalities and were previously addressed in this review.[1]

Currently it is recommended to measure glucose profile (fasting glucose and HbA1c) at diagnosis and annually in active disease.[67] Patients with controlled disease have no well-defined timeline screening but it should depend on age, weight, other comorbidities, and type of treatment.[1] Patients who use pasireotide should follow specific recommendations.[22]

Lipid

As previously mentioned (see **Fig. 2**), GH induces increase in serum free fat acids (FFA). This effect in combination with IR increases production of triglycerides (TG) and decrease high-density lipoprotein (HDL). In opposite, IGF-I reduces lipogenesis and increases FFA uptake into hepatocytes and adipose tissue.[1] Hypertriglyceridemia and reduced HDL are the main abnormalities of lipid metabolism.[74]

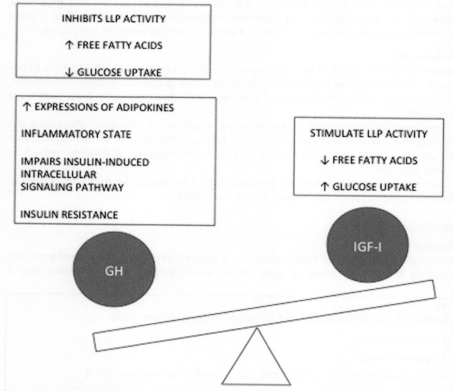

Fig. 2. Counterbalanced effects of GH and IGF-I on glucose and lipid metabolism. LLP, lipoprotein lipase.

The prevalence of hyperlipidemia varies on studies ranging from 13% to 51% depending on the series.[1] Different acromegaly treatment modalities have similar results in improving TG and HDL.[1]

Cancer

Recent studies suggested that neoplasia is currently the main cause of death in patients with acromegaly[75,76]; however, the direct link between acromegaly and cancer risk is still debatable.[77,78] In past decades, better treatment of acromegaly and better control of comorbidities provided an increase in life expectancy.[1] As cancer risk is age-dependent, it is still not clear if it is only a consequence of this improvement on treatment or if a direct relationship between acromegaly and cancer exists.[77,78]

That controversy can be illustrated by conflict results of recent studies: on a Danish nationwide study (n = 529), cancer incidence rate was only slightly elevated in comparison with national rates and cancer-specific mortality was not higher.[79] On the other hand, a recent review of prevalence and incidence of cancer in acromegaly, including 17 published series, demonstrated a significantly higher prevalence of cancer than in the global population (10.8% vs 0.59%, respectively).[80] Heterogeneity of studies and control population and different methodology could explain part of the different results.

From all types of neoplasia, colon cancer has more data in the literature showing a higher risk in patients with acromegaly.[79] Increased risk of colonic polyposis is well-defined.[1] Prevalence of colonic polyps is reported from 27% to 55%.[1] Incidence of colon cancer is 2.6 that of the general population.[79]

Current guidelines recommend at least 1 colonoscopy at diagnosis to screen for colon cancer and to repeat the examination depending on findings of initial colonoscopy and disease activity.[3,67]

Nodular thyroid disease is increased as a result of GH and IGF-I proliferation effects on thyroid cells.[1] Prevalence of nodular goiter is up to 75% in ultrasound studies but it is still controversial if there is higher risk of thyroid malignancy in acromegaly.[80–82] Nowadays, it is recommended to perform ultrasound only in presence of palpable thyroid nodule as recommended to the general population.[3]

Regarding other cancers, there are no conclusive data about increased risk, and screening should follow recommendations for the general population.[67,80]

SUMMARY

Acromegaly treatment has evolved considerably in the past decades, as well as knowledge of its long-term morbidities. An adequate disease control allows not only normalization of mortality, but also reduction of the considerable morbidity associated with the disease.

DISCLOSURE

M.R. Gadelha has received unrestricted research grants and lecture fees from Novartis, Ipsen, and Pfizer; has participated on advisory boards for Novartis and Ionis; and is a principal investigator in clinical trials by Novartis and Ipsen. L. Kasuki has received lecture fees from Novartis, Pfizer, and Ipsen and has participated as a coinvestigator in clinical trials by Novartis and Ipsen. The other authors have nothing to disclose.

REFERENCES

1. Gadelha MR, Kasuki L, Lim DST, et al. Systemic complications of acromegaly and the impact of the current treatment landscape: an update. Endocr Rev 2019; 40(1):268–332.
2. Casanueva FF, Barkan AL, Buchfelder M, et al. Criteria for the definition of pituitary tumor centers of excellence (PTCOE): a pituitary society statement. Pituitary 2017;20(5):489–98.
3. Katznelson L, Laws ER Jr, Melmed S, et al. Acromegaly: an endocrine society clinical practice guideline. J Clin Endocrinol Metab 2014;99(11):3933–51.
4. Giustina A, Bronstein MD, Chanson P, et al. Staging and managing patients with acromegaly in clinical practice: baseline data from the SAGIT(R) validation study. Pituitary 2019;22(5):476–87.
5. van der Lely AJ, Gomez R, Pleil A, et al. Development of ACRODAT((R)), a new software medical device to assess disease activity in patients with acromegaly. Pituitary 2017;20(6):692–701.
6. Melmed S, Bronstein MD, Chanson P, et al. A Consensus Statement on acromegaly therapeutic outcomes. Nat Rev Endocrinol 2018;14(9):552–61.
7. Nomikos P, Buchfelder M, Fahlbusch R. The outcome of surgery in 668 patients with acromegaly using current criteria of biochemical 'cure'. Eur J Endocrinol 2005;152(3):379–87.
8. Antunes X, Ventura N, Camilo GB, et al. Predictors of surgical outcome and early criteria of remission in acromegaly. Endocrine 2018;60(3):415–22.
9. Fathalla H, Cusimano MD, Di Ieva A, et al. Endoscopic versus microscopic approach for surgical treatment of acromegaly. Neurosurg Rev 2015;38(3): 541–8 [discussion: 8–9].
10. Gadelha MR, Wildemberg LE, Bronstein MD, et al. Somatostatin receptor ligands in the treatment of acromegaly. Pituitary 2017;20(1):100–8.
11. Colao A, Auriemma RS, Pivonello R, et al. Interpreting biochemical control response rates with first-generation somatostatin analogues in acromegaly. Pituitary 2016;19(3):235–47.
12. Melmed S, Colao A, Barkan A, et al. Guidelines for acromegaly management: an update. J Clin Endocrinol Metab 2009;94(5):1509–17.
13. Gadelha MR, Kasuki L, Korbonits M. Novel pathway for somatostatin analogs in patients with acromegaly. Trends Endocrinol Metab 2013;24(5):238–46.
14. Mattar P, Alves Martins MR, Abucham J. Short- and long-term efficacy of combined cabergoline and octreotide treatment in controlling IgF-I levels in acromegaly. Neuroendocrinology 2010;92(2):120–7.
15. Vilar L, Azevedo MF, Naves LA, et al. Role of the addition of cabergoline to the management of acromegalic patients resistant to longterm treatment with octreotide LAR. Pituitary 2011;14(2):148–56.
16. Higham CE, Atkinson AB, Aylwin S, et al. Effective combination treatment with cabergoline and low-dose pegvisomant in active acromegaly: a prospective clinical trial. J Clin Endocrinol Metab 2012;97(4):1187–93.
17. Bernabeu I, Alvarez-Escola C, Paniagua AE, et al. Pegvisomant and cabergoline combination therapy in acromegaly. Pituitary 2013;16(1):101–8.
18. Lesche S, Lehmann D, Nagel F, et al. Differential effects of octreotide and pasireotide on somatostatin receptor internalization and trafficking in vitro. J Clin Endocrinol Metab 2009;94(2):654–61.
19. Taboada GF, Luque RM, Neto LV, et al. Quantitative analysis of somatostatin receptor subtypes (1-5) gene expression levels in somatotropinomas and

correlation to in vivo hormonal and tumor volume responses to treatment with oc-treotide LAR. Eur J Endocrinol 2008;158(3):295–303.

20. Colao A, Bronstein MD, Freda P, et al. Pasireotide versus octreotide in acromegaly: a head-to-head superiority study. J Clin Endocrinol Metab 2014;99(3): 791–9.

21. Gadelha MR, Bronstein MD, Brue T, et al. Pasireotide versus continued treatment with octreotide or lanreotide in patients with inadequately controlled acromegaly (PAOLA): a randomised, phase 3 trial. Lancet Diabetes Endocrinol 2014;2(11): 875–84.

22. Samson SL. Management of hyperglycemia in patients with acromegaly treated with pasireotide LAR. Drugs 2016;76(13):1235–43.

23. Kopchick JJ. Discovery and mechanism of action of pegvisomant. Eur J Endocrinol 2003;148(Suppl 2):S21–5.

24. Tritos NA, Chanson P, Jimenez C, et al. Effectiveness of first-line pegvisomant monotherapy in acromegaly: an ACROSTUDY analysis. Eur J Endocrinol 2017; 176(2):213–20.

25. Kasuki L, Machado EO, Ogino LL, et al. Experience with pegvisomant treatment in acromegaly in a single Brazilian tertiary reference center: efficacy, safety and predictors of response. Arch Endocrinol Metab 2016;60(5):479–85.

26. Muhammad A, van der Lely AJ, Delhanty PJD, et al. Efficacy and safety of switching to pasireotide in patients with acromegaly controlled with pegvisomant and first-generation somatostatin analogues (PAPE Study). J Clin Endocrinol Metab 2018;103(2):586–95.

27. Chiloiro S, Bima C, Tartaglione T, et al. Pasireotide and pegvisomant combination treatment in acromegaly resistant to second-line therapies: a longitudinal study. J Clin Endocrinol Metab 2019;104(11):5478–82.

28. Buchfelder M, van der Lely AJ, Biller BMK, et al. Long-term treatment with pegvisomant: observations from 2090 acromegaly patients in ACROSTUDY. Eur J Endocrinol 2018;179(6):419–27.

29. Caron PJ, Petersenn S, Houchard A, et al. Glucose and lipid levels with lanreotide autogel 120 mg in treatment-naive patients with acromegaly: data from the PRIMARYS study. Clin Endocrinol (Oxf) 2017;86(4):541–51.

30. Fleseriu M, Rusch E, Geer EB, et al. Safety and tolerability of pasireotide long-acting release in acromegaly-results from the acromegaly, open-label, multi-center, safety monitoring program for treating patients who have a need to receive medical therapy (ACCESS) study. Endocrine 2017;55(1):247–55.

31. Feola T, Cozzolino A, Simonelli I, et al. Pegvisomant improves glucose metabolism in acromegaly: a meta-analysis of prospective interventional studies. J Clin Endocrinol Metab 2019;104(7):2892–902.

32. Kasuki L, Wildemberg LE, Gadelha MR. Management of endocrine disease: personalized medicine in the treatment of acromegaly. Eur J Endocrinol 2018; 178(3):R89–100.

33. Gheorghiu ML. Updates in outcomes of stereotactic radiation therapy in acromegaly. Pituitary 2017;20(1):154–68.

34. Iwai Y, Yamanaka K, Yoshimura M, et al. Gamma knife radiosurgery for growth hormone-producing adenomas. J Clin Neurosci 2010;17(3):299–304.

35. Losa M, Gioia L, Picozzi P, et al. The role of stereotactic radiotherapy in patients with growth hormone-secreting pituitary adenoma. J Clin Endocrinol Metab 2008; 93(7):2546–52.

36. Jenkins PJ, Bates P, Carson MN, et al. Conventional pituitary irradiation is effective in lowering serum growth hormone and insulin-like growth factor-I in patients with acromegaly. J Clin Endocrinol Metab 2006;91(4):1239–45.

37. Minniti G, Jaffrain-Rea ML, Osti M, et al. The long-term efficacy of conventional radiotherapy in patients with GH-secreting pituitary adenomas. Clin Endocrinol (Oxf) 2005;62(2):210–6.

38. Brada M, Burchell L, Ashley S, et al. The incidence of cerebrovascular accidents in patients with pituitary adenoma. Int J Radiat Oncol Biol Phys 1999;45(3):693–8.

39. Minniti G, Traish D, Ashley S, et al. Risk of second brain tumor after conservative surgery and radiotherapy for pituitary adenoma: update after an additional 10 years. J Clin Endocrinol Metab 2005;90(2):800–4.

40. Abu Dabrh A, Asi N, Farah W, et al. Radiotherapy vs. radiosurgery in treating patients with acromegaly: systematic review and meta-analysis. Endocr Pract 2015;1–33. https://doi.org/10.4158/EP14574.RA.

41. Bogazzi F, Lombardi M, Strata E, et al. High prevalence of cardiac hypertophy without detectable signs of fibrosis in patients with untreated active acromegaly: an in vivo study using magnetic resonance imaging. Clin Endocrinol (Oxf) 2008; 68(3):361–8.

42. dos Santos Silva CM, Gottlieb I, Volschan I, et al. Low frequency of cardiomyopathy using cardiac magnetic resonance imaging in an acromegaly contemporary cohort. J Clin Endocrinol Metab 2015;100(12):4447–55.

43. Maione L, Brue T, Beckers A, et al. Changes in the management and comorbidities of acromegaly over three decades: the French Acromegaly Registry. Eur J Endocrinol 2017;176(5):645–55.

44. Volschan ICM, Kasuki L, Silva CMS, et al. Two-dimensional speckle tracking echocardiography demonstrates no effect of active acromegaly on left ventricular strain. Pituitary 2017;20(3):349–57.

45. Puglisi S, Terzolo M. Hypertension and acromegaly. Endocrinol Metab Clin North Am 2019;48(4):779–93.

46. Kamenicky P, Mazziotti G, Lombes M, et al. Growth hormone, insulin-like growth factor-1, and the kidney: pathophysiological and clinical implications. Endocr Rev 2014;35(2):234–81.

47. Colao A, Spinelli L, Marzullo P, et al. High prevalence of cardiac valve disease in acromegaly: an observational, analytical, case-control study. J Clin Endocrinol Metab 2003;88(7):3196–201.

48. van der Klaauw AA, Bax JJ, Roelfsema F, et al. Uncontrolled acromegaly is associated with progressive mitral valvular regurgitation. Growth Horm IGF Res 2006; 16(2):101–7.

49. Warszawski L, Kasuki L, Sa R, et al. Low frequency of cardiac arrhythmias and lack of structural heart disease in medically-naive acromegaly patients: a prospective study at baseline and after 1 year of somatostatin analogs treatment. Pituitary 2016;19(6):582–9.

50. Dos Santos Silva CM, Lima GA, Volschan IC, et al. Low risk of coronary artery disease in patients with acromegaly. Endocrine 2015;50(3):749–55.

51. Schofl C, Petroff D, Tonjes A, et al. Incidence of myocardial infarction and stroke in acromegaly patients: results from the German Acromegaly Registry. Pituitary 2017;20(6):635–42.

52. Dal J, Feldt-Rasmussen U, Andersen M, et al. Acromegaly incidence, prevalence, complications and long-term prognosis: a nationwide cohort study. Eur J Endocrinol 2016;175(3):181–90.

53. Ayuk J, Clayton RN, Holder G, et al. Growth hormone and pituitary radiotherapy, but not serum insulin-like growth factor-I concentrations, predict excess mortality in patients with acromegaly. J Clin Endocrinol Metab 2004;89(4):1613–7.

54. Colao A, Ferone D, Marzullo P, et al. Systemic complications of acromegaly: epidemiology, pathogenesis, and management. Endocr Rev 2004;25(1):102–52.

55. Attal P, Chanson P. Endocrine aspects of obstructive sleep apnea. J Clin Endocrinol Metab 2010;95(2):483–95.

56. van Haute FR, Taboada GF, Correa LL, et al. Prevalence of sleep apnea and metabolic abnormalities in patients with acromegaly and analysis of cephalometric parameters by magnetic resonance imaging. Eur J Endocrinol 2008; 158(4):459–65.

57. Powlson AS, Gurnell M. Cardiovascular disease and sleep-disordered breathing in acromegaly. Neuroendocrinology 2016;103(1):75–85.

58. Davi MV, Dalle Carbonare L, Giustina A, et al. Sleep apnoea syndrome is highly prevalent in acromegaly and only partially reversible after biochemical control of the disease. Eur J Endocrinol 2008;159(5):533–40.

59. Mazziotti G, Lania A, Canalis E. Management of endocrine disease: bone disorders associated with acromegaly: mechanisms and treatment. Eur J Endocrinol 2019;81(2):R45–56.

60. Marazuela M, Astigarraga B, Tabuenca MJ, et al. Serum bone Gla protein as a marker of bone turnover in acromegaly. Calcif Tissue Int 1993;52(6):419–21.

61. Scillitani A, Chiodini I, Carnevale V, et al. Skeletal involvement in female acromegalic subjects: the effects of growth hormone excess in amenorrheal and menstruating patients. J Bone Miner Res 1997;12(10):1729–36.

62. Bonadonna S, Mazziotti G, Nuzzo M, et al. Increased prevalence of radiological spinal deformities in active acromegaly: a cross-sectional study in postmenopausal women. J Bone Miner Res 2005;20(10):1837–44.

63. Mazziotti G, Bianchi A, Porcelli T, et al. Vertebral fractures in patients with acromegaly: a 3-year prospective study. J Clin Endocrinol Metab 2013;98(8): 3402–10.

64. Claessen KM, Kroon HM, Pereira AM, et al. Progression of vertebral fractures despite long-term biochemical control of acromegaly: a prospective follow-up study. J Clin Endocrinol Metab 2013;98(12):4808–15.

65. Madeira M, Neto LV, Torres CH, et al. Vertebral fracture assessment in acromegaly. J Clin Densitom 2013;16(2):238–43.

66. Wassenaar MJ, Biermasz NR, Hamdy NA, et al. High prevalence of vertebral fractures despite normal bone mineral density in patients with long-term controlled acromegaly. Eur J Endocrinol 2011;164(4):475–83.

67. Giustina A, Barkan A, Beckers A, et al. A consensus on the diagnosis and treatment of acromegaly comorbidities: an update. J Clin Endocrinol Metab 2019; 105(4):dgz096.

68. Barkan AL. Acromegalic arthropathy. Pituitary 2001;4(4):263–4.

69. Kropf LL, Madeira M, Vieira Neto L, et al. Functional evaluation of the joints in acromegalic patients and associated factors. Clin Rheumatol 2013;32(7):991–8.

70. Colao A, Cannavo S, Marzullo P, et al. Twelve months of treatment with octreotide-LAR reduces joint thickness in acromegaly. Eur J Endocrinol 2003;148(1):31–8.

71. Frara S, Maffezzoni F, Mazziotti G, et al. Current and emerging aspects of diabetes mellitus in acromegaly. Trends Endocrinol Metab 2016;27(7):470–83.

72. Espinosa-de-los-Monteros AL, Gonzalez B, Vargas G, et al. Clinical and biochemical characteristics of acromegalic patients with different abnormalities in glucose metabolism. Pituitary 2011;14(3):231–5.

73. Fieffe S, Morange I, Petrossians P, et al. Diabetes in acromegaly, prevalence, risk factors, and evolution: data from the French Acromegaly Registry. Eur J Endocrinol 2011;164(6):877–84.
74. Vilar L, Naves LA, Costa SS, et al. Increase of classic and nonclassic cardiovascular risk factors in patients with acromegaly. Endocr Pract 2007;13(4):363–72.
75. Mercado M, Gonzalez B, Vargas G, et al. Successful mortality reduction and control of comorbidities in patients with acromegaly followed at a highly specialized multidisciplinary clinic. J Clin Endocrinol Metab 2014;99(12):4438–46.
76. Arosio M, Reimondo G, Malchiodi E, et al. Predictors of morbidity and mortality in acromegaly: an Italian survey. Eur J Endocrinol 2012;167(2):189–98.
77. Bolfi F, Neves AF, Boguszewski CL, et al. Mortality in acromegaly decreased in the last decade: a systematic review and meta-analysis. Eur J Endocrinol 2018;179(1):59–71.
78. Boguszewski CL, Boguszewski MC, Kopchick JJ. Growth hormone, insulin-like growth factor system and carcinogenesis. Endokrynol Pol 2016;67(4):414–26.
79. Dal J, Leisner MZ, Hermansen K, et al. Cancer incidence in patients with acromegaly: a cohort study and meta-analysis of the literature. J Clin Endocrinol Metab 2018;103(6):2182–8.
80. Boguszewski CL, Ayuk J. Management of endocrine disease: acromegaly and cancer: an old debate revisited. Eur J Endocrinol 2016;175(4):R147–56.
81. Wolinski K, Stangierski A, Gurgul E, et al. Thyroid lesions in patients with acromegaly—case-control study and update to the meta-analysis. Endokrynol Pol 2017;68(1):2–6.
82. Uchoa HB, Lima GA, Correa LL, et al. Prevalence of thyroid diseases in patients with acromegaly: experience of a Brazilian center. Arq Bras Endocrinol Metabol 2013;57(9):685–90.

Endoscopic Surgery for Pituitary Tumors

Wouter R. van Furth, MD, PhD[a],*, Friso de Vries, MD[b], Daniel J. Lobatto, MD[a], Maarten C. Kleijwegt, MD[c], Pieter J. Schutte, MD[a], Alberto M. Pereira, MD, PhD[b], Nienke R. Biermasz, MD, PhD[b,1], Marco J.T. Verstegen, MD[a,1]

KEYWORDS

- Endoscopic surgery • Pituitary adenoma • Tumor • Skull base surgery
- Center of excellence • Surgical video

KEY POINTS

- Endoscopic transsphenoidal surgery is first-line treatment of most pituitary adenomas.
- Multidisciplinary team work is key for all phases of treatment: indication, preparation, surgery, and postoperative care.
- Identification of anatomy and intraoperative risk assessment with adjustment of the surgical objective is essential for safe and effective surgery.
- Cushing's disease and giant adenomas often are highly complex surgeries.
- In addition to traditional outcome measures, like remission and complication rate, modern outcomes, like quality of life, accomplishment of the surgical goal, and health care usage, are important to monitor quality of care.

 Video content accompanies this article at http://www.endo.theclinics.com.

INTRODUCTION

Transsphenoidal surgery is the front-line treatment of most pituitary adenomas.[1] After the first transsphenoidal pituitary surgery in the Netherlands was performed in the authors' hospital, it remained a focus point.[2] The authors have invested in organizing pituitary patient care in a multidisciplinary way, adopting the value-based health care principles with clinician-reported and patient-reported outcome measures. The authors work in a large-volume center, taking care of the whole spectrum of pituitary

[a] Department of Neurosurgery, Leiden University Medical Center J11-86, Center for Endocrine Tumors Leiden, PO-Box 9600, Leiden 2300 RC, the Netherlands; [b] Department of Endocrinology, Leiden University Medical Center, PO-Box 9600, Leiden 2300 RC, the Netherlands; [c] Department of Ear Nose and Throat – Head and Neck Cancer, Leiden University Medical Center, PO-Box 9600, Leiden 2300 RC, the Netherlands
[1] Shared last authors.
* Corresponding author.
E-mail address: W.R.van_Furth@lumc.nl

Endocrinol Metab Clin N Am 49 (2020) 487–503
https://doi.org/10.1016/j.ecl.2020.05.011
0889-8529/20/© 2020 The Author(s). Published by Elsevier Inc.

endo.theclinics.com

patients, including last-resort options for patients with complex (functional) pituitary adenomas and other parasellar lesions. Patient preference and individual risk/benefit assumptions are discussed during preoperative consultations using shared decision making after weighing treatment choices. In select cases, innovative imaging is used to optimally identify this individual benefit/risk balance. The authors believe that, if feasible, total resection of functional tumors without compromising pituitary function is imperative to improving ultimate health outcome of patients. This article describes the authors' philosophy, surgical technique, outcomes, and complications.

In the past decades, a transition from microscopic transseptal to an endoscopic, 2-nostril approach has been made. The surgical microscope is still the most important tool for the neurosurgeon, allowing great illumination, magnification, 2-handed surgery, and 3-dimensional view. Endoscopy for pituitary adenomas finds its origin in functional endoscopic sinus surgery, performed by ear, nose, and throat (ENT) surgeons. It is no surprise that adoption of the endoscopic technique was slow, due to the steep learning curve and the not immediately clear advantages of endoscopy. Although for midline microadenomas endoscopy offers little benefit, the endoscopic panoramic view is superior in terms of efficacy and safety for macroadenomas and tumors near the cavernous sinus.[3–5]

In the authors' center, transsphenoidal surgery has been performed exclusively endoscopically from 2007 onward. The entire procedure is always performed by a pair of 2 dedicated surgeons, either an ENT/neurosurgeon couple or 2 neurosurgeons. Because of the large surgical volume, recently well over 100 cases a year, and limited ENT surgeon availability and proper training of the neurosurgeons, the majority of cases is performed by 2 neurosurgeons. Dedicated equipment is needed, which includes not only endoscopes (0° and 30°), high-definition (HD) cameras, and monitors but also, among others, specialized drills, curettes, and dissectors. A Doppler ultrasound probe is used to identify the carotid artery. Even a routine pituitary adenoma surgery is equipment intense. The authors have protocolized the operation, which has improved efficiency and benefitted teamwork for the whole operating room (OR) team. It is also the authors' experience that greater surgical volume benefits quality of care and efficiency. They are strongly in favor of centralization of pituitary adenoma surgery, with a limited number of centers of excellence,[6,7] connected to a wide network for endocrine diagnostics, follow-up, and treatment.

CLASSIC AND NONTRADITIONAL INDICATIONS FOR SURGERY

At the authors' center, the indication for surgery is always discussed by a multidisciplinary team (MDT), where treatment objectives, alternative treatments, and timing of surgery are considered. An individualized approach to advantages or disadvantages of either treatment is discussed with the patient. In most cases, complete adenoma resection benefits the patient best, but sometimes tumor extension makes complete resection uncertain or with raised risks (**Fig. 1**). Perhaps it is here where experience, a large surgical volume, and surgery performed by 2 surgeons have the most impact on quality of care through better preoperative and intraoperative risk assessment. The surgical goal and expectations are defined preoperatively and this evaluation is discussed with the patient.

There may be a situation of high chance of total resection with very low chance of complications in microadenoma and small noninvasive macroadenoma. In invasive adenoma and small nearly undetectable adenoma remnants, however, the chances for surgical success are lower, and risk assessment is crucial to deciding optimal

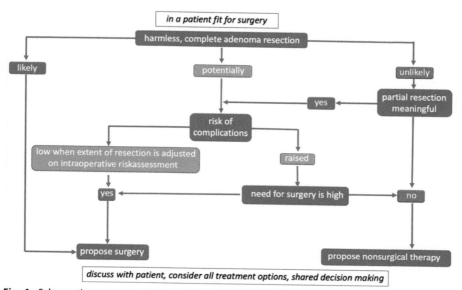

Fig. 1. Schematic representation of consideration of surgical therapy in a patient with a pituitary adenoma, who is fit to undergo surgery. If complete adenoma resection is likely and risks are low, surgery is proposed. When risks for complete resection are raised, surgery is proposed only when there is a high need for surgery (eg, Cushing's disease). Correspondingly when complete resection is possible, but uncertain, usually because of suspected cavernous sinus ingrowth or close relation to the stalk, surgery is proposed only when there is a high need for resection (eg, drug intolerance or resistance or decompression) and when it can be anticipated that risks can be kept low by adapting surgical strategy when faced with unfavorable adenoma consistency and unfavorable local anatomy. The planning of partial resection is based on a careful evaluation of anticipated risks and benefits (eg, preservation of pituitary function and risk of leaving remnant tissue) and the added value of surgery in the multimodality treatment algorithm.

treatment. When risk of complication is higher, alternative treatments (medication and radiotherapy) may be indicated. If, despite higher risks, there is a high need for surgery, the goal of treatment is defined explicitly and surgery planned accordingly.

In select cases, an incomplete adenoma resection is advised because it is expected that this is best for the patients, through lower complication rates and preserving pituitary function. Real cavernous sinus invasion[8] (Knosp classification grades 3B and 4) and certain growth patterns[9] are known to limit likeliness of complete resection. Surgery sometimes is offered, even when the chance of success is limited, for example, residual adenoma in cavernous sinus with uncertain invasion in functional tumors with severe symptoms or drug intolerance. In those cases, adjustment of the degree of resection to intraoperative risk assessment is key; for example, success may depend on the consistency of the tumor. Typically, intact pituitary gland function is deemed more important than residual adenoma. Repeat pituitary adenoma surgery has proved safe in the authors' hands and well tolerated by patients. The authors prefer repeat intervention instead of sella clean out in difficult Cushing's disease cases, trying to prevent irreversible hypopituitarism whenever possible.

There is a striking variance between centers in surgical indications for pituitary adenomas in different centers of excellence, depending on local experience and culture, availability of interventions, alternative strategies, and so forth (**Boxes 1** and **2** list authors'

Box 1

Classic surgical indications for pituitary adenoma and (para)sellar tumors

Nonfunctioning adenoma
- Nonfunctioning adenoma with compression of the optic chiasm and visual field defects
- Nonfunctional adenoma that shows consistent growth over time and close to, or touching, the optic chiasm

Cushing's disease
- Cushing's disease with a visible adenoma on the MRI, or positive petrosal sinus sampling
- Recurrent disease, with resectable adenoma

Acromegaly
- Acromegaly, with an adenoma that is likely to be completely resected
- Acromegaly, with a large adenoma, where debulking is likely to improve medical treatment

Prolactinoma
- Prolactinoma, medication refractory
- Prolactinoma, medication intolerance
- Prolactinoma with new CSF leakage after tumor shrinkage under medical therapy

Thyrotropinoma
- Thyrotropinoma, with thyrotoxicosis

General
- Apoplexy with visual deterioration
- Unknown pituitary, or sellar lesion necessitating histologic diagnosis
- Other (para)sellar tumors, such as craniopharyngioma, Rathke cleft cysts, meningioma, chordoma, pituicytoma, metastasis, and so forth

---

Box 2

Nontraditional surgical indications of pituitary adenoma

Nonfunctioning adenoma
- Recent onset of pituitary insufficiencies surgical objective: increasing the odds of restoration of pituitary gland function

Cushing's disease
- Second reoperation for small, identifiable adenoma remnant/recurrence surgical objective: remission of Cushing's disease, while maintaining pituitary gland function

Acromegaly
- Reoperation for acromegaly if visible remnant/recurrence is resectable surgical objective: remission of acromegaly, while maintaining pituitary gland function, and reducing need of, potentially side-effect inducing medical treatment

Prolactinoma
- Prolactinoma as initial treatment
- Prolactinoma after a short (6-month) trial period of dopaminergic medication
- Prolactinoma, with recurrence after 2 years of medical therapy, as alternative to lifelong medical treatment surgical objective: remission of prolactinoma, while maintaining pituitary gland function, and omitting need of, potentially side-effect inducing medical treatment

General
- Apoplexy with either extreme headache, and/or (partial) ophthalmoplegia
- (Small) sellar mass with debilitating headache surgical objective: resecting sellar lesion, while maintaining pituitary gland function, hereby optimizing chances of symptom reduction

indications). Although in most guidelines, surgery is considered the initial treatment in acromegaly patients if safe and complete resection can be achieved,[10,11] this is perhaps the group where treatment strategies differ the most. The authors' center always has been surgically oriented, with medical treatment and radiation reserved for secondary or tertiary therapy. Upfront medical treatment sometimes is initiated to make surgery safer or more likely to succeed. The authors advise on surgery and reoperations as long as there is a chance to achieve total resection with low chance of complications. Patient preferences and individual situations are taken into account, however, and alternative treatment options have proved their efficacy and added value in the multimodality treatment of this difficult-to treat disease. The authors make a plea for a multidisciplinary consultation of every new patient with acromegaly, because they have encountered several cases in which surgical chances were assumed optimal at diagnosis, but after many years of SRL treatment, the remnant tumor is less likely to be totally resected.

The authors' surgical attitude also is shown in surgical indications that are nontraditional (see **Box 2**). They recently started a study about surgery as initial treatment of patients with a small or medium-sized prolactinoma (Zandbergen IM, Najafabadi AHZ, Pelsma ICM, et al. The ProlaC & PRolaCT studies – a study protocol for a cohort and multiple Randomized Clinical Trials study design in Prolactinoma, submitted). Dopaminergic therapy, the traditional first-line treatment of prolactinoma, may have more side effects than previously recognized, at least in a substantial proportion of patients, whereas surgery has become safer; therefore, a comparison between the 2 treatment options is timely.[12,13]

Perhaps even more controversial is early surgery in non-functioning lesions not yet compressing the optic chiasm, with the main goal restoring pituitary gland function instead of accepting hypopituitarism and waiting for tumor growth and optic chiasm compression. Traditionally, restoration of gland function was an unexpected beneficial side effect of surgery,[14] not its aim. The authors have not yet properly investigated this indication, but initial clinical experiences support the concept that in select cases early surgical intervention can restore gland function. When surgery is considered anyways, in a patient with recent-onset pituitary gland dysfunction, the authors attempt to do the surgery with little delay in an attempt to maximize the chances of restoring gland function.

Another indication that has been a cause of debate is the optimal treatment strategy for apoplexy.[15] In a patient with extensive sellar bleeding/infarct and visual field defects, surgery is standard of care. The authors, however, treat almost all apoplexies as an emergency; patients often have severe headache, partial ophthalmoplegia, and loss of pituitary gland function. The authors aim to perform surgery within 24 hours after admission, reduce the headache, and optimize the odds of restoration of cranial nerves and pituitary gland function. In a patient with apoplexy, without headache, and only partial third nerve palsy, a conservative, careful, wait-and-observe approach (with hormone replacement for adrenal insufficiency when needed) usually also results in good recovery of the ophthalmoplegia. Headache, in a patient with pituitary adenoma or cyst, without accompanying apoplexy, is a symptom the authors encounter with some frequency. Predicting headache relief after surgery is unreliable[16] and as a solitary surgical goal often denied. In patients with daily, incapacitating headache and a sellar mass or cyst, however, the authors have offered surgery as a last-resort treatment and have obtained occasional good, lasting effects.

IMAGING

Imaging of the pituitary gland and stalk, optic nerves, chiasm, cavernous sinuses, sella turcica, sinuses, and nose is extremely important for a surgeon to assess surgical risks and likelihood of success. Modern imaging of the pituitary adenoma, with various magnetic resonance imaging (MRI) techniques, is key to identifying (residual) functional adenomas and tumor extensions.[17] A thin-sliced computed tomography (CT) scan of the skull base is performed to identify the exact bony anatomy, in particular the degree of pneumatization, optic canals, bony covering of carotids, sphenoid septations, septum deviation, and size of turbinates (**Fig. 2**). Postoperative imaging is done mainly for future referencing for the assessment of possible recurrence. Differentiating between normal postoperative changes in the resection cavity and residual adenoma can be difficult on initial postoperative MRI.

SURGICAL SETUP

Surgery is done under general anesthesia, in supine position, with the head elevated. An endotracheal tube is placed in the left corner of the mouth; usually, no gastric, arterial, or bladder catheter is placed. Intranasal decongestion and local anesthesia are achieved by applying a mixture of cocaine (dosage 4 mg/kg; maximum, 200 mg), adrenaline, xylometazoline, and lidocaine on 6 small gauzes (patty), which are placed on both sides adjacent to the nasal septum (upper, middle, and lower meatus) under direct vision.

Positioning of surgeons, OR nurse, and anesthesiology team in the OR is important to allow optimal, somewhat ergonomic, working posture for all. The authors perform the surgery with 2 standing surgeons positioned on the right side of the patient at the level of the shoulder (**Fig. 3**). They both look at a large HD monitor on the left side of the head of the patient. The OR nurse is on the left side of the patient, while anesthesiology is placed as far cranial on the left side as possible. At least 1 additional surgical monitor is placed for the OR nurse to follow the procedure. This setup works well for the authors and allows doing the surgery quickly and safely. A common variation in the setup is with 1 surgeon placed on the right side of the head and 1 surgeon on the left side.

A zero degree endoscope is used and fitted with a lens rinsing system. Endoscopes are used for visualization only; instruments are passed separately into the nose. Technically, therefore, this is endoscopic-assisted surgery and not endoscopic surgery.

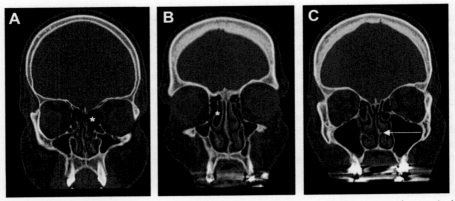

Fig. 2. Three different coronal CT scans with anatomic variations, which narrows the surgical access to the sphenoid sinus. (*A*) Strong pneumatized bulla ethmoidalis (*asterisk*). (*B*) Concha bullosa on the right side (*asterisk*). (*C*) Spur of the septum (*arrow*).

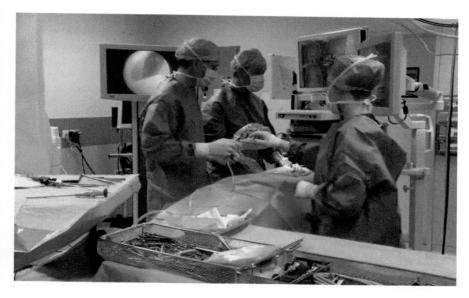

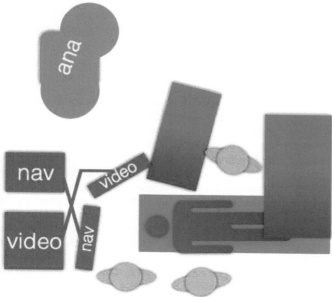

Fig. 3. Picture and schematic drawing of setup in the OR for endoscopic pituitary adenoma surgery. ana, machine of anesthesiologist; nav, navigation.

The initial steps of surgery are done with the surgeon holding the scope in 1 hand and an instrument in the other. Once the sphenoid sinus is opened on both sides and a posterior septectomy is performed, a 2-handed surgical technique is used. For this, 1 surgeon is the scope driver and the other is using both hands for surgery, similar to when a microscope is used for visualization. The endoscope is placed in the upper quadrant of the right nostril to provide ample space for surgery. The benefit of performing surgery with a handheld endoscope, compared with a rigid scope holding system, is dynamic visualization. Delicate movements of the scope, in and out, allow for better 3-dimensional understanding of anatomy. Furthermore, the scope driver can optimize visualization at all times, while allowing sufficient space for surgical instruments to maneuver. So-called sword-fighting can occur, when the endoscope and instruments compete for the narrow space in the sphenoid. Usually, this is easily solved by enlarging the opening of the anterior sphenoid wall. Magnification of the image is done simply by moving the endoscope closer to the object. With the HD scopes and monitors, the quality of the image is at least as good as with modern microscopes. Last, but not least, the authors favor surgery performed by 2 surgeons, because not infrequently it is the scope driver who identifies anatomic landmarks before the operating surgeon, which increases safety.

An electromagnetic (EM) neuronavigational system is used in all cases. Optic systems are less practical, because the line of sight often is obstructed by the endoscope. EM navigation systems have enough accuracy to be useful during surgery. The most important reason to always use the system is that it is hard to predict in which cases it can possibly have a benefit. Furthermore, the authors find that the reliability of the navigational system is better when used routinely.

APPROACH OF THE SELLA

Using the septum, nasal floor, turbinates, and choanae, the first surgical step is to identify the right sphenoid ostium. Usually, it is sufficient to carefully lateralize the middle turbinate, without the need to resect it. With a monopolar needle, an incision is made in the mucosa of the face of the sphenoid, just below the ostium, toward the septum. The length of this incision is arbitrary but should be at least as long as the length of the posterior septectomy. The mucosa inferior to this incision is reflected downward; the mucosa superiorly provides a free mucosa graft. This septal incision is always made, to always allow for mucoseptal flap harvesting. This so-called rescue flap[18] rarely is needed for pituitary adenoma surgery but the authors find it good practice to have this closure option available in all patients and in this way conserve the septal branches of the sphenopalatine artery. Injuries of these branches can result in (late) postoperative epistaxis.

The connection between the cartilaginous septum and the vomer is broken and the mucosa of the left face of the sphenoid elevated. A small chisel is used to break out the central part of the vomer and gain access to the sphenoid sinus. Next, the left nostril is entered and middle turbinate lateralized. As an option, another free mucosa flap is taken at the back of the nasal septum. A small strip of septal mucosa always is left superiorly, because of the olfactory nerve fibers, which may be recognized by a more orange color of the mucosa. The anterior wall of the sphenoid is opened extensively in all directions, tailored to the specific needs of the patient. In patients with adenomas with extensive suprasellar growth, superior opening of the anterior wall of the sphenoid is enlarged, whereas with cavernous sinus invasion, lateral opening is more extensive. When needed, the inferior one-third part of the superior turbinate is cut, allowing it to be reflected laterally for the duration of the surgery.

The bony septations in the sphenoid show a lot of variation, although often they are attached at the level of the carotid artery. This is why these septations are best drilled away carefully and not broken and removed. Force may cause carotid artery injury. Septations are removed and mucosa over the sella is opened as curtains, or fully removed, to allow for optimal bony anatomy identification. It is essential to identify on both sides the following structures, prior to commencing to the next phase (**Fig. 4**):

- Carotid artery
- Optic canal
- Medial opticocarotid recess
- Lateral opticocarotid recess
- Sella floor
- Tuberculum sellae
- Planum sphenoidale

SELLAR PHASE

To benefit from the panoramic view the endoscope offers, a larger bony opening of the sella is preferred. The authors have noticed that a major cause of incomplete adenoma resection was a too limited sellar bony opening. The technique is to outline the extend of the opening with a drill, until the cutline is eggshell thin and then break it and remove a small bone flap. Bony opening is tailored to pathology. When an adenoma is adjacent to the medial wall of the cavernous sinus, the bony opening on that side is extended over the cavernous sinus. This technique allows safe bony removal, even over the cavernous sinus and carotid artery. Correspondingly, tuberculum sellae, or even the first part of the planum sphenoidale bone, is removed for adenomas with suprasellar growth.

Before the dura is cut, anatomic reorientation is performed, and the location of both carotid arteries is confirmed. Doppler and neuronavigation may be useful for this. Dura opening is done with a disposable microblade, making sure to keep distance from the cavernous sinuses and carotid arteries. The intercavernous sinus inferior and/or superior sometimes may need bipolar coagulation. With the superior cuts, the authors try to avoid cutting into the cerebrospinal fluid (CSF) that often is here in a dural fold. The

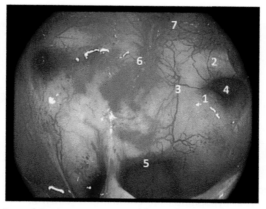

Fig. 4. Endoscopic view of the bony anatomy of face of sella in well-pneumatized sphenoid. 1, Carotid artery; 2, optic canal; 3, medial opticocarotid recess; 4, lateral opticocarotid recess; 5, sella floor; 6, tuberculum sellae; and 7, planum sphenoidale.

dura of the sella floor also is cut, to get wide exposure of the sellar content. Because of the wide bony opening, the dura edges can be mobilized, allowing direct visual intrasellar inspection.

Bleeding during resection of the pituitary adenoma is venous and, therefore, usually limited. This venous bleeding, however, does obstruct good visibility of the resection planes. Bleeding, usually from the cavernous sinus or intercavernous sinus, is best prevented or stopped before adenoma resection is continued. Packing with hemostatic agents works well and, in more persistent bleeding, injection with a specialized product Floseal (Baxter Health Care, Deerfield, IL, USA) or Surgiflo (Ethicon, New Brunswick, NJ, USA) may be needed to get full hemostasis.

In macroadenoma, the pituitary gland often is displaced laterally and superiorly, so that the adenoma is first encountered after dura opening (**Fig. 5**, Video 1). With dissectors and blunt ring curettes, the borders of the adenoma are dissected first and then the adenoma is removed in a piecemeal fashion. Early identification of the adenoma edges is crucial to limit the risk of damage to the pituitary gland and tearing of the arachnoid at the level of the diaphragm sellae. In some more firm adenomas, extracapsular resection is possible.[19] In this technique, the adenoma edge is dissected all around, without piecemeal removal. Although this surgical technique has a high chance of complete adenoma resection, it also has a higher chance of inadvertently removal or pituitary gland injury. After selective adenoma resection, intrasellar inspection is performed to assess completeness of tumor removal. In adenomas with large suprasellar components, a 30o endoscope is used to inspect the superior compartment. Placing the patient in Trendelenburg position raises the CSF pressure, which pushes the suprasellar compartment of the adenoma downward, sometimes allowing resection of residual adenoma.

In microadenoma, the exposed surface of the pituitary gland can look completely normal (**Fig. 6**, Video 2). Based on preoperative imaging, a small cut then is made in the gland at the location where the adenoma is expected. There currently are no techniques for intraoperative imaging of the gland, but neuronavigation (merging CT and MRI) can help based on preoperative imaging. Sometimes gentle palpation of the gland surface with an instrument also may provide information about the localization of the adenoma. After a cut is made in the pituitary gland, again the edges of the microadenoma are identified and dissected. Often the consistency of the microadenoma is

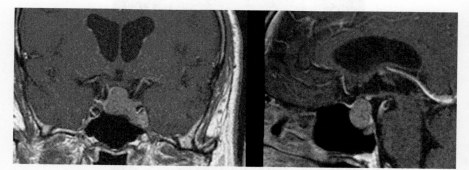

Fig. 5. A 68-year-old male patient with a growing macroadenoma that abuts the chiasm, with recent-onset partial hypopituitarism. Coronal (*left panel*) and sagittal (*right panel*) MRI show extension of the adenoma into the left cavernous sinus. The postoperative course was uneventful with recovery of pituitary function. A postoperative MRI showed small cavernous sinus residual adenoma on the left side. For surgical video, see Video 1.

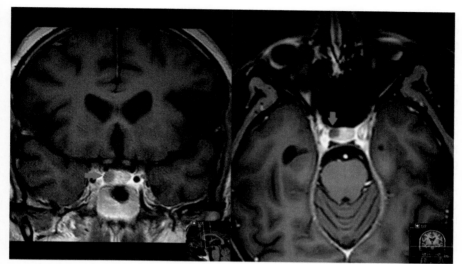

Fig. 6. An 18-year-old female patient with severe Cushing's disease (cortisol, 1376 nmol/L) due to a microadenoma located on the right side of the sella. Coronal (*left panel*) and axial (*right panel*) MRI show the location of the adenoma (*arrows*). Postoperative course was uneventful with recovery of symptoms, biochemical remission, without the need for hormone replacement except for hydrocortisone (10 mg, 5 mg, 5 mg over the day). Pathology showed ACTH positive adenoma. For surgical video, see Video 2.

soft, limiting the option of extracapsular dissection. With small ring curettes the adenoma is removed and the resection cavity explored. The authors try to visually inspect the entire cavity, to assess completeness of resection. It can be useful to fill the resection cavity with saline and dive into the cavity with the endoscope, rinsing continuously for detailed inspection.[20]

CLOSURE

When selective adenoma resection is performed without CSF leakage, closure can be simple. The authors normally place a collagen foam material in the opening of the resection cavity, to close it off. In macroadenoma with extensive exposure of the arachnoid, it is wise to be stricter about closure. The authors have had patients without CSF leakage during surgery, who started leaking a couple of days later, sometimes provoked by a sneeze or other activity causing rise in intracranial pressure. In these patients, CSF leakage is prevented by filling the resection cavity with autologous fat tissue, harvested from a paraumbilical 2-cm incision and held in place by fibrin glue. In all these cases, unless removed, the sphenoidal mucosa is draped over the sella to promote remucosalization.

In patients with a CSF leak during surgery, a more stringent closure technique is crucial. There are many variations in closing techniques; the authors rely mostly on the following technique. The arachnoidal tear is closed by placing a small piece of abdominal fat in the opening and secured by several drops of fibrin-glue. Subsequently, the closure is reinforced by filling the resection cavity with small pieces of abdominal fat, taking care not to overpack it. In larger CSF leaks, the next layer is 1 or 2 pieces of fascia lata. This can be an autograft or may be available from donor tissue. Finally, the free mucosa graft that was harvested at the beginning of the surgery is placed on top and again secured with drops of fibrin glue. Only in a patient with a larger defect and reconstruction are fatty gauzes placed in the sphenoid to hold the reconstruction in place. A mucoseptal flap is not used for pituitary adenomas. Lumbar drains are not placed and postoperative bedrest is refrained from.

PATHOLOGY-SPECIFIC SURGICAL ISSUES
Cushing's disease

Surgery for Cushing's disease almost always is complex. The adenoma can be invisible on MRI. Visible adenomas may have extensions that are not always visible on the MRI. In rare cases, there may be multiple adenomas present, which is why some surgeons place several vertical cuts in the nonadenomatous part of the pituitary gland. The sellar dura can be infiltrated and cause a recurrence.[21] A small remnant or recurrence eventually can cause reoccurrence of symptomatic Cushing's disease. Completeness of resection, therefore, is essential. Typically, the first surgical attempt is the most likely to succeed; therefore, this should be done only by experienced surgeons, after extensive preoperative imaging and with a low threshold to do a wide, bilateral inspection of the sella.

Acromegaly

Adenomas in patients with acromegaly usually are larger than in Cushing's disease, with a high number demonstrating an invasive growth pattern.[11] To allow better medical treatment, partial resection of the adenoma also can be beneficial and is something the authors often consider when treating invasive adenomas. For unknown reasons, acromegaly adenomas tend to grow more in the inferior than the superior direction. Surgeons, therefore, should be aware of the possibility of small adenoma remnants in the clivus.

Prolactinoma

Surgery for prolactinomas usually is straightforward as long as the adenoma is reasonable in size[22] (**Fig. 7**, Video 3). A recent report showed that prolactinomas next to the cavernous sinus had lower remission rates than more centrally located adenomas.[23] This has not yet been replicated, however, and is not the authors' experience.

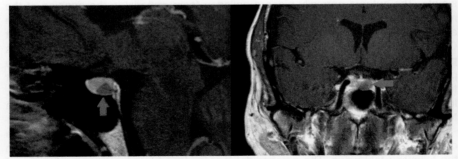

Fig. 7. A 45-year-old female patient with a microprolactinoma on the left side of the sella, treated medically for 4 years, with side effects and persistent disease. Sagittal (*left panel*) and coronal (*right panel*) MRI show location of adenoma (*red arrow*). Postoperative course was uneventful with complete recovery of symptoms, normal prolactin level, and normal pituitary function. Pathology showed a prolactin positive adenoma (growth hormone negative). For surgical video, see Video 3.

Giant Adenoma

Surgery for a giant adenoma (diameter >4 cm), is associated with a much higher risk profile compared with other pituitary adenoma operations. A feared complication is bleeding/apoplexy in tumor remnant, causing acute stretching of the optic chiasm and/or hypothalamus. Emergency surgical evacuation through a craniotomy often is required to try to reduce permanent damage. In an attempt to reduce this risk, the authors sometimes perform a combined approach,[24] through both endoscopic transsphenoidal and microscopic transcranial approach (**Fig. 8**) and/or endoscopic transventricular approach. Although the authors' experience with the combined approach is limited, they believe a combined approach in select, giant adenomas is safer than a staged combined approach or only transsphenoidal operation.

POSTOPERATIVE CARE

Careful postoperative monitoring is essential, because transient postoperative fluid disbalance occurs frequently. At day 2 after surgery, patients start rinsing the nose twice a day with saline solution, which is continued for 6 weeks. Recently, the authors introduced a short-stay protocol for preoperatively classified as low-risk patients, discharging patients 2 days after surgery under supervision of a trained pituitary case manager. Patients are screened daily to assess for potential complications. In this group, but also in the historical cohort, the reason encountered most frequently for readmission was syndrome of inappropriate antidiuretic hormone secretion (SIADH), which is present in 43% of readmissions (overall readmission rate was 17% vs 10%

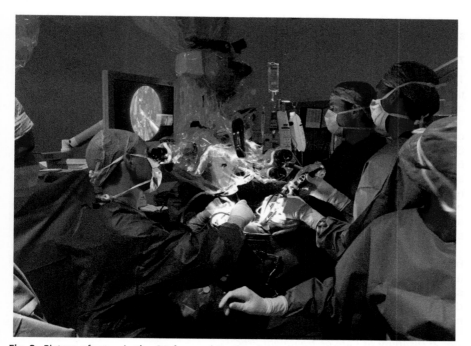

Fig. 8. Picture of setup in the OR for combined endoscopic transsphenoidal and microscopic transcranial pituitary adenoma surgery. Two surgeons perform the endoscopic transsphenoidal approach (*right*), while 1 surgeon does the microscopic cranial approach (*left*).

in the short stay and historical control group, respectively).[25] Recent studies show that a reduction of readmission can be achieved by introducing a strict postoperative fluid restriction (1–1.5 L) during the first 2 weeks after surgery.[26,27]

OUTCOMES

For the assessment of outcomes, it is important to periodically evaluate quality of care through plan-do-check-act cycles. At the authors' center, this is done through weekly case discussions with the pituitary MDT and by periodic result evaluations. The authors have published both retrospective[5,28] and prospective[29] analyses of the outcomes and are continuing prospective outcome measurements. For the periodic evaluations, 2 different approaches to address outcomes are used: the 3-tier model of value-based health care[30] and a surgical goal assessment (de Vries F, Lobatto DJ, Verstegen MJT, et al. Novel surgical outcome classification integrating efficacy and safety, as applied to functioning pituitary adenoma surgery, submitted for publication). Based on the authors' experiences with the prospective outcome measurement, they have developed a dedicated system in the electronic patient record, which enables registering and evaluating outcomes as a part of regular clinical and outpatient care. Outcomes all are registered and automatically extracted from the source. These include the more classic outcomes, such as endocrine function, remission, postoperative remnant, visual function, and so forth, but also postoperative complications as well as the innovative, patient-reported outcomes. A selection of results of a prospective cohort of 103 patients treated at the authors' center that were categorized through the 3-tier model of value-based health care are presented by Lobatto and colleagues[29]. These figures are a work in progress and will be adjusted with new data being entered in the database. Results are highly dependent on case mix (complexity of cases), as is specified in detail in the article by Lobatto and colleagues[29].

Tier 1: Health Status Achieved or Retained

Tier 1, health status achieved or retained, includes outcomes that matter most to patients and includes outcomes, such as mortality, remission, and degree of resection, and also patient-reported outcomes.[30] Mortality in pituitary adenoma surgery generally is low for pituitary adenoma surgery; however, it occasionally does occur. Degree of resection generally is high, with complete resection possible in 70% of cases. Short-term remission rates among all functioning tumors at the authors' center are 69%, with 93% of patients obtaining improvement of hormone excesses. After endoscopic surgery for Cushing's disease, 83% were in remission. Both 5-year and 10-year recurrence-free survival rates were 71% (95% CI, 55%–87%).[5] In patients with ophthalmologic manifestations, complete visual recovery was achieved among 46% and partial recovery in 52%, whereas only 1 patient (2%) did not improve after surgery.[29]

The authors found a clinically relevant self-perceived improvement on disease burden in 41% of patients, which lags behind other outcomes.[29] This indicates that although physician-reported outcomes are important, the patient-reported outcomes should complement the outcome set. It shows the impact of a pituitary tumor on the daily lives of patients for which targeted interventions could lead to greater improvement on the long term.

Tier 2: Disutility of Care or Treatment Process

Tier 2, disutility of care or treatment process, includes length of stay, return to activity, treatment-induced complaints, and complications (described later).[30] Median length of hospital stay was 3 days (interquartile range 2–5).[29] In total, short-term return to work was high (86%); however, work disability among patients with pituitary tumors is substantial.[31] Nasal disability after treatment initially is high, however, in general, returning to baseline after 6 weeks.[29]

Tier 3: Sustainability of Health

Tier 3, sustainability of health, includes the long-term effects of treatment.[30] When initial surgery does not lead to remission, the authors often explore the options of early reoperation, with extensive new imaging. The need for long-term hormone replacement for pituitary insufficiency is substantial among patients with pituitary adenomas, the majority of pituitary function loss already occurring due to the tumor and not due to the intervention. Most patients present with pituitary dysfunction preoperatively (51%), and long-term hormone replacement ultimately remains necessary in 51% of patients.[29]

COMPLICATIONS

Although complications frequently occur after pituitary tumor surgery, most complications are transient. The authors differentiate between neurosurgical complications and endocrine complications. Although neurosurgical complications potentially are more life-threatening, the incidence of major neurosurgical complications usually is very low and patients often are hampered more by the endocrine consequences of the disease/complications. A systematic review performed by the authors' group found an increased risks of complications for patients of older age as well as for those patients with larger, invasive, and previously irradiated tumors.[32]

In the authors' published series, the most common complication is transient diabetes insipidus (26.2%), followed by SIADH (12.6%). Permanent diabetes insipidus was present in 7.8% of patients. For the onset of new pituitary deficiencies, it is important to differentiate between tumor types, because larger/giant adenomas and craniopharyngiomas have a higher chance of manifesting with postoperative pituitary deficits compared with functioning tumors. As with outcomes, the complication rate is dependent on surgeon volume and experience[33] and also is based on the complexity of the condition (see also **Fig. 1**). Thanks to monitoring of the complication rates, outcomes, and baseline characteristics, the MDT now is able to better appraise surgical risks at the preoperative consultation and together with the patient decide the treatment strategy.

SUMMARY

Endoscopic transsphenoidal surgery for pituitary adenomas is a safe and highly effective first-line treatment that is well tolerated by patients. Reoperations are more complex but generally still well tolerated, but these procedures require optimal preoperative planning and intraoperative risk assessment to maximize chances of success and minimize risks. This article presents the authors' philosophy, surgical techniques, and outcomes in a high-volume pituitary adenoma center. Three surgical videos illustrate the different procedures. The authors' experience has reinforced their belief that a multidisciplinary approach, experience, and surgical volume are key to delivering high quality of care.

DISCLOSURE

The authors have nothing to disclose.

SUPPLEMENTARY DATA

Supplementary data related to this article can be found online at https://doi.org/10.1016/j.ecl.2020.05.011.

REFERENCES

1. Molitch ME. Diagnosis and treatment of pituitary adenomas: a review. JAMA 2017;317(5):516–24.
2. Roelfsema F, Van Dulken H, Frölich M. Long-term results of transsphenoidal pituitary microsurgery in 60 acromegalic patients. Clin Endocrinol (Oxf) 1985;23(5): 555–65.
3. Kuo JS, Barkhoudarian G, Farrell CJ, et al. Guidelines: congress of neurological surgeons systematic review and evidence-based guideline on surgical techniques and technologies for the management of patients with nonfunctioning pituitary adenomas. Neurosurgery 2016;79(4):E536–8.
4. McLaughlin N, Eisen berg AA, Cohan P, et al. Value of endoscopy for maximizing tumor removal in endonasal transsphenoidal pituitary adenoma surgery. J Neurosurg 2013;118(3):613–20.
5. Broersen LHA, Biermasz NR, van Furth WR, et al. Endoscopic vs. microscopic transsphenoidal surgery for Cushing's disease: a systematic review and meta-analysis. Pituitary 2018;21:524–34.
6. McLaughlin N, Laws ER, Oyesiku NM, et al. Pituitary centers of excellence. Neurosurgery 2012;71(5):916–26.
7. Casanueva FF, Barkan AL, Buchfelder M, et al. Criteria for the definition of Pituitary Tumor Centers of Excellence (PTCOE): a pituitary society statement. Pituitary 2017;20(5):489–98.
8. Micko ASG, Wöhrer A, Wolfsberger S, et al. Invasion of the cavernous sinus space in pituitary adenomas: endoscopic verification and its correlation with an MRI-based classification. J Neurosurg 2015;122:803–11.
9. Mooney MA, Sarris CE, Zhou JJ, et al. Proposal and validation of a simple grading scale (TRANSSPHER Grade) for predicting gross total resection of nonfunctioning pituitary macroadenomas after transsphenoidal surgery. Oper Neurosurg (Hagerstown) 2019;17(5):460–9.
10. Buchfelder M, Schlaffer SM. The surgical treatment of acromegaly. Pituitary 2017; 20(1):76–83.
11. Melmed S. Acromegaly pathogenesis and treatment. J Clin Invest 2009;119(11): 3189–202.
12. Honegger J, Nasi-Kordhishti I, Aboutaha N, et al. Surgery for prolactinomas: a better choice? Pituitary 2020;23(1):45–51.
13. Supplementary data to the paper: Surgery as a viable alternative first-line treatment for prolactinoma patients. A systematic review and meta-analysis. J Clin Endocrinol Metab 2020;105(3):e32–41.
14. Jr ERL, Iuliano SL, Cote DJ, et al. A benchmark for preservation of normal pituitary function after endoscopic transsphenoidal surgery for pituitary macroadenomas. World Neurosurg 2016;91:371–5.
15. Briet C, Salenave S, Bonneville JF, et al. Pituitary apoplexy. Endocr Rev 2015; 36(6):622–45.
16. Suri H, Dougherty C. Clinical presentation and management of headache in pituitary tumors. Curr Pain Headache Rep 2018;22(8):1–6.
17. MacFarlane J, Bashari WA, Senanayake R, et al. Advances in the imaging of pituitary tumours. Endocrinol Metab Clin North Am 2020;49(3):357–73.

18. Rivera-Serrano CM, Snyderman CH, Gardner P, et al. Nasoseptal "rescue" flap: A novel modification of the nasoseptal flap technique for pituitary surgery. Laryngoscope 2011;121(5):990–3.
19. Prevedello DM, Ebner FH, De Lara D, et al. Extracapsular dissection technique with the Cotton Swab for pituitary adenomas through an endoscopic endonasal approach - How i do it. Acta Neurochir (Wien) 2013;155(9):1629–32.
20. Locatelli D, Canevari FR, Acchiardi I, et al. The endoscopic diving technique in pituitary and cranial base surgery: Technical note. Neurosurgery 2010;66(2). https://doi.org/10.1227/01.NEU.0000363746.84763.A5.
21. Lonser RR, Ksendzovsky A, Wind JJ, et al. Prospective evaluation of the characteristics and incidence of adenoma-associated dural invasion in Cushing disease. J Neurosurg 2012;116(2):272–9.
22. Buchfelder M, Zhao Y, Schlaffer SM. Surgery for prolactinomas to date. Neuroendocrinology 2019;109(1):77–81.
23. Micko A, Vila G, Höftberger R, et al. Endoscopic transsphenoidal surgery of microprolactinomas: a reappraisal of cure rate based on radiological criteria. Clin Neurosurg 2019;85(4):508–15.
24. Nishioka H, Hara T, Usui M, et al. Simultaneous combined supra-infrasellar approach for giant/large multilobulated pituitary adenomas. World Neurosurg 2012;77(3–4):533–9.
25. Lobatto DJ, Vlieland TPMV, van den Hout WB, et al. Feasibility, safety and outcomes of a fast-track care trajectory in pituitary surgery. Endocrine 2020. https://doi.org/10.1007/s12020-020-02308-2.
26. Burke WT, Cote DJ, Iuliano SI, et al. A practical method for prevention of readmission for symptomatic hyponatremia following transsphenoidal surgery. Pituitary 2018;21(1):25–31.
27. Deaver KE, Catel CP, Lillehei KO, et al. Strategies to reduce readmissions for hyponatremia after transsphenoidal surgery for pituitary adenomas. Endocrine 2018;62(2):333–9.
28. Broersen LHA, Andela CD, Dekkers OM, et al. Improvement but no normalization of quality of life and cognitive functioning after treatment for Cushing's syndrome. J Clin Endocrinol Metab 2019;104:5325–37.
29. Lobatto DJ, Zamanipoor Najafabadi AH, de Vries F, et al. Towards value-based health care in pituitary surgery: application of a comprehensive outcome set in perioperative care. Eur J Endocrinol 2019. https://doi.org/10.1530/EJE-19-0344.
30. Porter ME, Lee TH. The strategy that will fix health care. Harv Bus Rev 2013;91: 50–70.
31. Lobatto DJ, Steffens ANV, Zamanipoor Najafabadi AH, et al. Work disability and its determinants in patients with pituitary tumor-related disease. Pituitary 2018; 21(6):593–604.
32. Lobatto DJ, de Vries F, Zamanipoor Najafabadi AH, et al. Preoperative risk factors for postoperative complications in endoscopic pituitary surgery: a systematic review. Pituitary 2017. https://doi.org/10.1007/s11102-017-0839-1.
33. Honegger J, Grimm F. The experience with transsphenoidal surgery and its importance to outcomes. Pituitary 2018;21(5):545–55.

Aggressive Pituitary Adenomas and Carcinomas

Mirela Diana Ilie, MD, MSc[a], Emmanuel Jouanneau, MD, PhD[b],
Gérald Raverot, MD, PhD[c],*

KEYWORDS

- Aggressive pituitary tumor • Pituitary carcinoma • Definition • Diagnosis
- Treatment • Tumor growth • Temozolomide • Stupp protocol

KEY POINTS

- A subset of pituitary tumors present an aggressive behavior that remains difficult to predict, and, in very rare cases, they metastasize.
- From 2018, there are guidelines for the management of aggressive pituitary tumors and carcinomas, but several issues remain unaddressed because of the scarcity of available data.
- This article defines clinically relevant tumor growth based on signs and symptoms, whereas unusually rapid tumor growth rate refers to the tumor increasing by 20% in less than 6 to 12 months.
- Temozolomide and the Stupp protocol might have a place earlier in the management of aggressive pituitary tumors and carcinomas, and not only as a salvage therapy.
- Despite temozolomide efficacy in about 40% of cases, a need for alternative therapies exists, and immunotherapy should be considered.

INTRODUCTION

Pituitary adenomas and carcinomas are neoplasms derived from the endocrine cells of the adenohypophysis. Most are benign, and either they remain clinically inapparent[1] or they are easily treatable with the currently available conventional therapies (medical treatments, surgery, and in some cases radiotherapy).[2] However, some of these

[a] Endocrinology Department VI, "C.I.Parhon" National Institute of Endocrinology, 34-36 Avi-atorilor Boulevard, Bucharest 011863, Romania; [b] Neurosurgery Department, Reference Center for Rare Pituitary Diseases HYPO, "Groupement Hospitalier Est" Hospices Civils de Lyon, "Claude Bernard" Lyon 1 University, Hôpital Pierre Wertheimer, 59 Pinel Boulevard, Lyon, Bron 69677, France; [c] Endocrinology Department, Reference Center for Rare Pituitary Diseases HYPO, "Groupement Hospitalier Est" Hospices Civils de Lyon, "Claude Bernard" Lyon 1 University, Hôpital Louis Pradel, 59 Pinel Boulevard, Lyon, Bron 69677, France
* Corresponding author.
E-mail address: gerald.raverot@chu-lyon.fr
Twitter: @the_hormone_doc (M.D.I.); @GeraldRaverot (G.R.)

Endocrinol Metab Clin N Am 49 (2020) 505–515
https://doi.org/10.1016/j.ecl.2020.05.008
0889-8529/20/© 2020 Elsevier Inc. All rights reserved.

tumors show an aggressive behavior that is difficult to predict, and, in very rare cases, they metastasize.[3] The prevalence of pituitary adenomas and carcinomas is presented in **Fig. 1**.[4,5] Both aggressive pituitary adenomas and carcinomas are difficult to manage and are responsible for increased morbidity and mortality. The recently published European Society of Endocrinology (ESE) guidelines[2] provide valuable guidance, but at the same time leave some unaddressed issues because of the scarcity of the data available in the literature. This article presents key clinical aspects from definition to diagnosis, treatment, and follow-up. It also discusses some of the unanswered questions of the ESE guidelines (eg, how to define a clinically relevant tumor growth) and the potential place of temozolomide (TMZ) earlier in the management of aggressive pituitary tumors and pituitary carcinomas, instead of using it only as a salvage therapy.

Current Definitions

- Aggressive pituitary adenomas are defined by the ESE guidelines as radiologically invasive tumors with unusually rapid tumor growth rate or as tumors presenting clinically relevant tumor growth in spite of optimal use of standard therapies (conventional medical treatments, surgery, and radiotherapy).[2] However, there is no definition proposed for clinically relevant tumor growth or for unusually rapid tumor growth rate.
- Pituitary carcinomas are defined exclusively based on the presence of metastases (craniospinal and/or systemic), because so far there are no histologic characteristics distinguishing carcinomas from adenomas before metastasis.[6] Moreover, clinical and histologic data from the ESE survey on aggressive pituitary tumors and carcinomas, because of similarities between the 2 groups, made Trouillas and colleagues[5] question whether aggressive pituitary tumors and pituitary carcinomas are 2 sides of the same coin, and propose that aggressive pituitary tumors be considered tumors with malignant potential. However, despite the similarity between the two groups, pituitary carcinomas more frequently showed a mitotic count greater than 2 per high-power field (90% vs 63%) and had higher mortality in comparison with aggressive pituitary tumors (43% vs 28%).[5]

Diagnosis

From a practical point of view, the diagnosis of these tumors should comprise:

- Imaging studies
- Full endocrine laboratory evaluation
- Ophthalmologic evaluation
- Histopathologic analysis[2]

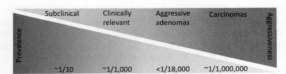

Fig. 1. Prevalence of pituitary adenomas and carcinomas. (*Data from* Ho, KKY, Fleseriu M, Wass J, et al. A tale of pituitary adenomas: to NET or not to NET: Pituitary Society position statement. Pituitary. 2019; 22:569-573 and Trouillas J, Burman P, McCormack A, et al. Aggressive pituitary tumours and carcinomas: two sides of the same coin? *Eur J Endocrinol.* 2018;178(6):C7-C9.)

Imaging studies

The imaging studies are performed mainly to assess tumor dimension, invasion, and growth. MRI is the preferred option; thin slices are needed and the sequences should include sagittal T1-weighted native; coronal T1-weighted native; and contrast-enhanced, coronal T2-weighted native ± axial T1-weighted native sequences. Other than the MRI, computed tomography (CT) scan should be performed when the assessment of bone invasion is needed,[2] and clinicians should screen for metastases as discussed later.

Invasion Regarding invasion, the ESE guidelines note that invasiveness alone is not synonymous with aggressiveness, but that nonetheless the invasion is a determinant of incomplete resection.[2] Another point concerns the assertion of tumor invasion based on the MRI findings, which could be misleading because the extension into the cavernous sinus can result from both tumor invasion and/or tumor expansion.[7,8] It has become common practice to label tumors as invasive when they are classified as Knosp grade 3A, 3B, or 4 on the MRI. However, initially, the modified Knosp classification (grades 1, 2, 3A, 3B, and 4) was meant to predict the likelihood of surgically observed invasion into the cavernous sinus (and therefore to predict the surgical outcome) and not to define invasion per se. The investigators showed important differences in the parasellar invasion found during endoscopic transsphenoidal surgery between grades 3A, 3B, and 4 (26.5%, 70.6%, and 100%, respectively). Moreover, tumors classified as Knosp grade 2 were found to be invasive during endoscopic transsphenoidal surgery in 10% of the cases.[7] The authors recently confirmed the difference in the surgically observed invasion into the cavernous sinus between grade 3A and 3B tumors. The rate of intraoperative invasion of grade 3A tumors was higher (61.5%) than in the original study (26.5%),[7] but still lower than for grade 3B tumors (78.6%). Moreover, gross total resection was negatively associated with the Knosp grade, with a 56% rate for grade 3A tumors and a 25% rate for grade 3B tumors. It has to be noted that, for functioning pituitary tumors, the postoperative remission rate did not differ between grade 3A and 3B tumors, suggesting persistent residual tumor not visible on MRI.[9]

Tumor growth How the tumor growth should be measured and classified in order to assess the treatment response is an important issue. Imber and colleagues[10] recently showed that although pituitary tumors are irregularly shaped (especially after treatment), a 1D approach (ie, the longest diameter, as governed by the revised Response Evaluation Criteria in Solid Tumors [RECIST] guideline 1.1, used in most cancers outside of the central nervous system[11,12]) was in general adequately correlated with the volumetric assessment. The investigators warn that, in particular cases of pituitary tumors, such as multiloculated pituitary tumors, multifocal and bony invasive tumors, small recurrences, and small areas of residual tumor, the three-dimensional volumetric assessment might be more accurate than the one-dimensional assessment and add value, but this seemed to be true especially in diagnosing partial remission versus stable disease, and not in cases of tumor progression.[10]

RECIST 1.1 define progressive disease as a 20% increase in the sum of the longest diameters (compared with the smallest sum of the longest diameters recorded since a particular treatment was started), with a 5-mm absolute increase in the sum required, and/or as the appearance of new lesions. The term sum of diameters is used to account for the multiple lesions that may be present. The 5-mm absolute increase in the sum is in order to avoid overdiagnosing progressive disease when the sum of the longest diameters is very small and a 20% increase would be within measurement error. It is also important to note that the RECIST guideline is based mainly on CT scans and, for consistency and ease, it recommends to measure the longest diameter on the axial plane (even though the true longest diameter may be on another plane); moreover, to be consider measurable, a lesion must be initially greater than or equal to 1 cm.[11,12]

However, in the case of pituitary tumors, given that the lesion is unique (and therefore there is a sole longest diameter and not a sum of diameters), increases of less than 5 mm might be accurately measured, depending also on how well delineated is the tumor and, on the MRI machine, sequence and slice thickness. The authors suggest that it should be discussed with the radiologist within each pituitary team what represents the smallest accurately measurable increase, but that a 20% increase in the longest diameter should usually suffice to call it progressive disease.

Returning to the definition of an aggressive pituitary tumor, the guidelines do not define clinically relevant tumor growth or unusually rapid tumor growth rate because not enough data exist in the literature to allow a clear and evidence-based definition. Therefore, studies of this matter are most needed, but, until these are available, based on our own experience, we propose the following. For the first term, in the case of pituitary tumors, because of their location, even when a tumor does not show progressive disease (ie, increasing its longest diameter by 20%), it may still show clinically relevant tumor growth. These situations include a tumor starting to approach or to compress the optical chiasm, aggravation of the optical field defects, and compression of the cranial nerves bypassing the cavernous sinuses. In these cases, as the name states, it is really the signs and symptoms (present, or anticipated if the tumor is in contact with the optical chiasm) that should make the diagnosis of a clinically relevant tumor growth independent of the absolute or relative increase in the tumor diameters (especially because it may not be the longest diameter that causes the complications). Alternatively, a tumor should be considered as progressive when its longest diameter increases by more than 20% even if the growth is not clinically relevant (eg, tumors expanding in the sphenoid sinus). Unusually rapid tumor growth rate is more difficult to define. Normally, pituitary tumors grow slowly and it is necessary to compare the last imaging study not only with the penultimate one but also with older imaging studies in order to evaluate the tumor growth, as recommended by the ESE guidelines,[2] and as shown in **Fig. 2**. Therefore, if the tumor increases by 20% in less

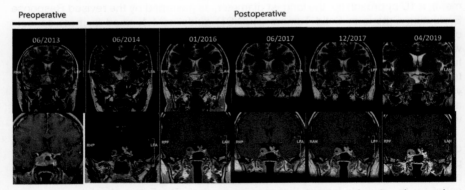

Fig. 2. Radiological follow-up of a slowly growing pituitary tumor, showing the need to compare the last imaging study not only with the penultimate one but also with older imaging studies in order to evaluate the tumor growth. (*Top*) Coronal T2-weighted native MRI sequences. (*Bottom*) Coronal T1-weighted contrast-enhanced MRI sequences.

than 6 months (or even in <12 months if only annual MRI is available), the growth rate is classified as unusually rapid. **Fig. 3** shows a rapidly growing pituitary tumor.

Histopathologic analysis and prediction of aggressiveness

The aggressive behavior may manifest even more than 10 years after the primary diagnosis of a pituitary tumor, and, so far, no single marker is capable of accurately predicting it.[2] This fact is of particular importance because it allows for an earlier and more intensive management of these tumors. At present, the ESE guidelines recommend, at a minimum, to perform immunohistochemistry for pituitary hormones and to determine the Ki-67 index, and state that the mitotic count and p53 immunodetection should be envisioned at least in cases with a Ki-67 index greater than or equal to 3%.[2] In contrast, the European Pituitary Pathology Group (EPPG) has recently proposed a standardized diagnostic approach for these tumors, in which both the Ki-67 index and the mitotic count are listed to be performed systematically, with a cutoff for the mitotic count of greater than 2 mitoses per high-power field.[13] For the prediction of aggressiveness, the EPPG also suggested the introduction in the routine clinical practice of the 5-tiered classification of Trouillas and colleagues[14] (1a, noninvasive and nonproliferative; 1b, proliferative and noninvasive; 2a, invasive and nonproliferative; 2b, invasive and proliferative; 3, pituitary carcinoma) given that its ability to predict the risk of progression and recurrence after surgery was validated by multiple independent studies.[13,15–17]

Treatment

Temozolomide

TMZ is an oral alkylating agent that led to a remarkable improvement in the 5-year overall and progression-free survival rates in patients with aggressive pituitary tumors

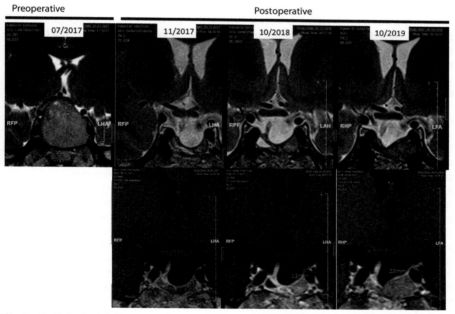

Fig. 3. Radiological follow-up of a rapidly growing pituitary tumor. (*Top*) Coronal T2-weighted native MRI sequences. (*Bottom*) Coronal T1-weighted contrast-enhanced MRI sequences.

and carcinomas that respond to TMZ.[18,19] TMZ monotherapy is now recommended by the ESE guidelines as the first-line chemotherapy after the failure of standard therapies and following documented tumor growth.[2] However, in the largest series to date, a radiological response was seen in only about 40% of cases treated with a first course of TMZ, with clinically functioning tumors showing a better response to TMZ than the nonfunctioning ones (the former were 3.3 times more likely to regress). Moreover, after TMZ was stopped, 25% to 48% of tumors progressed after a median of 1-year follow-up,[20] and the response to a second course of TMZ was rarely effective.[20,21] Therefore, other treatment options are clearly needed.

Because of insufficient data in the literature, the ESE guidelines only suggest, in patients with rapid tumor growth in whom maximal doses of radiotherapy have not been previously reached, the use of the Stupp protocol[2] (ie, radiotherapy with concomitant and adjuvant TMZ[22]). However, in glioblastomas, in which the Stupp protocol was first validated (before the Stupp protocol, newly diagnosed glioblastoma was treated by surgical resection, followed by adjuvant radiotherapy), adding to radiotherapy concomitant and adjuvant TMZ resulted in a survival benefit with minimal additional toxicity.[22] In aggressive pituitary tumors and carcinomas, data from the ESE survey on 157 patients treated with TMZ as first-line chemotherapy, of which 14 patients received concomitant radiotherapy, showed that first-line TMZ plus concomitant radiotherapy was associated with an increased response rate (complete or partial radiological response in 71% of the cases) compared with TMZ monotherapy (complete or partial radiological response in 34% of the cases). Although the investigators state that there were no evident clinicopathologic differences between these two treatment groups, they also note that most patients treated with first-line TMZ plus concomitant radiotherapy had not received radiotherapy previously,[20] and therefore this increase in the response rate may also reflect a selection bias. Nonetheless, TMZ was shown to have radiosensitizer properties in vitro and in vivo,[23] and, in an Italian study in which 27 patients with aggressive pituitary tumor or carcinomas were treated with radiotherapy, the tumor recurred after the last radiotherapy in all but 3 patients who were given TMZ concomitantly with radiotherapy or 1 month thereafter.[24] In our clinical practice, we tried the Stupp protocol in 2 patients not previously treated with radiotherapy, and achieved partial response in both cases (a male patient with a prolactinoma described in Ref.[25] and a male patient with a silent corticotroph carcinoma). We think that, in selected cases of pituitary tumors, the Stupp protocol may represent an option instead of using radiotherapy alone. However, doing so not only implies using a Stupp protocol instead of TMZ monotherapy, it also implies using it before the failure of radiotherapy alone. This option leads to a second point, that of using TMZ solely as a salvage therapy (ie, after the failure of all conventional therapies). So far, this is how TMZ was mainly used, and how it is recommended by the ESE guidelines. However, there are several investigators who argue that TMZ might have a place earlier in the management of aggressive pituitary tumors.[26–28] As long as the benefits are evaluated to be greater than the risks (the most commonly described side effects of TMZ when used in pituitary tumors were fatigue, nausea/vomiting, and cytopenias, but other side effects, including abnormal liver function, headache, hearing loss, edema, hypotension, and adrenal crisis, have also been noted[2,20]; in other cancers, although rarely, secondary hematological malignancies have been described[29]), the authors agree that TMZ might be worth trying earlier in the management of selected cases, and not only as a salvage therapy, but a stronger level of evidence would be welcomed.

Another point when it comes to TMZ is the duration of treatment. The ESE guidelines recommend that, in responders, TMZ should be administered for at least 6 months, and that longer duration of treatment should be considered in the case of continued therapeutic benefit.[2] It is not currently known whether continuing the treatment for a longer period improves the chances of a sustained remission in responders,[2] but it is known that, after stopping TMZ, an important percentage of responders show progressive disease and that the response to a second course of TMZ is poor.[20] In contrast, an argument in favor of a shorter duration of treatment is the cumulative bone marrow toxicity caused by TMZ, especially because patients with pituitary tumors are more probable long-term survivors.[26] Therefore, prospective studies analyzing the optimal duration of treatment with TMZ would be most welcomed. In our practice, we usually continue TMZ for as long as an antitumoral and hormonal effect is observed and the treatment is tolerated. However, we try to decrease TMZ to a half-dose after 24 cycles in order to limit the potential cumulative toxicity.

Other treatment options

The main other treatment options have been recently reviewed by our team[30] and involve a limited number of patients: 20 patients treated with peptide receptor radionuclide therapy (PRRT),[19,20,28,31–37] 12 treated with bevacizumab (a vascular endothelial growth factor receptor–targeted therapy),[2,20,38–42] 10 treated with tyrosine kinase inhibitors,[20,43,44] 6 treated with everolimus (a mammalian target of rapamycin inhibitor),[20,45–47] and 2 patients treated with immune checkpoint inhibitors.[48,49] Not enough data are available to draw any definitive conclusion, but, based on the radiological response, the therapies currently showing the most promise are bevacizumab, PRRT, and immune checkpoint inhibitors.[30] **Fig. 4** shows the radiological response of these 50 patients on the aforementioned treatments.[30,49]

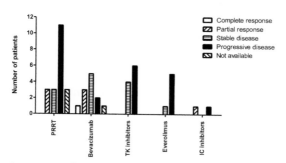

Fig. 4. Radiological response of the aggressive pituitary tumors and carcinomas treated so far with peptide receptor radionuclide therapy (PRRT), bevacizumab, tyrosine kinase (TK) inhibitors, everolimus, and immune checkpoint (IC) inhibitors. Note that some of these patients were previously treated with temozolomide, and that, in some patients, the mentioned treatment was administered concomitantly with other treatments (including temozolomide). Regarding the 2 cases treated so far with IC inhibitors, partial response was seen in a patient with corticotroph carcinoma treated with combined ipilimumab and nivolumab, whereas progressive disease was seen in a patient with an aggressive corticotroph adenoma treated with pembrolizumab. Complete response = no visible tumor; partial response = greater than 30% decrease in tumor size; stable disease = less than 10% increase and less than 30% decrease in tumor size; progressive disease = new metastases or greater than 10% increase in tumor size. (*Data from* Ilie MD, Lasolle H, Raverot G. Emerging and Novel Treatments for Pituitary Tumors. *J Clin Med*. 2019; 8(8):1107:1-17; and Caccese M, Barbot M, Ceccato F, et al. Rapid disease progression in patient with mismatch-repair deficiency pituitary ACTH-secreting adenoma treated with checkpoint inhibitor pembrolizumab: *Anticancer Drugs*. 2020; 31(2):199-204.)

Follow-up

Imaging (usually MRI) and full endocrine evaluation are recommended every 3 to 12 months, depending on the location of the tumor, the previous growth rate, and the clinical context. The follow-up should be lifelong, because the acceleration of the growth rate and metastasis may appear many years after the diagnosis of an aggressive pituitary tumor.[2]

The average latency period from the primary diagnosis of a pituitary tumor to metastasis was 9 years in a recent review of 72 cases of pituitary carcinomas. The metastases were most frequently intracranial and spinal, followed by liver, cervical lymph nodes, and bone metastases (lung, endolymphatic sac, and orbit metastases were rare).[50] In patients with aggressive pituitary tumors, it is currently recommended to screen for metastases either in case of discordant biochemical and radiological findings (ie, when hormone levels increase without a corresponding increase in tumor dimension) or in case of site-specific symptoms (neck pain, back pain, and/or neurologic complaints). In these cases, the guidelines recommend structural (MRI and CT scans) and/or functional imaging studies, such as fluorodeoxyglucose and/or somatostatin receptor PET-CT scans, as appropriate. Regarding the treatment of metastases, the same guidelines suggest locoregional therapies in cases of isolated metastases/localized disease and low metastatic disease burden.[2]

SUMMARY

Especially given the rarity of aggressive pituitary tumors and carcinomas, and the scarcity of available data, the ESE guidelines are of tremendous help, providing clinicians with vital guidance in the management of such tumors. However, several important points regarding both diagnosis (how to classify the tumor growth velocity, how to predict an aggressive behavior, and so forth) and treatment (should TMZ be used earlier in selected cases of aggressive tumors, should a Stupp protocol sometimes be used instead of radiotherapy alone, and so forth) remain unanswered or only partially answered. Studies on these matters are therefore urgently needed in order to enable evidence-based answers and recommendations, and would be of most help to the patients bearing such tumors and to the clinicians caring for them.

DISCLOSURE

The authors have nothing to disclose.

REFERENCES

1. Dudziak K, Honegger J, Bornemann A, et al. Pituitary carcinoma with malignant growth from first presentation and fulminant clinical course—case report and review of the literature. J Clin Endocrinol Metab 2011;96(9):2665–9.

2. Raverot G, Burman P, McCormack A, et al. European Society of Endocrinology Clinical Practice Guidelines for the management of aggressive pituitary tumours and carcinomas. Eur J Endocrinol 2018;178(1):G1–24.

3. Asa SL, Casar-Borota O, Chanson P, et al. From pituitary adenoma to pituitary neuroendocrine tumor (PitNET): an International Pituitary Pathology Club proposal. Endocr Relat Cancer 2017;24(4):C5–8.

4. Ho KKY, Fleseriu M, Wass J, et al. A tale of pituitary adenomas: to NET or not to NET: Pituitary Society position statement. Pituitary 2019. https://doi.org/10.1007/s11102-019-00988-2.

5. Trouillas J, Burman P, McCormack A, et al. Aggressive pituitary tumours and carcinomas: two sides of the same coin? Eur J Endocrinol 2018;178(6):C7–9.
6. Lopes MBS. The 2017 World Health Organization classification of tumors of the pituitary gland: a summary. Acta Neuropathol 2017;134(4):521–35.
7. Micko ASG, Wöhrer A, Wolfsberger S, et al. Invasion of the cavernous sinus space in pituitary adenomas: endoscopic verification and its correlation with an MRI-based classification. J Neurosurg 2015;122(4):803–11.
8. Saeger W, Petersenn S, Schöfl C, et al. Emerging histopathological and genetic parameters of pituitary adenomas: clinical impact and recommendation for future WHO classification. Endocr Pathol 2016;27(2):115–22.
9. Buchy M, Lapras V, Rabilloud M, et al. Predicting early post-operative remission in pituitary adenomas: evaluation of the modified knosp classification. Pituitary 2019;22(5):467–75.
10. Imber BS, Lin AL, Zhang Z, et al. Comparison of radiographic approaches to assess treatment response in pituitary adenomas: is RECIST or RANO Good enough? J Endocr Soc 2019;3(9):1693–706.
11. Schwartz LH, Litière S, de Vries E, et al. RECIST 1.1—Update and clarification: From the RECIST committee. Eur J Cancer 2016;62:132–7.
12. Eisenhauer EA, Therasse P, Bogaerts J, et al. New response evaluation criteria in solid tumours: Revised RECIST guideline (version 1.1). Eur J Cancer 2009;45(2): 228–47.
13. Villa C, Vasiljevic A, Jaffrain-Rea ML, et al. A standardised diagnostic approach to pituitary neuroendocrine tumours (PitNETs): a European Pituitary Pathology Group (EPPG) proposal. Virchows Arch 2019. https://doi.org/10.1007/s00428-019-02655-0.
14. Trouillas J, Roy P, Sturm N, et al. A new prognostic clinicopathological classification of pituitary adenomas: a multicentric case–control study of 410 patients with 8 years post-operative follow-up. Acta Neuropathol 2013;126(1):123–35.
15. Asioli S, Righi A, Iommi M, et al. Validation of a clinicopathological score for the prediction of post-surgical evolution of pituitary adenoma: retrospective analysis on 566 patients from a tertiary care centre. Eur J Endocrinol 2019;127–34. https://doi.org/10.1530/EJE-18-0749.
16. Lelotte J, Mourin A, Fomekong E, et al. Both invasiveness and proliferation criteria predict recurrence of non-functioning pituitary macroadenomas after surgery: a retrospective analysis of a monocentric cohort of 120 patients. Eur J Endocrinol 2018;237–46. https://doi.org/10.1530/EJE-17-0965.
17. Raverot G, Dantony E, Beauvy J, et al. Risk of recurrence in pituitary neuroendocrine tumors: a prospective study using a five-tiered classification. J Clin Endocrinol Metab 2017;102(9):3368–74.
18. Ji Y, Vogel RI, Lou E. Temozolomide treatment of pituitary carcinomas and atypical adenomas: systematic review of case reports. Neurooncol Pract 2016;3(3): 188–95.
19. Lasolle H, Cortet C, Castinetti F, et al. Temozolomide treatment can improve overall survival in aggressive pituitary tumors and pituitary carcinomas. Eur J Endocrinol 2017;176(6):769–77.
20. McCormack A, Dekkers OM, Petersenn S, et al. Treatment of aggressive pituitary tumours and carcinomas: results of a European Society of Endocrinology (ESE) survey 2016. Eur J Endocrinol 2018;265–76. https://doi.org/10.1530/EJE-17-0933.

21. Bengtsson D, Schrøder HD, Berinder K, et al. Tumoral MGMT content predicts survival in patients with aggressive pituitary tumors and pituitary carcinomas given treatment with temozolomide. Endocrine 2018;62(3):737–9.

22. Stupp R, Mason WP, van den Bent MJ, et al. Radiotherapy plus Concomitant and Adjuvant Temozolomide for Glioblastoma. N Engl J Med 2005;352(10):987–96.

23. Kil WJ, Cerna D, Burgan WE, et al. In vitro and In vivo Radiosensitization Induced by the DNA Methylating Agent Temozolomide. Clin Cancer Res 2008;14(3): 931–8.

24. Losa M, Bogazzi F, Cannavo S, et al. Temozolomide therapy in patients with aggressive pituitary adenomas or carcinomas. J Neurooncol 2016;126(3): 519–25.

25. Lasolle H, Ilie MD, Raverot G. Aggressive prolactinomas: how to manage? Pituitary 2019. https://doi.org/10.1007/s11102-019-01000-7.

26. Lin AL, Sum MW, DeAngelis LM. Is there a role for early chemotherapy in the management of pituitary adenomas? Neurooncol 2016;18(10):1350–6.

27. Whitelaw BC. How and when to use temozolomide to treat aggressive pituitary tumours. Endocr Relat Cancer 2019;26(9):R545–52.

28. Bengtsson D, Schrøder HD, Andersen M, et al. Long-Term Outcome and MGMT as a predictive marker in 24 patients with atypical pituitary adenomas and pituitary carcinomas given treatment with temozolomide. J Clin Endocrinol Metab 2015;100(4):1689–98.

29. Momota H, Narita Y, Miyakita Y, et al. Secondary hematological malignancies associated with temozolomide in patients with glioma. Neurooncol 2013;15(10): 1445–50.

30. Ilie MD, Lasolle H, Raverot G. Emerging and Novel Treatments for Pituitary Tumors. J Clin Med 2019;8(8):1107, 1-17.

31. Giuffrida G, Ferraù F, Laudicella R, et al. Peptide receptor radionuclide therapy for aggressive pituitary tumors: a monocentric experience. Endocr Connect 2019;8(5):528–35.

32. Baldari S, Ferraù F, Alafaci C, et al. First demonstration of the effectiveness of peptide receptor radionuclide therapy (PRRT) with 111In-DTPA-octreotide in a giant PRL-secreting pituitary adenoma resistant to conventional treatment. Pituitary 2012;15(S1):57–60.

33. Komor J, Reubi JC, Christ ER. Peptide receptor radionuclide therapy in a patient with disabling non-functioning pituitary adenoma. Pituitary 2014;17(3):227–31.

34. Maclean J, Aldridge M, Bomanji J, et al. Peptide receptor radionuclide therapy for aggressive atypical pituitary adenoma/carcinoma: variable clinical response in preliminary evaluation. Pituitary 2014;17(6):530–8.

35. Kovács GL, Góth M, Rotondo F, et al. ACTH-secreting Crooke cell carcinoma of the pituitary: crooke cell carcinoma of the pituitary. Eur J Clin Invest 2013; 43(1):20–6.

36. Waligórska-Stachura J, Gut P, Sawicka-Gutaj N, et al. Growth hormone–secreting macroadenoma of the pituitary gland successfully treated with the radiolabeled somatostatin analog 90Y-DOTATATE: case report. J Neurosurg 2016;125(2): 346–9.

37. Priola SM, Esposito F, Cannavò S, et al. Aggressive pituitary adenomas: the dark side of the moon. World Neurosurg 2017;97:140–55.

38. Ortiz LD, Syro LV, Scheithauer BW, et al. Anti-VEGF therapy in pituitary carcinoma. Pituitary 2012;15(3):445–9.

39. Kurowska M, Nowakowski A, Zieliński G, et al. Temozolomide-Induced Shrinkage of Invasive Pituitary Adenoma in Patient with Nelson's Syndrome: A Case Report and Review of the Literature. Case Rep Endocrinol 2015;2015:1–8.

40. Touma W, Hoostal S, Peterson RA, et al. Successful treatment of pituitary carcinoma with concurrent radiation, temozolomide, and bevacizumab after resection. J Clin Neurosci 2017;41:75–7.

41. Rotman LE, Vaughan TB, Hackney JR, et al. Long-term survival after transformation of an adrenocorticotropic hormone–secreting pituitary macroadenoma to a silent corticotroph pituitary carcinoma. World Neurosurg 2019;122:417–23.

42. O'Riordan LM, Greally M, Coleman N, et al. Metastatic ACTH-producing pituitary carcinoma managed with combination pasireotide and bevacizumab following failure of temozolamide therapy: A case report. J Clin Oncol 2013; 31(15_suppl):e13022.

43. Cooper O, Mamelak A, Bannykh S, et al. Prolactinoma ErbB receptor expression and targeted therapy for aggressive tumors. Endocrine 2014;46(2):318–27.

44. Cooper O, Bonert V, Rudnick J, et al. SUN-442 EGFR/ErbB2 targeted therapy for aggressive prolactinomas. J Endocr Soc 2019;3(Supplement_1). https://doi.org/ 10.1210/js.2019-SUN-442.

45. Donovan LE, Arnal AV, Wang S-H, et al. Widely metastatic atypical pituitary adenoma with mTOR pathway STK11(F298L) mutation treated with everolimus therapy. CNS Oncol 2016;5(4):203–9.

46. Jouanneau E, Wierinckx A, Ducray F, et al. New targeted therapies in pituitary carcinoma resistant to temozolomide. Pituitary 2012;15(1):37–43.

47. Zhang D, Way JS, Zhang X, et al. Effect of everolimus in treatment of aggressive prolactin-secreting pituitary adenomas. J Clin Endocrinol Metab 2019;104(6): 1929–36.

48. Lin AL, Jonsson P, Tabar V, et al. Marked Response of a hypermutated ACTH-secreting pituitary carcinoma to ipilimumab and nivolumab. J Clin Endocrinol Metab 2018;103(10):3925–30.

49. Caccese M, Barbot M, Ceccato F, et al. Rapid disease progression in patient with mismatch-repair deficiency pituitary ACTH-secreting adenoma treated with checkpoint inhibitor pembrolizumab. Anticancer Drugs 2019. https://doi.org/10. 1097/CAD.0000000000000856.

50. Yoo F, Kuan EC, Heaney AP, et al. Corticotrophic pituitary carcinoma with cervical metastases: case series and literature review. Pituitary 2018;21(3):290–301.

Diabetes Insipidus
An Update

Julie Refardt, MD[a,b], Bettina Winzeler, MD[a,b],
Mirjam Christ-Crain, MD, PhD[a,b,*]

KEYWORDS

- Polyuria polydipsia syndrome • Diabetes insipidus • Primary polydipsia

KEY POINTS

- There are 3 main types of polyuria polydipsia syndrome, namely, central diabetes insipidus, nephrogenic diabetes insipidus and primary polydipsia.
- In addition, gestational diabetes insipidus can occur owing to increased arginine vasopressin metabolism during pregnancy.
- Copeptin, the C-terminal segment of the arginine vasopressin prohormone, is an easy-to-measure arginine vasopressin surrogate.
- Copeptin measurement upon osmotic stimulation with hypertonic saline or upon nonosmotic stimulation improves the differential diagnosis of diabetes insipidus.
- Treatment of central diabetes insipidus has not changed significantly. Desmopressin is the treatment of choice, in oral or nasal form.

INTRODUCTION

Diabetes insipidus is one of the main causes of the polyuria polydipsia syndrome and is characterized by a high hypotonic urinary output of more than 50 mL/kg body weight per 24 hours, accompanied by polydipsia of more than 3 L/d.[1] After exclusion of osmotic diuresis (such as uncontrolled diabetes mellitus), the differential diagnosis of diabetes insipidus involves the distinction between primary forms (with central or renal origin) and secondary forms of polyuria (resulting from primary polydipsia). Central diabetes insipidus, also called hypothalamic or neurogenic diabetes insipidus, results from inadequate secretion and usually deficient synthesis of arginine vasopressin (AVP) in the hypothalamic neurohypophyseal system in response to osmotic stimulation. It is mostly acquired owing to disorders that disrupt the neurohypophysis. Less

^a Division of Endocrinology, Diabetes and Metabolism, Department of Clinical Research, University Hospital Basel, University of Basel, Basel, Switzerland; ^b Department of Endocrinology, University Hospital Basel, University of Basel, Petersgraben 4, Basel 4031, Switzerland
* Corresponding author. Department of Endocrinology, University Hospital Basel, University of Basel, Petersgraben 4, Basel 4031, Switzerland.
E-mail address: mirjam.christ@usb.ch

Endocrinol Metab Clin N Am 49 (2020) 517–531
https://doi.org/10.1016/j.ecl.2020.05.012
0889-8529/20/© 2020 Elsevier Inc. All rights reserved.

endo.theclinics.com

commonly, it is congenital by genetic mutations of the AVP gene.[2] Nephrogenic diabetes insipidus can be congenital owing to mutations in the gene for the AVP V2R or the aquaporin 2 (AQP2) water channel.[3] More common, however, it presents as an adverse effect of certain drugs, most prominently lithium, or owing to electrolyte disorders, that is, hypercalcemia or hypokalemia. Last, primary polydipsia is characterized by excessive fluid intake leading to polyuria in the presence of intact AVP secretion and appropriate antidiuretic renal response. The chronic polydipsia eventually leads to a decreased concentration ability of the kidneys—the so-called wash out phenomenon—which makes it difficult to differentiate it from diabetes insipidus.[4]

Differentiation between the 3 mentioned entities is important because the treatment strategies vary and application of the wrong treatment can be dangerous.[5] Reliable differentiation is, however, often difficult to achieve,[6] especially in patients with primary polydipsia or partial, mild forms of diabetes insipidus.[1,7]

This review describes the different types and etiologies of diabetes insipidus and then focuses on new procedures in the differential diagnosis of diabetes insipidus. Treatment is discussed briefly as well.

POLYURIA POLYDIPSIA SYNDROME

Diabetes insipidus is a rare disease with a prevalence of approximately 1:25,000.[8] The disorder can manifest at any age, and the prevalence is similar among males and females. The clinical manifestation of diabetes insipidus, characterized by excessive excretion of large volumes of diluted urine, is caused by a decrease in the secretion or action of AVP. There are 3 main types of polyuria polydipsia, which are characterized by a different defect. In addition, gestational diabetes insipidus can occur owing to increased AVP metabolism during pregnancy (**Fig. 1, Table 1**).

The most common type is central diabetes insipidus, and is caused by inadequate AVP production and secretion from the posterior pituitary in response to osmotic stimulation. In most cases, this effect is due to destruction of the neurohypophysis by a variety of acquired causes, for example, trauma, surgery, vascular or granulomatous etiologies (see **Table 1**). It can also be of congenital origin, in which case it is most often owing to an autosomal dominant AVP gene mutation.[9]

A second variant of diabetes insipidus is caused by decreased renal sensitivity to the antidiuretic effect of physiologic levels of AVP.[3] This AVP insensitivity leads to a deficiency of AQP-mediated water reabsorption in the collecting duct. This nephrogenic variant of the diabetes insipidus can be due to mutations of the key proteins AVP V2 receptor and AQP2; however, it can also be secondary to drug exposure (especially lithium), infiltrating lesions of the kidneys or vascular disorders, among others (see **Table 1**).

A third mechanism of the clinical syndrome is due to physiologic suppression of AVP secretion by excessive, osmotically independent fluid intake plus loss of the renal concentration ability owing to the washout phenomenon described elsewhere in this article.[4] This type is referred to as primary polydipsia to distinguish it from the secondary polydipsia that occurs in response to water loss in other types of diabetes insipidus. In addition to psychiatric patients and health enthusiasts, there is a small subgroup of patients with primary polydipsia commonly referred to as having dipsogenic diabetes insipidus, in which polydipsia seems to be due to an abnormally low thirst threshold.[10]

A final type of defect, gestational diabetes insipidus, is caused by an increased degradation of AVP by the placenta enzyme vasopressinase,[11,12] thus presenting similar to the abnormalities in central diabetes insipidus. In some cases, patients

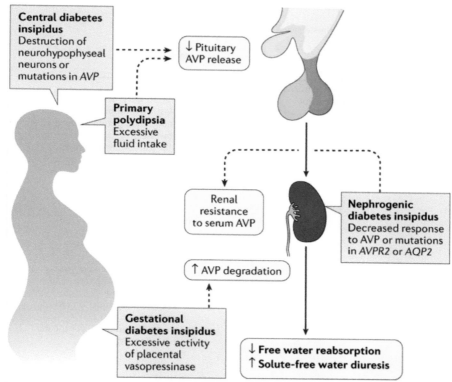

Fig. 1. Different etiologies of polyuria polydipsia syndrome. (*From* Christ-Crain M, Bichet DG, Fenske WK, et al. Diabetes insipidus. Nat Rev Dis Primers. 2019; 8;5(1):54; with permission.)

may be predisposed to its development by preexisting, subclinical deficiency in AVP.[13,14] All etiologies are summarized in **Table 1** and in **Fig. 1**.

DIABETES INSIPIDUS: AN UPDATE ON DIAGNOSIS
Clinical Manifestations

The lead symptoms of diabetes insipidus are increased thirst, polyuria, and polydipsia, which are not necessarily different in their specific manifestation between diabetes insipidus and primary polydipsia.[15] Patients with central diabetes insipidus more often describe nocturia and a sudden onset of symptoms. This results from the fact that urinary concentration can often be maintained fairly well until the residual neuronal capacity of the hypothalamus to synthesize AVP decreases to less than 10% to 15% of normal, after which urine output increases dramatically.

Patients with diabetes insipidus, especially those with underlying osmoreceptor defect syndromes, can manifest with varying degrees of dehydration and hyperosmolality, if renal water losses cannot be fully compensated by fluid intake. Resulting symptoms can be divided into those produced by dehydration, which are largely cardiovascular (including hypotension, acute tubular necrosis secondary to renal hypoperfusion, and shock)[16,17] and those caused by hyperosmolality. The latter are mainly neurologic and reflect the degree of brain dehydration as a result of osmotic

Table 1
Etiology of polyuria polydipsia syndrome

Type of Hypotonic Polyuria	Basic Defect	Causes
Central diabetes insipidus	Deficiency in AVP synthesis or secretion	Acquired Trauma (surgery, deceleration injury) Neoplastic (craniopharyngioma, meningioma, germinoma, metastases) Vascular (cerebral/hypothalamic hemorrhage, infarction or ligation of anterior communicating artery aneurysm) Granulomatous (histiocytosis, sarcoidosis) Infectious (meningitis, encephalitis, tuberculosis) Inflammatory/autoimmune (lymphocytic infundibuloneurohypophysitis, IgG4 neurohypophysitis) Drug/toxin induced Osmoreceptor dysfunction (adipsic diabetes insipidus) Others (hydrocephalus, ventricular/suprasellar cyst, trauma, degenerative disease) Idiopathic Congenital Autosomal dominant: AVP gene mutation Autosomal recessive: Wolfram syndrome (diabetes insipidus, diabetes mellitus, optic atrophy, and deafness) X-linked recessive
Nephrogenic diabetes insipidus	Reduced renal sensitivity to antidiuretic effect of physiologic AVP levels	Acquired Drug exposure (lithium, demeclocyclin, cisplatin, etc) Hypercalcemia, hypokalemia Infiltrating lesions (sarcoidosis, amyloidosis, multiple myeloma, etc) Vascular disorders (sickle cell anemia) Mechanical (polycystic kidney disease, urethral obstruction) Congenital X-linked *AVPR2* gene mutations Autosomal recessive or dominant *AQP2* gene mutations

(continued on next page)

Table 1 (continued)		
Type of Hypotonic Polyuria	**Basic Defect**	**Causes**
Primary polydipsia	Excessive osmotically unregulated fluid intake	Dipsogenic (downward resetting of the thirst threshold; idiopathic or similar lesions as with central diabetes insipidus) Psychosis intermittent hyponatremia polydipsia (psychosis, intermittent hyponatremia, and polydipsia syndrome) Compulsive water drinking Health enthusiasts
Gestational diabetes insipidus	Increased enzymatic metabolism of circulating AVP hormone	Increased AVP metabolism Pregnancy

water shifts from the intracellular compartment. Manifestations may range from nonspecific symptoms such as irritability and cognitive dysfunction to more severe manifestations such as disorientation, reduced consciousness, seizure, coma, focal neurologic deficits, and cerebral infarction.[16,18]

Radiologic Findings

Sometimes useful information in the differential diagnosis of diabetes insipidus may derive from unenhanced brain MRI via assessment of the posterior pituitary and the pituitary stalk. An area of hyperintensity, often referred to as the pituitary "bright spot," is normally observed in the posterior part of the sella turcica in sagittal views on T1-weighted images,[19] and is thought to result from the T1-shortening effects of stored AVP in neurosecretory granules of the posterior lobe of the pituitary.[20] Although earlier small-scale studies demonstrated the presence of the bright spot in normal subjects and its absence in patients with central diabetes insipidus,[21] subsequent larger studies reported an age-related absence of the bright spot in up to 52% to 100% of normal subjects.[22] Conversely, individual cases with persistent bright spot have been reported in patients with central diabetes insipidus,[23,24] possibly owing to an early stage of disease or a reflection of oxytocin stores rather than AVP. In nephrogenic diabetes insipidus, the bright spot has been reported to be absent in some patients, but present in others.[25] A recent large prospective observation of 92 patients with polyuria polydipsia syndrome receiving brain MRI revealed absence of the bright spot in 70% of patients with central diabetes insipidus but also in 39% of patients with primary polydipsia.[15] Consequently, the presence or absence of the bright spot on MRI seems not to be qualified as a diagnostic test in patients with diabetes insipidus.

A similar conclusion seems to apply to the assessment of the pituitary stalk, whose enlargement beyond 2 to 3 mm is generally considered to be pathognomonic,[26] but is not necessarily specific for idiopathic central diabetes insipidus.[15,27] The situation is quite different if scans reveal thickening of the stalk with an absence of the bright spot; in this case, a diligent search for neoplastic or infiltrative lesions of the hypothalamus or pituitary gland is indicated.[28]

Tests for Differential Diagnosis of Diabetes Insipidus

Differentiation between the 3 main entities (ie, central diabetes insipidus, nephrogenic diabetes insipidus, and primary polydipsia) is important because the treatment strategies vary and application of the wrong treatment can be dangerous.[5] However, reliable differentiation has proved difficult in the past,[6] because many available tests are unsatisfactory[29] and often result in false diagnoses, especially in patients with primary polydipsia or partial, mild forms of diabetes insipidus.[1,7]

The water deprivation test

The accepted gold standard for many years for differential diagnosis of polyuria polydipsia syndrome was the indirect water deprivation test. This test is based on the concept that AVP activity is indirectly assessed by measurement of the urine concentration capacity during a prolonged period of dehydration, and again after a subsequent injection of an exogenous synthetic AVP variant (desmopressin).[30–32] Interpretation of the test results is based on recommendations from Miller and colleagues.[33] Nephrogenic diabetes insipidus is diagnosed if urinary osmolality remains below 300 mOsm/kg with water deprivation and does not increase by more than 50% after exogenous synthetic AVP injection. If the respective increase upon exogenous synthetic AVP is more than 50%, complete diabetes insipidus is diagnosed. In partial central diabetes insipidus and primary polydipsia, urinary concentration increases to 300 to 800 mOsm/kg, with an increase upon desmopressin of more than 9% (in partial central diabetes insipidus) and less than 9% (in primary polydipsia).

However, these criteria from Miller and colleagues are based on data from only 36 patients, showing a wide overlap in urinary osmolalities. Furthermore, the diagnostic criteria for this test are derived from a single study with post hoc assessment[33] and have not been prospectively validated on a larger scale (for details see[5]). Consequently, the indirect water deprivation test has been shown to have considerable diagnostic limitations, with an overall diagnostic accuracy of 70%, and an accuracy of only 41% in patients with primary polydipsia.[7] These findings have been confirmed in a recent large prospective observation on 156 patients with polyuria polydipsia syndrome.[15]

There are several reasons for the disappointing diagnostic outcome of the indirect water deprivation test. First, chronic polyuria itself can affect renal concentration capacity through renal washout or downregulation of expression of AQP2 water channels in the kidney.[4] This process may lead to a reduced renal response to osmotic stimulation or to exogenous desmopressin[4] in different forms of chronic polyuria.[33] Second, in patients with a deficiency of AVP, urine concentration can be higher than expected,[34,35] especially in patients with impaired glomerular function,[29,36,37] or as a result of a compensatory increase in AVPR2 gene expression in chronic central diabetes insipidus.[38] Finally, patients with acquired nephrogenic diabetes insipidus often exhibit only a partial resistance to AVP leading to a higher than expected increase in urine osmolality upon exogeneous desmopressin administration.

Arginine vasopressin measurement

To overcome these limitations of the indirect water deprivation test, direct measurement of AVP has been proposed to improve the differential diagnosis of polyuria polydipsia syndrome. Indeed, first data published in 1981[39] reported that patients with central diabetes insipidus showed AVP levels of less than a calculated normal area (defining the normal relationship between plasma osmolality and AVP levels), whereas patients with nephrogenic diabetes insipidus showed levels above the normal area, and patients with primary polydipsia demonstrated concentrations within the normal range. However, despite these promising first results, AVP measurement failed to enter routine clinical use. The main reason for this are the technical limitations of the AVP assay resulting in a high preanalytical instability.[35,40,41] Second, the results of studies using commercially available AVP assays have been disappointing, with a diagnostic accuracy of only 38% and particularly poor differentiation between partial central diabetes insipidus and primary polydipsia.[5,7] Third, an accurate definition of the normal physiologic area defining the relationship between plasma AVP and osmolality is still lacking, especially for commercially available assays.[39,42,43] This, however, is a crucial prerequisite for the identification of inadequate AVP secretion in patients suspected of diabetes insipidus.[7]

Copeptin-based new diagnostic algorithms

Copeptin, the C-terminal segment of the AVP prohormone, is an easy-to-measure AVP surrogate with high ex vivo stability.[41] Despite a possible involvement in the folding of the AVP precursor,[44,45] no physiologic role for copeptin has yet been found. However, copeptin shows a strong correlation with AVP and plasma osmolality, the latter correlation being even stronger than for AVP.[46] The observation that copeptin reflects osmosensitive circulating AVP concentrations makes copeptin a promising biomarker for the differential diagnosis of polyuria polydipsia syndrome.

Two studies have shown that a basal copeptin level greater than 21.4 pmol/L without prior thirsting unequivocally identifies nephrogenic diabetes insipidus, rendering a further water deprivation unnecessary in these patients.[7,47] However, for the more challenging differentiation between patients with primary polydipsia and central diabetes insipidus osmotically stimulated copeptin values are needed because baseline levels show a large overlap in those patient groups.[47] The use of osmotically stimulated copeptin levels as a diagnostic tool for diabetes insipidus has recently been confirmed in the so far largest study including 156 patients with diabetes insipidus or primary polydipsia.[15] Osmotic stimulation was achieved using a body weight–adapted hypertonic (3%) saline infusion aimed at a plasma sodium level of 150 mmol/L or greater, at which time copeptin was measured. In a head-to-head comparison, osmotically stimulated copeptin at a cut-off level of greater than 4.9 pmol/L showed a greater diagnostic accuracy of 97% (93% sensitivity and 100% specificity) to distinguish patients with primary polydipsia from patients with central diabetes insipidus compared with the classical water deprivation test with an accuracy of 77% (86% sensitivity and 70% specificity).[15] Copeptin taken at the end of the water deprivation test did not improve its diagnostic accuracy. This finding is best explained by the insufficient osmotic stimulus achieved by water deprivation alone.[15] The diagnostic accuracy of the 2 tests in comparison is shown in **Fig. 2**.

In addition to its superior diagnostic accuracy, the hypertonic saline stimulation test comes with the advantage that it can be performed in the out-patient clinic, whereas in most countries patients have to be hospitalized for the water deprivation test. Also, despite the adverse symptoms associated with osmotic stimulation, patients seem to prefer it over the water deprivation test.[15]

According to these data, copeptin can be used as a reliable biomarker to discriminate between different forms of the polyuria polydipsia syndrome, therefore the osmotic stimulated copeptin levels will probably replace the classical water deprivation test in the future. However, it has to be noted that the hypertonic saline infusion test requires close monitoring of sodium levels to ascertain a diagnostically meaningful increase of plasma sodium within the hyperosmotic range,[48,49] while preventing a marked increase.

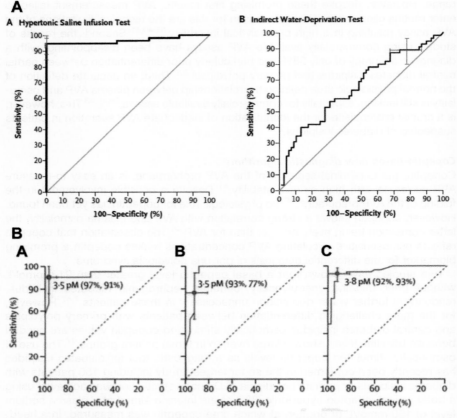

Fig. 2. (*A*) ROC analysis of hypertonic saline test plus copeptin measurement (panel A) as compared to the indirect water deprivation test (panel B). (*B*) ROC analysis of arginine-stimulated copeptin level (panel A-C). (panel A) ROC for the derivation cohort, (panel B) validation cohort, (panel C) whole cohort. ([*A*] *From* Fenske W, Refardt J, Chifu I, et al. A copeptin-based approach in the diagnosis of Diabetes insipidus. N Engl J Med 2018;379:428-39; with permission; and [*B*] Winzeler B, Cesana-Nigro N, Refardt J, et al. Arginine-stimulated copeptin measurements in the differential diagnosis of diabetes insipidus: a prospective diagnostic study. Lancet 2019;394(10198):587-95; with permission.)

An easier approach to stimulate copeptin—without inducing high sodium levels—is via arginine infusion. Indeed, arginine infusion, which has widely been used to stimulate growth hormone and therefore to test for growth hormone deficiency,[50] is also a potent nonosmotic stimulus of the posterior pituitary gland. Arginine-stimulated copeptin values were evaluated in a prospective diagnostic study with 98 patients with central diabetes insipidus or primary polydipsia.[51] A copeptin cutoff of 3.8 pmol/L at 60 minutes after arginine infusion had an accuracy of 93% (sensitivity 93%, specificity 92%) to diagnose diabetes insipidus[51] (see **Fig. 2**). The test was safe and well-tolerated, although nausea was a frequently reported symptom. Importantly, other adverse effects such as vertigo, headache, or malaise (previously described in ≥70% of patients during the hypertonic saline infusion test)[15] were negligible during arginine stimulation. Further advantages of the arginine test over the hypertonic saline infusion test and the water deprivation test are the shorter test duration (a single copeptin measurement after 60 minutes is sufficient) and the improved feasibility without the need for sodium monitoring.

Accordingly, this proof-of-concept study offers the promise of a simple and convenient test that may become the standard diagnostic approach for diabetes insipidus. A definitive head-to-head study comparing the diagnostic accuracy of hypertonic saline-stimulated versus arginine-stimulated copeptin measurement is currently ongoing (NCT03572166). Pending those results, we suggest a stepwise approach: a diagnostic workflow favoring copeptin as a critical diagnostic marker in the differentiation of polyuria polydipsia syndrome, as shown in **Fig. 3**.

Copeptin has also been evaluated as a predictive marker for the development of diabetes insipidus in the setting of sellar region operations. The manipulation or damage of the pituitary gland during surgery may lead to postoperative diabetes insipidus and severe hypernatremia in the early postoperative period if fluid is not adequately replenished. A prospective multicenter study including 205 patients undergoing pituitary surgery showed that patients who did not exhibit a pronounced stress-induced copeptin increase after surgery (reflecting a damaged neurohypophysis) were at risk for postoperative central diabetes insipidus.[52] In this cohort, 50 patients (24%) developed postoperative central diabetes insipidus, which was predicted by a postoperative (measured within the first 12 hours after surgery) copeptin value of less than 2.5 pmol/L with a high specificity of 97% (positive predictive value of 81%). In contrast, a high postoperative copeptin value of greater than 30 pmol/L was predictive of an uneventful postoperative course and excluded the development of central diabetes insipidus with a negative predictive value of 95% and a sensitivity of 94%.

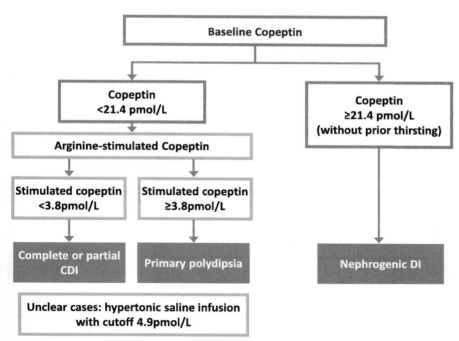

Fig. 3. Suggested copeptin-based 2-step algorithm in the differential diagnosis of polyuria polydipsia syndrome.

A recent smaller study evaluating 66 patients undergoing pituitary surgery suggested using copeptin values 1 hour after extubation to predict central diabetes insipidus.[53] In this study, a copeptin value of less than or equal to 12.8 pmol/L indicated patients at risk for central diabetes insipidus. Moreover, a copeptin level of 4.2 pmol/L or greater excluded permanent forms. Although the reliability of their proposed cut offs is limited by the small number of affected patients (n = 8), their results confirmed postoperative copeptin measurements as a useful tool for risk stratification of the development of postoperative central diabetes insipidus. Additionally, the extent of stress-induced AVP/copeptin release at this early time point after extubation may distinguish between transient and permanent forms of diabetes insipidus.

DIABETES INSIPIDUS: AN UPDATE ON MANAGEMENT

In contrast with the diagnostic evaluation, treatment of diabetes insipidus did not significantly change over the last decades. Therefore, we briefly summarize the current treatment options for central and nephrogenic diabetes insipidus.

Untreated central and nephrogenic diabetes insipidus may lead to hyperosmolar dehydration. The general goals of treatment of all forms of diabetes insipidus are therefore a correction of any preexisting water deficits and a reduction in ongoing excessive urinary water losses (for details please see[54]).

Specific replacement therapy for central diabetes insipidus treatment is usually straightforward and primarily aims at ameliorating symptoms (polyuria and polydipsia) by replacing antidiuretic hormone. Desmopressin, an AVP analogue, is the preferred drug for almost all patients. To avoid the risk of hyponatremia, patients should be instructed to avoid excessive fluid intake and it is suggested to measure the serum sodium within the first days after the initiation of desmopressin therapy. Patients should be educated about hyponatremia symptoms like nausea, vomiting, headache, lethargy, or seizures. Once a stable dose of desmopressin is achieved, annual monitoring of the serum sodium should be performed.

Desmopressin is dosed empirically. The initial aim of therapy is to reduce nocturia and therefore the first dose is usually given at bedtime and, if needed, a daytime dose is added. In most cases, diabetes insipidus is permanent and therefore requires lifelong treatment. However, after neurosurgery, diabetes insipidus is mostly only transient.[55] Therefore, patients with diabetes insipidus after trans-sphenoidal surgery should not receive a fixed dose of desmopressin, but the degree of polyuria should be monitored and if polyuria becomes less pronounced or ceases, desmopressin can be tapered or withdrawn. If diabetes insipidus is still present 2 weeks after surgery, permanent diabetes insipidus becomes more likely. Desmopressin can be administered intranasally, orally, subcutaneously, or intravenously (**Table 2**).

Usually, starting with an intranasal preparation is recommended because not all patients respond to oral therapy. For the intranasal preparation, an initial dose of 10 μg at bedtime can be titrated upward in 10 μg increments. The usual daily maintenance

Table 2				
Different forms and administrations of desmopressin treatment				
Application	**IV/SC/ IM**	**Intranasal**	**Per Os**	**Sublingual**
Concentration	4 μg/mL	0.1 mg/mL 10 μg/dosage	100/200 μg tablets	60/120/240 μg tablets
Starting dosage	1 μg	10 μg	50 μg	60 μg

dose is 10 to 20 μg once or twice per day. For the oral preparation, the initial dose is 0.05 mg at bedtime with titration upward until 0.10 mg to 0.80 mg (maximum of 1.2 mg) in divided doses. Because the oral dose cannot be precisely predicted from a previous nasal dose, transfer of patients from nasal to oral therapy usually requires some dose retitration.

For intravenous administration, 1 to 2 μg of desmopressin acetate may be given over 2 minutes; the duration of action is 12 hours or more.

A special challenge in treatment are patients with osmoreceptor dysfunction. The long-term management of these patients requires measures to prevent dehydration and at the same time to prevent water intoxication. Because loss of thirst perception mostly cannot be cured, the focus of management is based on education of the patient about the importance of regulating their fluid intake according to their hydration status.[56] This monitoring can be accomplished most efficaciously by a fixed daily fluid intake regardless of the patient's thirst, which can be adjusted in response to changes in body weight. If the patient has polyuria, desmopressin should also be prescribed. The success of the fluid prescription should be monitored periodically by measuring serum sodium concentration. If treated accordingly, central diabetes insipidus is associated with a fairly normal quality of life, particularly when oral or nasal desmopressin is prescribed.

Nephrogenic diabetes insipidus is more difficult to treat because these patients have at least partial resistance to AVP agents. Response to (sub)maximal doses of desmopressin is, however, possible in some patients. Of course, the underlying disorder (eg, hypercalcemia) should be corrected if possible.

Patients should be instructed to follow a low-sodium diet, leading to modest hypovolemia, which stimulates isotonic proximal tubular reabsorption and thereby reduces solute delivery to the distal parts of the nephron.[3] Thiazide diuretics are sometimes efficient owing to induced natriuresis, mainly if combined with a low sodium diet. Nonsteroidal anti-inflammatory agents can also be used because they block prostaglandin synthesis, thereby increasing non–AVP-dependent water reabsorption.

Amiloride is the preferred drug to prevent progression or possibly improve lithium-induced diabetes insipidus in patients in whom lithium is continued. Usually, nephrogenic diabetes insipidus is reversible after lithium withdrawal. However, in some cases it takes several months or years for the full recovery of the renal ability to concentrate urine and very few patients have irreversible nephrogenic diabetes insipidus, even with discontinuation of lithium.

Treatment options for primary polydipsia patients are limited. A stepwise voluntary reduction of fluid intake is the treatment of choice, but often fails owing to the strong thirst perception in those patients.[57] Accordingly, most treatment recommendations aim at the prevention of hyponatremia occurrence. This goal might be achieved through patient education, recommending a balanced diet, and body weight monitoring to avoid water retention. Furthermore, any drugs with dry mouth effects should be avoided whenever possible. Supportive measures such as behavioral therapy or antipsychotics have been evaluated. However, success rates vary and these interventions are best implemented on an individual patient basis.

SUMMARY

In the diagnosis and differential diagnosis of diabetes insipidus, new test methods have shown greater diagnostic accuracy than the classical water deprivation test. These diagnostic algorithms are based on the measurement of copeptin measured either after osmotic stimulation by hypertonic saline infusion or after nonosmotic stimulation by arginine. A head-to-head study comparing these 2 test methods is currently ongoing.

Treatment of diabetes insipidus has not significantly changed within the last years and involves correction of any preexisting water deficits, if present, and exogeneous desmopressin for patients with central diabetes insipidus, which most often is given as an oral or nasal application. Most important, patients have to be instructed about the risk for hyponatremia.

COMPETING INTERESTS

M. Christ-Crain received speaking honoraria from Thermo Fisher AG, the manufacturer of the copeptin assay.

REFERENCES

1. Robertson GL. Diabetes insipidus. Endocrinol Metab Clin North Am 1995;24(3): 549–72.
2. Babey M, Kopp P, Robertson GL. Familial forms of diabetes insipidus: clinical and molecular characteristics. Nat Rev Endocrinol 2011;7(12):701–14.
3. Bockenhauer D, Bichet DG. Pathophysiology, diagnosis and management of nephrogenic diabetes insipidus. Nat Rev Nephrol 2015;11(10):576–88.
4. Cadnapaphornchai MA, Summer SN, Falk S, et al. Effect of primary polydipsia on aquaporin and sodium transporter abundance. Am J Physiol Renal Physiol 2003; 285(5):F965–71.
5. Fenske W, Allolio B. Clinical review: current state and future perspectives in the diagnosis of diabetes insipidus: a clinical review. J Clin Endocrinol Metab 2012;97(10):3426–37.
6. Carter AC, Robbins J. The use of hypertonic saline infusions in the differential diagnosis of diabetes insipidus and psychogenic polydipsia. J Clin Endocrinol Metab 1947;7(11):753–66.
7. Fenske W, Quinkler M, Lorenz D, et al. Copeptin in the differential diagnosis of the polydipsia-polyuria syndrome–revisiting the direct and indirect water deprivation tests. J Clin Endocrinol Metab 2011;96(5):1506–15.
8. Di Iorgi N, Napoli F, Allegri AE, et al. Diabetes insipidus–diagnosis and management. Horm Res Paediatr 2012;77(2):69–84.
9. Rutishauser J, Kopp P, Gaskill MB, et al. Clinical and molecular analysis of three families with autosomal dominant neurohypophyseal diabetes insipidus associated with a novel and recurrent mutations in the vasopressin-neurophysin II gene. Eur J Endocrinol 2002;146(5):649–56.
10. Robertson GL. Dipsogenic diabetes insipidus: a newly recognized syndrome caused by a selective defect in the osmoregulation of thirst. Trans Assoc Am Physicians 1987;100:241–9.
11. Barron WM, Cohen LH, Ulland LA, et al. Transient vasopressin-resistant diabetes insipidus of pregnancy. N Engl J Med 1984;310(7):442–4.
12. Durr JA, Hoggard JG, Hunt JM, et al. Diabetes insipidus in pregnancy associated with abnormally high circulating vasopressinase activity. N Engl J Med 1987; 316(17):1070–4.
13. Iwasaki Y, Oiso Y, Kondo K, et al. Aggravation of subclinical diabetes insipidus during pregnancy. N Engl J Med 1991;324(8):522–6.

14. Hashimoto M, Ogura T, Otsuka F, et al. Manifestation of subclinical diabetes insipidus due to pituitary tumor during pregnancy. Endocr J 1996;43(5): 577–83.

15. Fenske W, Refardt J, Chifu I, et al. A copeptin-based approach in the diagnosis of diabetes insipidus. N Engl J Med 2018;379(5):428–39.

16. Adrogue HJ, Madias NE. Hypernatremia. N Engl J Med 2000;342(20):1493–9.

17. Palevsky PM, Bhagrath R, Greenberg A. Hypernatremia in hospitalized patients. Ann Intern Med 1996;124(2):197–203.

18. Riggs JE. Neurologic manifestations of fluid and electrolyte disturbances. Neurol Clin 1989;7(3):509–23.

19. Fujisawa I, Nishimura K, Asato R, et al. Posterior lobe of the pituitary in diabetes insipidus: MR findings. J Comput Assist Tomogr 1987;11(2):221–5.

20. Arslan A, Karaarslan E, Dincer A. High intensity signal of the posterior pituitary. A study with horizontal direction of frequency-encoding and fat suppression MR techniques. Acta Radiol 1999;40(2):142–5.

21. Moses AM, Clayton B, Hochhauser L. Use of T1-weighted MR imaging to differentiate between primary polydipsia and central diabetes insipidus. AJNR Am J Neuroradiol 1992;13(5):1273–7.

22. Cote M, Salzman KL, Sorour M, et al. Normal dimensions of the posterior pituitary bright spot on magnetic resonance imaging. J Neurosurg 2014;120(2): 357–62.

23. Maghnie M, Cosi G, Genovese E, et al. Central diabetes insipidus in children and young adults. N Engl J Med 2000;343(14):998–1007.

24. Hannon M, Orr C, Moran C, et al. Anterior hypopituitarism is rare and autoimmune disease is common in adults with idiopathic central diabetes insipidus. Clin Endocrinol (Oxf) 2012;76(5):725–8.

25. Maghnie M, Villa A, Arico M, et al. Correlation between magnetic resonance imaging of posterior pituitary and neurohypophyseal function in children with diabetes insipidus. J Clin Endocrinol Metab 1992;74(4):795–800.

26. Bonneville JF. MRI of hypophysitis. Ann Endocrinol (Paris) 2012;73(2):76–7 [in French].

27. Leger J, Velasquez A, Garel C, et al. Thickened pituitary stalk on magnetic resonance imaging in children with central diabetes insipidus. J Clin Endocrinol Metab 1999;84(6):1954–60.

28. Verbalis JG. Disorders of water balance. In: Taal MW, Chertow GM, Marsden PA, et al, editors. Brenner and Rector's the kidney. 9th edition. Philadelphia: Saunders; 2011. p. 552–69. Chapter 15.

29. Barlow ED, De Wardener HE. Compulsive water drinking. Q J Med 1959;28(110): 235–58.

30. Baumann G, Dingman JF. Distribution, blood transport, and degradation of antidiuretic hormone in man. J Clin Invest 1976;57(5):1109–16.

31. Robertson GL. Posterior pituitary. In: Felig P, Baxter J, Frohman L, editors. Endocrinology and metabolism. New York: McGraw-Hill; 1995. p. 385–432.

32. Verbalis JG. Disorders of body water homeostasis. Best Pract Res Clin Endocrinol Metab 2003;17(4):471–503.

33. Miller M, Dalakos T, Moses AM, et al. Recognition of partial defects in antidiuretic hormone secretion. Ann Intern Med 1970;73(5):721–9.

34. Berliner RW, Davidson DG. Production of hypertonic urine in the absence of pituitary antidiuretic hormone. J Clin Invest 1957;36(10):1416–27.

35. Robertson GL, Mahr EA, Athar S, et al. Development and clinical application of a new method for the radioimmunoassay of arginine vasopressin in human plasma. J Clin Invest 1973;52(9):2340–52.
36. Dies F, Rangel S, Rivera A. Differential diagnosis between diabetes insipidus and compulsive polydipsia. Ann Intern Med 1961;54:710–25.
37. Harrington AR, Valtin H. Impaired urinary concentration after vasopressin and its gradual correction in hypothalamic diabetes insipidus. J Clin Invest 1968;47(3): 502–10.
38. Block LH, Furrer J, Locher RA, et al. Changes in tissue sensitivity to vasopressin in hereditary hypothalamic diabetes insipidus. Klin Wochenschr 1981;59(15): 831–6.
39. Zerbe RL, Robertson GL. A comparison of plasma vasopressin measurements with a standard indirect test in the differential diagnosis of polyuria. N Engl J Med 1981;305(26):1539–46.
40. Czaczkes JW, Kleeman CR. The effect of various states of hydration and the plasma concentration on the turnover of antidiuretic hormone in mammals. J Clin Invest 1964;43:1649–58.
41. Morgenthaler NG, Struck J, Alonso C, et al. Assay for the measurement of copeptin, a stable peptide derived from the precursor of vasopressin. Clin Chem 2006; 52(1):112–9.
42. Baylis PH, Gaskill MB, Robertson GL. Vasopressin secretion in primary polydipsia and cranial diabetes insipidus. Q J Med 1981;50(199):345–58.
43. Baylis PH. Diabetes insipidus. J R Coll Physicians Lond 1998;32(2):108–11.
44. Parodi AJ. Protein glucosylation and its role in protein folding. Annu Rev Biochem 2000;69:69–93.
45. Barat C, Simpson L, Breslow E. Properties of human vasopressin precursor constructs: inefficient monomer folding in the absence of copeptin as a potential contributor to diabetes insipidus. Biochemistry 2004;43(25):8191–203.
46. Fenske WK, Schnyder I, Koch G, et al. Release and decay kinetics of copeptin vs AVP in response to osmotic alterations in healthy volunteers. J Clin Endocrinol Metab 2018;103(2):505–13.
47. Timper K, Fenske W, Kuhn F, et al. Diagnostic accuracy of copeptin in the differential diagnosis of the polyuria-polydipsia syndrome: a prospective multicenter study. J Clin Endocrinol Metab 2015;100(6):2268–74.
48. Robertson GL. The regulation of vasopressin function in health and disease. Recent Prog Horm Res 1976;33:333–85.
49. Robertson GL, Shelton RL, Athar S. The osmoregulation of vasopressin. Kidney Int 1976;10(1):25–37.
50. Growth Hormone Research S. Consensus guidelines for the diagnosis and treatment of growth hormone (GH) deficiency in childhood and adolescence: summary statement of the GH Research Society. GH Research Society. J Clin Endocrinol Metab 2000;85(11):3990–3.
51. Winzeler B, Cesana-Nigro N, Refardt J, et al. Arginine-stimulated copeptin measurements in the differential diagnosis of diabetes insipidus: a prospective diagnostic study. Lancet 2019;394(10198):587–95.
52. Winzeler B, Zweifel C, Nigro N, et al. Postoperative copeptin concentration predicts diabetes insipidus after pituitary surgery. J Clin Endocrinol Metab 2015; 100(6):2275–82.
53. Berton AM, Gatti F, Penner F, et al. Early copeptin determination allows prompt diagnosis of post-neurosurgical central diabetes insipidus. Neuroendocrinology 2020;110(6):525–34.

54. Christ-Crain M, Bichet DG, Fenske WK, et al. Diabetes insipidus. Nat Rev Dis Primers 2019;5(1):54.
55. Garrahy A, Sherlock M, Thompson CJ. Management of endocrine disease: neuroendocrine surveillance and management of neurosurgical patients. Eur J Endocrinol 2017;176(5):R217–33.
56. Eisenberg Y, Frohman LA. Adipsic diabetes insipidus: a review. Endocr Pract 2016;22(1):76–83.
57. Sailer C, Winzeler B, Christ-Crain M. Primary polydipsia in the medical and psychiatric patient: characteristics, complications and therapy. Swiss Med Wkly 2017;147:w14514.

Management of Hypothalamic Obesity

Hermann L. Müller, MD

KEYWORDS

- Craniopharyngioma • Hypothalamus • Obesity • Pituitary • Bariatric surgery

KEY POINTS

- No pharmaceutical agent for treatment of hypothalamic obesity (HO) in craniopharyngioma has been proved efficient in controlled randomized trials.
- Sleeve gastrectomy and Roux-en-Y gastric bypass are the most efficient bariatric procedures for HO therapy, but are controversial in the pediatric age group because of ethical and legal considerations.
- Because no effective treatment of HO is currently available, prevention of treatment-associated hypothalamic lesions is recommended; that is, hypothalamus-sparing surgical and radio-oncological strategies.
- New interventions targeting the hypothalamus are required to improve future HO treatment.

INTRODUCTION

The functional disruption of the hypothalamic networks that regulate body composition causes hypothalamic obesity (HO) (**Fig. 1**).[1–4] Hypothalamic involvement of craniopharyngioma (CP) and/or damage to hypothalamic structures caused by surgical and/or radio-oncological interventions are associated with severe sequelae, mainly HO, with negative impact on quality of life in survivors of childhood-onset CP.[5–11]

HYPOTHALAMIC DYSFUNCTION

Thirty-five percent of patients with CP present with clinical manifestations associated with hypothalamic dysfunction, such as HO, neuropsychological deficits, and disturbances of circadian rhythms at the time of diagnosis.[2] The incidence of hypothalamic dysfunction increases up to 65% to 80% following radical surgical treatment.[2]

Treatment of suprachiasmatic lesions with hypothalamic involvement is challenging and associated with high morbidity.[12] HO is caused mainly by surgical damage of posterior hypothalamic structures, including the mammillary bodies.[13,14] Several reports

Department of Pediatrics and Pediatric Hematology/Oncology, University Children's Hospital, Klinikum Oldenburg AöR, Rahel-Straus-Strasse 10, Oldenburg 26133, Germany
E-mail address: mueller.hermann@klinikum-oldenburg.de

Endocrinol Metab Clin N Am 49 (2020) 533–552
https://doi.org/10.1016/j.ecl.2020.05.009
0889-8529/20/© 2020 Elsevier Inc. All rights reserved.

endo.theclinics.com

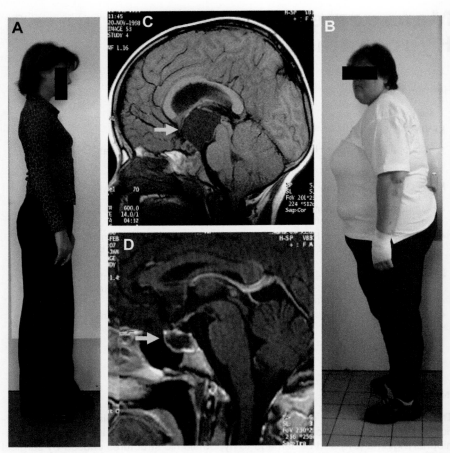

Fig. 1. Degree of obesity with regard to location of childhood CP. In both patients, CP (as indicated by the arrows on MRI before surgery) could be completely resected. Both patients had complete hypopituitarism after surgery, requiring endocrine substitution of all hypothalamic-pituitary axes. The patient in (*B*) developed severe obesity because of hypothalamic lesions of suprasellar parts of CP (*C*). The patient in (*A*) presented with a small tumor confined to the sellar region (*D*). After complete resection she kept normal weight without any eating disorders (*A*). (*From* Müller HL, Kaatsch P, Warmuth-Metz M, et al. Kraniopharyngeom im Kindes- und Jugendalter – Diagnostische und therapeutische Strategien. Monatsschr Kinderheilkd 2003; 151:1056-63; with permission.)

have shown that the degree of HO is clearly associated with the grade of hypothalamic damage in patients with CP.[14,15]

OBESITY AND EATING DISORDERS

Postoperative weight gain and morbid long-term HO are among the complications caused by hypothalamic involvement and/or treatment-related hypothalamic damage in CP. From 12% to 19% of patients are obese at the time of diagnosis.[16] Despite adequate endocrine replacement of pituitary hormone deficiencies, weight gain starts in most patients with CP during the early postoperative period (6–12 months after surgery) leading to HO, which stabilizes at a high plateau during long-term follow-up[17–19] **(Fig. 2)**. Factors limiting physical activity, such as neurologic deficits and disturbances of circadian rhythms, are further risk factors exacerbating the development of severe HO.[20] As a consequence of HO and eating disorders, prognosis after CP is associated with increased risk of cardiovascular disease[15] and metabolic syndrome,[18] including increased multisystem morbidity,[21] sudden death events,[22] and increased mortality.[23]

Although the association between HO and hypothalamic lesions is obvious,[15,24] the pathogenic mechanisms leading to increased cardiometabolic risk after CP are still less well understood. Hypothalamic nuclei synchronize circadian rhythms and biological clock mechanisms, thereby stabilizing the internal environment Accordingly, an equilibrium of the autonomic nervous system is important for metabolic function. Parasympathetic innervation of adipose tissue originating from separate sympathetic and parasympathetic neurons in the suprachiasmatic nucleus and the periventricular nucleus plays a major role in regulation of lipogenesis. It is reasonable to conclude

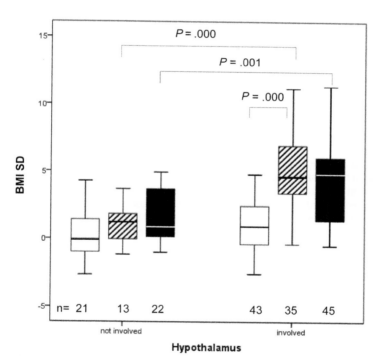

Fig. 2. Weight development in patients with childhood-onset CP recruited in the German observational trial on childhood-onset craniopharyngioma HIT Endo according to hypothalamic involvement. Body mass index (BMI) standard deviation (SD) is shown at time of diagnosis and at 2 intervals after diagnosis (8–12 years and more than 12 years). White boxes indicate BMI at diagnosis; hatched boxes indicate 8-year to 12-year follow-up; black boxes indicate more than 12-year follow-up. The horizontal lines in the middle of the boxes depict the median. The top and bottom edges of the boxes respectively mark the 25th and 75th percentiles. Whiskers indicate the range of values that are within 1.5 box lengths. (*From* Sterkenburg AS, Hoffmann A, Gebhardt U, et al. Survival, hypothalamic obesity, and neuropsychological/psychosocial status after childhood-onset craniopharyngioma: newly reported long-term outcomes. *Neuro Oncol.* 2015;17(7):1029-1038; with permission.)

that, in cases of suprasellar CP extension involving these nuclei, their regulatory function will be compromised and will remain compromised to a certain extent when treated surgically or with irradiation.

Roth and colleagues[25] observed increased serum leptin concentrations with regard to body mass index (BMI) in patients with CP with a suprasellar tumor extension and hypothesized that normal appetite inhibition did not occur because of disruption of hypothalamic receptors regulating the negative feedback loop in which leptin of adipocyte origin binds to hypothalamic leptin receptors. However, Harz and colleagues[26] analyzed self-assessment of caloric intake and observed that patients with CP with HO had similar caloric intake compared with healthy BMI-matched controls.

PHYSICAL ACTIVITY AND ENERGY EXPENDITURE

A study on physical activity as assessed by accelerometry found that the level of physical activity was significantly decreased in patients with CP compared with healthy BMI-matched controls.[26] In addition, markedly increased daytime sleepiness was observed in patients with severe HO caused by CP.[20] Decreased early morning and nocturnal melatonin saliva concentrations were associated with increased daytime sleepiness and the degree of HO in patients with CP. Hypothalamic dysregulation of circadian melatonin secretion was hypothesized as a relevant pathogenic mechanism. Although first experiences with melatonin medication (6 mg/d) were promising in patients with CP, based on normalization of melatonin saliva concentrations and short-term improvements of daytime sleepiness and physical activity,[27] data on the long-term effect on daytime sleepiness and HO have not been published.

Sleep patterns typical for secondary narcolepsy and hypersomnia (ie, frequent sleep-onset rapid eye movement phases) were found by polysomnography in patients with CP with HO and severe daytime sleepiness.[28–30] Pharmaceutical therapy with central stimulating agents (modafinil, methylphenidate) significantly reduced daytime sleepiness in these patients.[29] Mason and colleagues[31] treated 5 patients with CP with the central stimulating agent dextroamphetamine. The patients' parents observed marked improvements in their children's alertness and physical activity levels.

Changes in metabolic rate have been hypothesized to play a major role in weight gain and development of HO in patients with CP. A decreased resting energy expenditure (REE), not associated with differences in terms of body composition, has been shown in patients with CP compared with controls.[32,33] Lower energy intake/REE ratios were associated with third ventricle involvement of CP. Reduced levels of physical activity are also likely to contribute to observed overall reductions of total energy expenditure.[15,26,32]

AUTONOMIC NERVOUS SYSTEM

Hypothalamic disinhibition of vagal output resulting in increased pancreatic β-cell stimulation and hyperinsulinism was hypothesized by Lustig and colleagues[34,35] as a pathogenic mechanism for HO in CP caused by hypothalamic lesions. The investigators conducted a trial with octreotide, a somatostatin analogue, which decreases pancreatic β-cell activity.[34] Reduced central sympathetic output in terms of urine concentrations of catecholamine metabolites was observed to be associated with morbid HO in patients with CP and decreased levels of physical activity.[36,37]

APPETITE REGULATION

Roth and colleagues[38,39] showed that decreased ghrelin secretion and reduced postprandial suppression of ghrelin leads to disturbed regulation of appetite and satiety in patients with CP with severe HO. Comparing normal-weight, obese, and severely obese patients with CP, differences in terms of serum peptide YY concentrations were not observed. Furthermore, a potential role of peripheral α-melanocyte–stimulating hormone for HO in CP has been shown.[40]

Hoffmann and colleagues[6] found that patients with CP with HO presented with pathologic eating behavior and higher rates of eating disorders, compared with obese and normal or overweight patients with CP. However, patients with CP with severe HO showed similar or even less pathologic findings for eating behavior compared with BMI-matched normal controls.

Premeal and postmeal responses to visual food cues were assessed by functional MRI.[41] BMI-matched controls presented with suppression of activation by high-calorie food cues of a test meal. Patients with CP with HO showed a trend toward higher activation, supporting the hypothesis that in HO the perception of food cues may be altered after food intake.

Even though HO is a frequent sequela after CP,[38] diencephalic syndrome (DS) associated with significant weight loss is rarely diagnosed as a hypothalamic disturbance of body composition in patients with CP.[42] Hoffmann and colleagues[42] analyzed a small cohort of patients with CP with DS and observed that DS at diagnosis does not preclude subsequent HO during long-term follow-up.

TREATMENT OF HYPOTHALAMIC OBESITY
Lifestyle Interventions

Because of disturbances in satiety regulation, central sympathetic output, and energy expenditure, patients with CP often develop morbid HO that is mostly nonresponsive to conventional lifestyle modification (diet and exercise)[43–47] (**Table 1**).

Dietary Interventions

Only 1 case report observed a clinically significant effect of a dietary intervention by a protein-sparing modified fast program.[48] However, after discontinuation weight gain occurred.

PHARMACOLOGIC TREATMENT OF HYPOTHALAMIC OBESITY
Endocrine Substitution of Hypopituitarism

Hypopituitarism should be treated with substitution of the deficient hormones according to existing guidelines (**Table 2**).[49] Although safe with regard to the risk of CP recurrence, beneficial effects of growth hormone (GH) substitution on long-term body composition after CP are controversial.[50–53] Glucocorticoid overreplacement should be avoided and levothyroxine should be substituted in a dose sufficient to achieve free T4 levels in the mid to upper half of the reference range.[49]

TRIIODOTHYRONINE SUPPLEMENTATION

Triiodothyronine (T3) increases energy expenditure by induction of thermogenesis. In a case series, Fernandes and colleagues[54] reported on improved daytime lethargy and weight reduction under T3 supplementation for up to 24 months. van Santen and colleagues[55] analyzed metabolic brown adipose tissue activity in a T3-treated patient with CP with HO. Presumably because of damage to hypothalamic pathways, no changes in brown adipose tissue activity or energy expenditure were observed by the investigators, suggesting that adjunct therapy with T3 had no beneficial effects.

Table 1
Lifestyle interventions for treatment of hypothalamic obesity

Intervention	CP Cohorts	BMI (kg/m²)/Weight (kg) Before Intervention (Range)	Duration of Intervention (Range)	BMI (kg/m²)/Weight (kg) at Last Visit After Intervention (Range)	Follow-up Interval (Range)	Investigators
Pediatric hospital	1 ped CP	BMI 51.8	Not reported	41.8 kg	2 mo	Meijneke et al,[45] 2015
Psychiatry hospital	2 ped CP	Weight 64.0 kg / Weight 59.0 kg	2 y / 7 y	Weight 97.0 kg / Weight 97.7 kg	8 y	Skorzewska et al,[46] 1989
Rehabilitation program	31 ped CP	Median BMI 1.32 SD (1.1–7.0 SD)	Median 39 d (20–135 d)	Median BMI 4.92 SD (0.2–13.1 SD)	10.8 y (10–27 y)	Sterkenburg et al,[44] 2014
Specialized outpatient clinic	39 ped pts (84% CP)	Median BMI 1.93 SD (0–3.2 SD) / Median weight gain/y 21.4% (15.8%–32%)	Mean 3.3 visits (1–8) during 3–41 mo	Median BMI 2.03 SD (0.2–2.6 SD) / Median weight gain/y 8.5% (3.4%–14.0%)	Mean 0.97 y (3–41 mo)	Rakhshani et al,[43] 2010
Specialized outpatient clinic	77 adult pts	Median BMI 28.1 (IQR: 24.3–32.4)	Not reported	Median BMI 32.0 (IQR: 27.7–38.4)	Median 9 y	Steele et al,[47] 2013

Abbreviations: IQR, interquartile range; ped, pediatric; pts, patients; SD, standard deviation.
Data from Refs.[43–47]

Table 2
Pharmacologic treatment approaches for hypothalamic obesity

Pharmaceutical Agent	Mechanism of Action	Patient Cohorts	Outcomes	Investigators
Dextroamphetamine	Central stimulant, stimulation of noradrenalin, dopamine secretion, and dopamine reuptake inhibition	5 ped CP	Increase in physical activity, reduction in continuous weight gain, stabilization of BMI	Mason et al,[31] 2002
		9 ped CP, 2 ped astrocytoma, 1 ped glioma	Reduction in continuous weight gain and stabilization of BMI in 10 of 12 pts, improved daytime sleepiness in 11 of 12 pts	Ismail et al,[58] 2006
		4 CP (3 ped), 1 ped astrocytoma, 1 ped ganglioglioma, 1 ped meningitis	Reduction in continuous weight gain and stabilization of BMI	Denzer et al,[59] 2019
Caffeine and ephedrine-HCl	Methamphetamine analogue with sympathicomimetic effect	2 ped CP	Mean weight loss 13.9%, 6 mo after 2.6–5.5 y intervention	Greenway & Bray,[61] 2008
Mazindol	Sympathicomimetic amine similar to amphetamine	1 adult CP	Weight reduction from 70 kg to 60 kg after 3 wk intervention	Sadatomo et al,[60] 2001
Methyl-phenidate	Central stimulant, dopamine reuptake inhibition	1 ped CP	Beneficial against weight gain	Elfers & Roth,[62] 2011
Octreotide	Somatostatin analogue, reduced β-cell activation	13 ped CP, 4 ped astrocytoma, 1 ped germinoma, 2 ped ALL	Reduced insulin secretion, moderate to no improvement in BMI, increased risk of gallstone formation	Lustig et al,[34] 2003
Diazoxide	Potassium channel activator, inhibition of insulin secretion	18 pts	No BMI change	Brauner et al,[66] 2016
Diazoxide and metformin	Reduced insulin secretion, reduced hyperglycemia, improved insulin sensitivity	9 ped CP	Reduced weight gain, weight loss, peripheral edema, emesis, increased hepatic enzyme levels	Hamilton et al,[67] 2011
Fenofibrate and metformin	PPARa agonist, improved insulin sensitivity	10 ped CP	Improved insulin resistance and lipid profiles, no effect on BMI	Kalina et al,[68] 2015

(continued on next page)

Table 2
(continued)

Pharmaceutical Agent	Mechanism of Action	Patient Cohorts	Outcomes	Investigators
Exenatide	GLP-1 receptor agonists, improved insulin sensitivity, increased satiety feeling, reduced speed of gastric emptying	5 adult CP 1 ped hamartoma 1 adult astrocytoma 1 adult germinoma	Improved cardiovascular profile, improved metabolic profile, sustained weight reduction	Zoicas et al,[70] 2013
		4 ped CP 2 adult CP	No significant weight loss in total cohort, stable or decreased weight in responders (60%)	Lomenick et al,[69] 2016
Liraglutide		1 adult CP	BMI reduction from 41.8 to 35.3 after 8 mo intervention	Zoicas et al,[70] 2013
Beloranib	METAP2 inhibitor, angiogenesis inhibitor (removed from the market)	8 adult CP	Significant weight loss after 4 wk compared with placebo in RCT	Shoemaker et al,[75] 2017
Oxy and naltraxone	Naltrexone (opiate antagonist) decreases appetite and potentiates anorexigenic Oxy effects	1 ped CP	Improvement of hyperphagia and weight loss	Hsu et al,[81] 2018
Supraphysiologic supplementation of T3	T3 increases energy expenditure by induction of thermogenesis	1 adult pt (no CP) 3 ped pts (no CP)	Weight reduction under 3 × 10 µg T3/d for 11–27 mo	Fernandes et al,[54] 2002
		1 ped CP	No weight reduction under 3 × 12.5 µg T3/d for 2 mo	Van Santen et al,[55] 2015
Substitution with recombinant GH	Beneficial effects of GH on body composition and metabolism	199 ped CP	No reduction of BMI during 3 y GH substitution	Geffner et al,[51] 2004
		260 ped CP	No reduction of BMI during 5 y of GH substitution	Yuen et al,[52] 2013
		47 ped CP	No BMI reduction under GH during the first 3 y after diagnosis	Heinks et al,[53] 2018
		79 ped CP	Beneficial long-term effect of GH on BMI when substituted during pediatric and adult age	Boekhoff et al,[50] 2018

Abbreviations: GH, growth hormone; GLP-1, glucagonlike peptide receptor-1; METAP2, methionine aminopeptidase 2; Oxy, oxytocin; PPARa, peroxisome proliferator activated receptor alpha; RCT, randomized controlled trial; T3, triiodothyronine.
Data from Refs.[31,34,50–55,58–62,66–70,75,81]

CENTRAL STIMULATING AGENTS

Based on the observed reduction of epinephrine secretion and sympathoadrenal activation manifesting as an impaired endocrine response to hypoglycemia, pharmaceutical therapy with amphetamine derivatives has been analyzed.[31,56–62] Dextroamphetamine medication for 24 months, starting 10 months after surgery, stabilized BMI, diminished continuous weight gain, and increased spontaneous physical activity level.[31] Improvement in daytime sleepiness was observed even after shorter-term dextroamphetamine medication.[58] Elfers and Roth[62] observed beneficial methylphenidate effects on weight development after CP.

SOMATOSTATIN ANALOGUES

Lustig[63] hypothesized that morbidly obese patients with CP present with a parasympathetic predominance of the autonomic nervous system caused by vagal activation. Activation of pancreatic β cells by parasympathetic stimulation results in insulin hypersecretion promoting adipogenesis. The somatostatin analogue octreotide reduces insulin secretion. Lustig and colleagues[34] analyzed octreotide effects on HO in a double-blinded randomized controlled trial on children with HO and reported moderate reductions in weight gain. A larger trial was conducted using octreotide LAR (long-acting repeatable) in 60 patients with HO.[64] A 6-month medication of octreotide LAR was shown to have no effect on changes of BMI. The trial was terminated because of an increased risk of adverse side effects. Reported octreotide side effects are cholesterol gallstone or sludge formation, abdominal discomfort, mild glucose intolerance, peripheral edema, and diabetic hyperosmolar nonketotic coma.[34,65] Octreotide is currently not recommended by the US Food and Drug Administration and European Medicines Agency for treatment of HO.

ANTIDIABETIC AGENTS

Several trials analyzed effects of antidiabetic agents on weight development in patients with HO.[66–74]

GLUCAGONLIKE PEPTIDE 1 RECEPTOR AGONISTS

Zoicas and colleagues[70] analyzed effects of treatment with glucagonlike peptide 1 (GLP-1) receptor agonists on weight development in 8 patients (6 CP) with HO and reported on a sustained weight loss and improvements in cardiovascular and metabolic risk profiles. Simmons and colleagues[71] confirmed these findings in a patient with hypothalamic germ cell tumour.

METFORMIN AND DIAZOXIDE

Hamilton and colleagues[67] hypothesized that a combination therapy of diazoxide and metformin reduces insulin secretion and the risk for hyperglycemia. Insulin secretion is decreased by diazoxide binding to the KATP channel of the β cell. Metformin improves insulin sensitivity by decreasing hepatic gluconeogenesis. A combination therapy of diazoxide and metformin was studied in 9 patients with CP with HO. The synergism of lower insulin levels and enhanced insulin action led to an improved weight gain of +1.2 ± 5.9 kg compared with +9.5 ± 2.7 kg weight gain during 6 months before therapy. High pretreatment insulin levels were associated with the most robust weight reduction.[67] Limitations of the trial were small cohort size and adverse events in 1 patient withdrawing because of development of peripheral edema, and another because of emesis and increased hepatic enzyme levels.

BELORANIB

Methionine aminopeptidase 2 (MetAP2) inhibitors were initially developed as antiangiogenesis agents for oncological therapy. Subsequently, MetAP2 inhibitors were found to induce weight loss, decrease leptin concentrations, and increase adiponectin concentrations, which results in decreased lipogenesis and increased fat oxidation and lipolysis. Shoemaker and colleagues[75] treated 14 adult patients with HO with the MetAP2 inhibitor beloranib for 8 weeks and reported on an average weight loss of 3.2 kg in the first 4 weeks, and 6.2 kg at 8 weeks of treatment. Although consistent weight reduction was observed under beloranib medication, further development of the pharmaceutical agent was stopped because of venous thromboembolic complications occurring in clinical studies on patients with Prader-Willi syndrome treated with beloranib for HO.[76]

SIBUTRAMINE

Sibutramine, a serotonin and noradrenaline uptake inhibitor, reduces appetite and prevents reduced energy expenditure. However, sibutramine-induced weight reduction in children with HO was observed to be less efficient compared with nonhypothalamic obesity.[56] Future trials with sibutramine are not expected because sibutramine was withdrawn from the market in 2010 because of concerns over increased cardiovascular risk.[77]

FENOFIBRATE AND METFORMIN

Kalina and colleagues[68] treated 22 pediatric patients with CP with a combination of fenofibrate and metformin. Fenofibrate is a peroxisome proliferator activated receptor alpha (PPARa) agonist that has been hypothesized to improve insulin sensitivity and to reduce triglyceride serum concentrations. Improved insulin resistance and lipid profiles were reported under metformin and fenofibrate medication. However, treatment with these agents did not result in improvements of BMI development.[68]

OXYTOCIN

Patients with CP and surgical damage limited to specific anterior hypothalamic structures were recently reported to present with reduced fasting oxytocin levels.[78] Furthermore, changes in oxytocin saliva concentrations before and after standardized breakfast showed a significant correlation with BMI. Patients with CP and HO presented with impaired variation of oxytocin secretion caused by nutrition. The investigators hypothesized that oxytocin medication might exert beneficial effects on neuropsychological deficiencies in patients with CP with specific surgical lesions of anterior hypothalamic structures. In a small pilot study on 11 patients with CP, Hoffmann and colleagues[79] tested their hypothesis by single nasal application of 24 IU of oxytocin. Before single nasal administration of oxytocin, all patients with CP presented with detectable oxytocin saliva concentrations. Oxytocin medication was very well tolerated and resulted in increases of oxytocin concentration in saliva and urine. After oxytocin administration, patients with CP and surgical hypothalamic lesions limited to anterior hypothalamic areas presented improvements with regard to emotional identification compared with patients with CP and anterior plus posterior hypothalamic lesions.

Table 3
Surgical interventions for treatment of hypothalamic obesity

Intervention	CP pts Cohort	BMI (kg/m²)/Weight (kg) Before Intervention (Range)	BMI (kg/m²)/Weight (kg) at Last Visit After Intervention (Range)	Median Follow-up Interval (Range)	Complications and Side Effects Caused by Intervention	Investigators
Laparoscopic adjustable gastric banding	4 ped	BMI 46.4 BMI 44.9 BMI 51.9 BMI 40.0	BMI 49.6 BMI 53.6 BMI 53.6 BMI 42.7	7.1 y, (5.3–9.1 y)	None reported	Müller et al,[87] 2011
	6 ped	Median BMI 40.2 (44.7–61.6)	No weight and BMI change	5.5 y, (1–9 y)	Band readjustment, explantation of device	Weismann et al,[82] 2013
Sleeve gastrectomy	3 ped	Mean BMI 49.2 (41.6–58.1)	Mean BMI 35.3, (31.2–40.6)	2 y	Minor bleeding, folic acid and vitamin D deficiency	Trotta et al,[91] 2017
	2 pts	BMI 51.0 BMI 37.6	BMI 41.0 BMI 34.0	30 mo	None reported	Gatta et al,[88] 2016
	2 ped	BMI 55.6 BMI 43.3	No BMI change	2 y (0.5–4 y)	Vomiting, impaired effectiveness of desmopressin	Weismann et al,[82] 2013
	3 pts	Mean BMI 31.1	Mean weight loss 10%	24 mo	None reported	Wijnen et al,[83] 2017
RYGB	1 ped 1 ped	BMI 51.5 BMI 65.0	BMI 39 BMI 43.0	9 mo 4 y	None reported Diarrhea, dumping syndrome, psychological deterioration	Page-Wilson et al,[85] 2012 Rottembourg et al,[86] 2009
	3 pts	BMI 59.6 BMI 42.3	Mean weight loss 20 kg	18 mo	None	Bretault et al,[89] 2016
	5 pts	Mean BMI 43.4, +5.2 SD	Mean weight loss 25%	24 mo	None reported	Wijnen et al,[83] 2017
RYGB with vagotomy	1 ped	Weight 223 kg	Weight loss of 49 kg	2.5 y	Mild iron deficiency	Inge et al,[84] 2007

(continued on next page)

Table 3
(continued)

Intervention	CP pts Cohort	BMI (kg/m²)/Weight (kg) Before Intervention (Range)	BMI (kg/m²)/Weight (kg) at Last Visit After Intervention (Range)	Median Follow-up Interval (Range)	Complications and Side Effects Caused by Intervention	Investigators
Biliopancreatic diversion plus duodenal switch	1 ped	BMI 45.0	BMI 32.0	2 y	Bradycardia, pacemaker, intestinal stenosis	Rottembourg et al,[86] 2009
Gastric bypass	4 pts	BMI 49.2 BMI 59.5 BMI 41.0 BMI 46.1	BMI 29.4 BMI 53.6 BMI 32.5 BMI 28.7	33 mo 65 mo 17 mo 13 mo	None reported	Wolf et al,[90] 2016
	2 pts	BMI 43.7 BMI 37.7	BMI 37.5 BMI 49.0	48 mo 64 mo	Septicemia, esophagus ulceration	Gatta et al,[88] 2013
	1 ped	BMI 48.6	Loss of weight	36 mo	None reported	Weismann et al,[82] 2013
Truncal vagotomy	1 ped	Weight 106 kg	Weight 76 kg	27 mo	Occasional foul smelling	Smith et al,[96] 1983
Deep brain stimulation	1 ped	BMI 52.9	BMI 48.3	14 mo	None	Harat et al,[97] 2016

Abbreviation: RYGB, Roux-en-Y gastric bypass.
Data from Refs.[82–91,96,97]

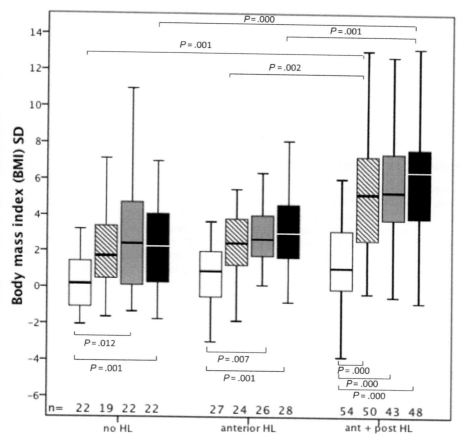

Surgical hypothalamic lesion (HL)

Fig. 3. Weight development in 109 patients with childhood-onset CP, recruited with primary involvement of anterior and posterior (ant + post) hypothalamus in the trial KRANIOPHAR-YNGEOM 2007, with regard to surgical hypothalamic lesions (HL) graded as previously described[14]: no HL; HL of the anterior hypothalamus not involving mammillary bodies and hypothalamic areas dorsal of mammillary bodies; and HL of anterior and posterior hypothalamic areas (ie, involving mammillary bodies and areas dorsal of mammillary bodies). BMI SD is shown at time of diagnosis and at 3 intervals after diagnosis (1 and 3 years after diagnosis, last visit). White boxes, BMI SD at diagnosis; hatched boxes, BMI SD at 1-year follow-up; gray boxes, BMI SD at 3-year follow-up; and black boxes, BMI SD at last visit. The horizontal line in the middle of the box depicts the median. The top and bottom edges of the box respectively mark the 25th and 75th percentiles. Whiskers indicate the range of values that are within 1.5 box lengths. (*From* Bogusz A, Boekhoff S, Warmuth-Metz M, et al. Posterior hypothalamus-sparing surgery improves outcome after childhood craniopharyngioma. *Endocr Connect.* 2019; 2019; 8(5):481-492; with permission.)

Daubenbüchel and colleagues[78,80] analyzed the association between oxytocin saliva concentrations and eating behavior in patients with CP and healthy controls. Patients with CP and anterior hypothalamic lesions and patients with CP and anterior plus posterior hypothalamic lesions presented with specific patterns of eating behavior. Reduced postprandial compared with fasting oxytocin saliva concentrations were associated with HO in patients with CP and with adverse eating behavior and eating disorders in both patients with CP and controls. Current knowledge on the effects of long-term oxytocin medication in CP is mainly based on rare case reports. Hsu and colleagues[81] reported that 10 weeks of oxytocin therapy induced improvement of hyperphagia and weight loss followed by a combined 38 weeks of therapy with oxytocin and naltrexone in a pediatric patient. A controlled randomized trial (ClinicalTrials.gov identifier: NCT 02849743) in patients with HO is currently testing whether nasal administration of oxytocin promotes weight loss.

BARIATRIC TREATMENT OF HYPOTHALAMIC OBESITY

Several reports on the effects of bariatric interventions on weight development in HO have been published with mixed results (**Table 3**).[82–91] First experiences with bariatric surgery in patients with CP with HO showed good tolerability.[84,92,93] After laparoscopic adjustable gastric banding (LAGB), an immediate improvement of binge-eating behavior was reported in patients with CP. However, long-term effects of LAGB in terms of weight reduction were not observed.[87] Bretault and colleagues[94] analyzed 12-month outcomes after bariatric surgery for HO caused by CP treatment in their systematic review. At 1 year, 6 of 18 cases presented with a greater than 20% loss of their initial weight; all of them were treated by Roux-en-Y gastric bypass (n = 3), sleeve gastrectomy, (n = 2) or biliopancreatic diversion (n = 1). Accordingly, sleeve gastrectomy, Roux-en-Y gastric bypass, and biliopancreatic diversion are the most efficient bariatric interventions for treatment of HO after CP. Bariatric treatment with invasive, nonreversible methods is controversial in pediatric patients with CP because of ethical, medical, and legal concerns.[86,87,95]

OTHER SURGICAL INTERVENTIONS FOR TREATMENT OF HYPOTHALAMIC OBESITY

Case reports on the effects of truncal vagotomy[96] and the implantation of deep brain stimulating electrodes to bilaterally stimulate the nucleus accumbens[97] have been published, with only limited effects observed (see **Table 3**).

SUMMARY

Although novel therapeutic approaches provide promising perspectives, in the studies published to date no bariatric or pharmacologic therapy for HO in patients with CP has been proved to be effective based on randomized trials. Treatment approaches with combinations of pharmaceutical agents seem most promising. Prevention of HO is recommended[1] with special regard to hypothalamus-sparing therapeutic approaches,[98] respecting the integrity of essential nuclei located in posterior hypothalamic areas (**Fig. 3**).[19]

DISCLOSURES

The author has received reimbursement of participation fees for scientific meetings and continuing medical education events from the following companies: Ferring, Lilly, Pfizer, Sandoz/Hexal, Novo Nordisk, Ipsen, and Merck Serono. He has received reimbursement of travel expenses from Ipsen and lecture honoraria from Pfizer. The author is supported by a grant (DKS 2014.13) of the German Childhood Cancer Foundation, Bonn, Germany.

REFERENCES

1. Muller HL, Merchant TE, Puget S, et al. New outlook on the diagnosis, treatment and follow-up of childhood-onset craniopharyngioma. Nat Rev Endocrinol 2017; 13(5):299–312.
2. van Iersel L, Brokke KE, Adan RAH, et al. Pathophysiology and Individualized Treatment of Hypothalamic Obesity Following Craniopharyngioma and Other Suprasellar Tumors: A Systematic Review. Endocr Rev 2019;40(1):193–235.
3. Bogusz A, Muller HL. Childhood-onset craniopharyngioma: latest insights into pathology, diagnostics, treatment, and follow-up. Exp Rev Neurother 2018; 18(10):793–806.
4. Castro DC, Cole SL, Berridge KC. Lateral hypothalamus, nucleus accumbens, and ventral pallidum roles in eating and hunger: interactions between homeostatic and reward circuitry. Front Syst Neurosci 2015;9:90.
5. Muller HL. Craniopharyngioma. Endocr Rev 2014;35(3):513–43.
6. Hoffmann A, Postma FP, Sterkenburg AS, et al. Eating behavior, weight problems and eating disorders in 101 long-term survivors of childhood-onset craniopharyngioma. J Pediatr Endocrinol Metab 2015;28(1–2):35–43.
7. Sterkenburg AS, Hoffmann A, Gebhardt U, et al. Survival, hypothalamic obesity, and neuropsychological/psychosocial status after childhood-onset craniopharyngioma: newly reported long-term outcomes. Neuro Oncol 2015;17(7):1029–38.
8. Daubenbuchel AM, Hoffmann A, Gebhardt U, et al. Hydrocephalus and hypothalamic involvement in pediatric patients with craniopharyngioma or cysts of Rathke's pouch: impact on long-term prognosis. Eur J Endocrinol 2015;172(5): 561–9.
9. Muller HL. Craniopharyngioma and hypothalamic injury: latest insights into consequent eating disorders and obesity. Curr Opin Endocrinol Diabetes Obes 2016;23(1):81–9.
10. Muller HL. MANAGEMENT OF ENDOCRINE DISEASE: Childhood-onset Craniopharyngioma: state of the art of care in 2018. Eur J Endocrinol 2019;180(4): R159–74.
11. Karavitaki N. Management of craniopharyngiomas. J Endocrinol Invest 2014; 37(3):219–28.
12. Muller HL. Hypothalamic involvement in craniopharyngioma-Implications for surgical, radiooncological, and molecularly targeted treatment strategies. Pediatr Blood Cancer 2018;65(5):e26936.
13. Muller HL. Consequences of craniopharyngioma surgery in children. J Clin Endocrinol Metab 2011;96(7):1981–91.
14. Muller HL, Gebhardt U, Teske C, et al. Post-operative hypothalamic lesions and obesity in childhood craniopharyngioma: results of the multinational prospective trial KRANIOPHARYNGEOM 2000 after 3-year follow-up. Eur J Endocrinol 2011; 165(1):17–24.
15. Holmer H, Ekman B, Bjork J, et al. Hypothalamic involvement predicts cardiovascular risk in adults with childhood onset craniopharyngioma on long-term GH therapy. Eur J Endocrinol 2009;161(5):671–9.
16. Muller HL, Emser A, Faldum A, et al. Longitudinal study on growth and body mass index before and after diagnosis of childhood craniopharyngioma. J Clin Endocrinol Metab 2004;89(7):3298–305.
17. Muller HL, Bueb K, Bartels U, et al. Obesity after childhood craniopharyngioma– German multicenter study on pre-operative risk factors and quality of life. Klin Padiatr 2001;213(4):244–9.

18. Srinivasan S, Ogle GD, Garnett SP, et al. Features of the metabolic syndrome after childhood craniopharyngioma. J Clin Endocrinol Metab 2004;89(1):81–6.

19. Bogusz A, Boekhoff S, Warmuth-Metz M, et al. Posterior hypothalamus-sparing surgery improves outcome after childhood craniopharyngioma. Endocr Connect 2019;8(5):481–92.

20. Muller HL, Handwerker G, Wollny B, et al. Melatonin secretion and increased daytime sleepiness in childhood craniopharyngioma patients. J Clin Endocrinol Metab 2002;87(8):3993–6.

21. Pereira AM, Schmid EM, Schutte PJ, et al. High prevalence of long-term cardiovascular, neurological and psychosocial morbidity after treatment for craniopharyngioma. Clin Endocrinol 2005;62(2):197–204.

22. Mong S, Pomeroy SL, Cecchin F, et al. Cardiac risk after craniopharyngioma therapy. Pediatr Neurol 2008;38(4):256–60.

23. Visser J, Hukin J, Sargent M, et al. Late mortality in pediatric patients with craniopharyngioma. J Neurooncol 2010;100(1):105–11.

24. Sterkenburg AS, Hoffmann A, Reichel J, et al. Nuchal Skinfold Thickness: A Novel Parameter for Assessment of Body Composition in Childhood Craniopharyngioma. J Clin Endocrinol Metab 2016;101(12):4922–30.

25. Roth C, Wilken B, Hanefeld F, et al. Hyperphagia in children with craniopharyngioma is associated with hyperleptinaemia and a failure in the downregulation of appetite. Eur J Endocrinol 1998;138(1):89–91.

26. Harz KJ, Muller HL, Waldeck E, et al. Obesity in patients with craniopharyngioma: assessment of food intake and movement counts indicating physical activity. J Clin Endocrinol Metab 2003;88(11):5227–31.

27. Muller HL, Handwerker G, Gebhardt U, et al. Melatonin treatment in obese patients with childhood craniopharyngioma and increased daytime sleepiness. Cancer Causes Control 2006;17(4):583–9.

28. O'Gorman CS, Simoneau-Roy J, Pencharz P, et al. Sleep-disordered breathing is increased in obese adolescents with craniopharyngioma compared with obese controls. J Clin Endocrinol Metab 2010;95(5):2211–8.

29. Muller HL, Muller-Stover S, Gebhardt U, et al. Secondary narcolepsy may be a causative factor of increased daytime sleepiness in obese childhood craniopharyngioma patients. J Pediatr Endocrinol Metab 2006;19(Suppl 1):423–9.

30. Muller HL. Increased daytime sleepiness in patients with childhood craniopharyngioma and hypothalamic tumor involvement: review of the literature and perspectives. Int J Endocrinol 2010;2010:519607.

31. Mason PW, Krawiecki N, Meacham LR. The use of dextroamphetamine to treat obesity and hyperphagia in children treated for craniopharyngioma. Arch Pediatr Adolesc Med 2002;156(9):887–92.

32. Shaikh MG, Grundy RG, Kirk JM. Reductions in basal metabolic rate and physical activity contribute to hypothalamic obesity. J Clin Endocrinol Metab 2008;93(7):2588–93.

33. Kim RJ, Shah R, Tershakovec AM, et al. Energy expenditure in obesity associated with craniopharyngioma. Childs Nerv Syst 2010;26(7):913–7.

34. Lustig RH, Hinds PS, Ringwald-Smith K, et al. Octreotide therapy of pediatric hypothalamic obesity: a double-blind, placebo-controlled trial. J Clin Endocrinol Metab 2003;88(6):2586–92.

35. Lustig RH. Hypothalamic obesity after craniopharyngioma: mechanisms, diagnosis, and treatment. Front Endocrinol 2011;2:60.

36. Roth CL, Hunneman DH, Gebhardt U, et al. Reduced sympathetic metabolites in urine of obese patients with craniopharyngioma. Pediatr Res 2007;61(4): 496–501.

37. Cohen M, Syme C, McCrindle BW, et al. Autonomic nervous system balance in children and adolescents with craniopharyngioma and hypothalamic obesity. Eur J Endocrinol 2013;168(6):845–52.

38. Roth CL, Gebhardt U, Muller HL. Appetite-regulating hormone changes in patients with craniopharyngioma. Obesity (Silver Spring) 2011;19(1):36–42.

39. Roth CL, Elfers C, Gebhardt U, et al. Brain-derived neurotrophic factor and its relation to leptin in obese children before and after weight loss. Metabolism 2013;62(2):226–34.

40. Roth CL, Enriori PJ, Gebhardt U, et al. Changes of peripheral alpha-melanocyte-stimulating hormone in childhood obesity. Metabolism 2010;59(2):186–94.

41. Roth CL, Aylward E, Liang O, et al. Functional neuroimaging in craniopharyngioma: a useful tool to better understand hypothalamic obesity? Obes Facts 2012;5(2):243–53.

42. Hoffmann A, Gebhardt U, Sterkenburg AS, et al. Diencephalic Syndrome in Childhood Craniopharyngioma-Results of German Multicenter Studies on 485 Long-term Survivors of Childhood Craniopharyngioma. J Clin Endocrinol Metab 2014;99(11):3972–7.

43. Rakhshani N, Jeffery AS, Schulte F, et al. Evaluation of a comprehensive care clinic model for children with brain tumor and risk for hypothalamic obesity. Obesity (Silver Spring) 2010;18(9):1768–74.

44. Sterkenburg AS, Hoffmann A, Gebhardt U, et al. Childhood craniopharyngioma with hypothalamic obesity - no long-term weight reduction due to rehabilitation programs. Klin Padiatr 2014;226(6–7):344–50 [in German].

45. Meijneke RW, Schouten-van Meeteren AY, de Boer NY, et al. Hypothalamic obesity after treatment for craniopharyngioma: the importance of the home environment. J Pediatr Endocrinol Metab 2015;28(1–2):59–63.

46. Skorzewska A, Lal S, Waserman J, et al. Abnormal food-seeking behavior after surgery for craniopharyngioma. Neuropsychobiology 1989;21(1):17–20.

47. Steele CA, Cuthbertson DJ, MacFarlane IA, et al. Hypothalamic obesity: prevalence, associations and longitudinal trends in weight in a specialist adult neuroendocrine clinic. Eur J Endocrinol 2013;168(4):501–7.

48. Lee YJ, Backeljauw PF, Kelly PD, et al. Successful weight loss with protein-sparing modified fast in a morbidly obese boy with panhypopituitarism, diabetes insipidus, and defective thirst regulation. Clin Pediatr 1992;31(4):234–6.

49. Fleseriu M, Hashim IA, Karavitaki N, et al. Hormonal Replacement in Hypopituitarism in Adults: An Endocrine Society Clinical Practice Guideline. J Clin Endocrinol Metab 2016;101(11):3888–921.

50. Boekhoff S, Bogusz A, Sterkenburg AS, et al. Long-term Effects of Growth Hormone Replacement Therapy in Childhood-onset Craniopharyngioma: Results of the German Craniopharyngioma Registry (HIT-Endo). Eur J Endocrinol 2018; 179(5):331–41.

51. Geffner M, Lundberg M, Koltowska-Haggstrom M, et al. Changes in height, weight, and body mass index in children with craniopharyngioma after three years of growth hormone therapy: analysis of KIGS (Pfizer International Growth Database). J Clin Endocrinol Metab 2004;89(11):5435–40.

52. Yuen KC, Koltowska-Haggstrom M, Cook DM, et al. Clinical characteristics and effects of GH replacement therapy in adults with childhood-onset

craniopharyngioma compared with those in adults with other causes of childhood-onset hypothalamic-pituitary dysfunction. Eur J Endocrinol 2013; 169(4):511–9.

53. Heinks K, Boekhoff S, Hoffmann A, et al. Quality of life and growth after childhood craniopharyngioma: results of the multinational trial KRANIOPHARYNGEOM 2007. Endocrine 2018;59(2):364–72.

54. Fernandes JK, Klein MJ, Ater JL, et al. Triiodothyronine supplementation for hypothalamic obesity. Metabolism 2002;51(11):1381–3.

55. van Santen HM, Schouten-Meeteren AY, Serlie M, et al. Effects of T3 treatment on brown adipose tissue and energy expenditure in a patient with craniopharyngioma and hypothalamic obesity. J Pediatr Endocrinol Metab 2015;28(1–2):53–7.

56. Schofl C, Schleth A, Berger D, et al. Sympathoadrenal counterregulation in patients with hypothalamic craniopharyngioma. J Clin Endocrinol Metab 2002; 87(2):624–9.

57. Coutant R, Maurey H, Rouleau S, et al. Defect in epinephrine production in children with craniopharyngioma: functional or organic origin? J Clin Endocrinol Metab 2003;88(12):5969–75.

58. Ismail D, O'Connell MA, Zacharin MR. Dexamphetamine use for management of obesity and hypersomnolence following hypothalamic injury. J Pediatr Endocrinol Metab 2006;19(2):129–34.

59. Denzer C, Denzer F, Lennerz BS, et al. Treatment of Hypothalamic Obesity with Dextroamphetamine: A Case Series. Obes Facts 2019;12(1):91–102.

60. Sadatomo T, Sakoda K, Yamanaka M, et al. Mazindol administration improved hyperphagia after surgery for craniopharyngioma–case report. Neurol Med Chir (Tokyo) 2001;41(4):210–2.

61. Greenway FL, Bray GA. Treatment of hypothalamic obesity with caffeine and ephedrine. Endocr Pract 2008;14(6):697–703.

62. Elfers CT, Roth CL. Effects of methylphenidate on weight gain and food intake in hypothalamic obesity. Front Endocrinol (Lausanne) 2011;2:78.

63. Lustig RH. Hypothalamic obesity: causes, consequences, treatment. Pediatr Endocrinol Rev 2008;6(2):220–7.

64. Available at: http://clinicaltrials.gov/ct2/show/NCT00076362. Accessed May 30, 2020.

65. Lustig RH, Rose SR, Burghen GA, et al. Hypothalamic obesity caused by cranial insult in children: altered glucose and insulin dynamics and reversal by a somatostatin agonist. J Pediatr 1999;135(2 Pt 1):162–8.

66. Brauner R, Serreau R, Souberbielle JC, et al. Diazoxide in Children With Obesity After Hypothalamic-Pituitary Lesions: A Randomized, Placebo-Controlled Trial. J Clin Endocrinol Metab 2016;101(12):4825–33.

67. Hamilton JK, Conwell LS, Syme C, et al. Hypothalamic Obesity following Craniopharyngioma Surgery: Results of a Pilot Trial of Combined Diazoxide and Metformin Therapy. Int J Pediatr Endocrinol 2011;2011:417949.

68. Kalina MA, Wilczek M, Kalina-Faska B, et al. Carbohydrate-lipid profile and use of metformin with micronized fenofibrate in reducing metabolic consequences of craniopharyngioma treatment in children: single institution experience. J Pediatr Endocrinol Metab 2015;28(1–2):45–51.

69. Lomenick JP, Buchowski MS, Shoemaker AH. A 52-week pilot study of the effects of exenatide on body weight in patients with hypothalamic obesity. Obesity (Silver Spring) 2016;24(6):1222–5.

70. Zoicas F, Droste M, Mayr B, et al. GLP-1 analogues as a new treatment option for hypothalamic obesity in adults: report of nine cases. Eur J Endocrinol 2013; 168(5):699–706.

71. Simmons JH, Shoemaker AH, Roth CL. Treatment with glucagon-like Peptide-1 agonist exendin-4 in a patient with hypothalamic obesity secondary to intracranial tumor. Horm Res Paediatr 2012;78(1):54–8.

72. Thondam SK, Cuthbertson DJ, Aditya BS, et al. A glucagon-like peptide-1 (GLP-1) receptor agonist in the treatment for hypothalamic obesity complicated by type 2 diabetes mellitus. Clin Endocrinol 2012;77(4):635–7.

73. Castro-Dufourny I, Carrasco R, Pascual JM. Hypothalamic obesity after craniopharyngioma surgery: Treatment with a long acting glucagon like peptide 1 derivated. Endocrinol Diabetes Nutr 2017;64(3):182–4.

74. Igaki N, Tanaka M, Goto T. Markedly improved glycemic control and enhanced insulin sensitivity in a patient with type 2 diabetes complicated by a suprasellar tumor treated with pioglitazone and metformin. Intern Med 2005;44(8):832–7.

75. Shoemaker A, Proietto J, Abuzzahab MJ, et al. A randomized, placebo-controlled trial of beloranib for the treatment of hypothalamic injury-associated obesity. Diabetes Obes Metab 2017;19(8):1165–70.

76. McCandless SE, Yanovski JA, Miller J, et al. Effects of MetAP2 inhibition on hyperphagia and body weight in Prader-Willi syndrome: A randomized, double-blind, placebo-controlled trial. Diabetes Obes Metab 2017;19(12):1751–61.

77. James WP, Caterson ID, Coutinho W, et al. Effect of sibutramine on cardiovascular outcomes in overweight and obese subjects. N Engl J Med 2010;363(10): 905–17.

78. Daubenbüchel AM, Hoffmann A, Eveslage M, et al. Oxytocin in survivors of childhood-onset craniopharyngioma. Endocrine 2016;54(2):524–31.

79. Hoffmann A, Ozyurt J, Lohle K, et al. First experiences with neuropsychological effects of oxytocin administration in childhood-onset craniopharyngioma. Endocrine 2017;56(1):175–85.

80. Daubenbüchel AM, Ozyurt J, Boekhoff S, et al. Eating behaviour and oxytocin in patients with childhood-onset craniopharyngioma and different grades of hypothalamic involvement. Pediatr Obes 2019;14:e12527.

81. Hsu EA, Miller JL, Perez FA, et al. Oxytocin and Naltrexone Successfully Treat Hypothalamic Obesity in a Boy Post-Craniopharyngioma Resection. J Clin Endocrinol Metab 2018;103(2):370–5.

82. Weismann D, Pelka T, Bender G, et al. Bariatric surgery for morbid obesity in craniopharyngioma. Clin Endocrinol 2013;78(3):385–90.

83. Wijnen M, Olsson DS, van den Heuvel-Eibrink MM, et al. Efficacy and safety of bariatric surgery for craniopharyngioma-related hypothalamic obesity: a matched case-control study with 2 years of follow-up. Int J Obes (Lond) 2017;41(2):210–6.

84. Inge TH, Pfluger P, Zeller M, et al. Gastric bypass surgery for treatment of hypothalamic obesity after craniopharyngioma therapy. Nat Clin Pract Endocrinol Metab 2007;3(8):606–9.

85. Page-Wilson G, Wardlaw SL, Khandji AG, et al. Hypothalamic obesity in patients with craniopharyngioma: treatment approaches and the emerging role of gastric bypass surgery. Pituitary 2012;15(1):84–92.

86. Rottembourg D, O'Gorman CS, Urbach S, et al. Outcome after bariatric surgery in two adolescents with hypothalamic obesity following treatment of craniopharyngioma. J Pediatr Endocrinol Metab 2009;22(9):867–72.

87. Müller HL, Gebhardt U, Maroske J, et al. Long-term follow-up of morbidly obese patients with childhood craniopharyngioma after laparoscopic adjustable gastric banding (LAGB). Klin Padiatr 2011;223(6):372–3.

88. Gatta B, Nunes ML, Bailacq-Auder C, et al. Is bariatric surgery really inefficient in hypothalamic obesity? Clin Endocrinol 2013;78(4):636–8.

89. Bretault M, Laroche S, Lacorte JM, et al. Postprandial GLP-1 Secretion After Bariatric Surgery in Three Cases of Severe Obesity Related to Craniopharyngiomas. Obes Surg 2016;26(5):1133–7.

90. Wolf P, Winhofer Y, Smajis S, et al. Hormone Substitution after Gastric Bypass Surgery in Patients with Hypopituitarism Secondary to Craniopharyngioma. Endocr Pract 2016;22(5):595–601.

91. Trotta M, Da Broi J, Salerno A, et al. Sleeve gastrectomy leads to easy management of hormone replacement therapy and good weight loss in patients treated for craniopharyngioma. Updates Surg 2017;69(1):95–9.

92. Muller HL, Gebhardt U, Wessel V, et al. First experiences with laparoscopic adjustable gastric banding (LAGB) in the treatment of patients with childhood craniopharyngioma and morbid obesity. Klin Padiatr 2007;219(6):323–5.

93. Bingham NC, Rose SR, Inge TH. Bariatric surgery in hypothalamic obesity. Front Endocrinol (Lausanne) 2012;3:23.

94. Bretault M, Boillot A, Muzard L, et al. Bariatric surgery following treatment for craniopharyngioma: a systematic review and individual-level data meta-analysis. J Clin Endocrinol Metab 2013;98(6):2239–46.

95. Schultes B, Ernst B, Schmid F, et al. Distal gastric bypass surgery for the treatment of hypothalamic obesity after childhood craniopharyngioma. Eur J Endocrinol 2009;161(1):201–6.

96. Smith DK, Sarfeh J, Howard L. Truncal vagotomy in hypothalamic obesity. Lancet 1983;1(8337):1330–1.

97. Harat M, Rudas M, Zielinski P, et al. Nucleus accumbens stimulation in pathological obesity. Neurol Neurochir Pol 2016;50(3):207–10.

98. Elowe-Grau E, Beltrand J, Brauner R, et al. Childhood craniopharyngioma: hypothalamus-sparing surgery decreases the risk of obesity. J Clin Endocrinol Metab 2013;98(6):2376–82.

Pituitary Tumors Centers of Excellence

Stefano Frara, MD[a,1], Gemma Rodriguez-Carnero, MD[b,1], Ana M. Formenti, MD[a], Miguel A. Martinez-Olmos, MD[b,c], Andrea Giustina, MD[a], Felipe F. Casanueva, MD, PhD[b,c],*

KEYWORDS

- Acromegaly • Cushing disease • Hypopituitarism • Pituitary adenoma
- Transsphenoidal surgery • Pituitary radiotherapy

KEY POINTS

- Pituitary tumors centers of excellence (PTCOE) are organizations of multidisciplinary, integrated, updated, and highly trained professionals to provide high-level medical care in a patient-centric organization, and to develop pituitary science.
- Expert clinical endocrinologists plus expert neurosurgeons are the core of PTCOE, with the contribution of different specialties such as neuroradiology, neuropathology, radiation oncology, neuro-ophthalmology, otorhinolaryngology, and trained nursing.
- Experience in pituitary surgery is based on excellent training plus maintaining of high workloads, and regional centers may be a solution to increase experience in a given PTCOE.

INTRODUCTION

In recent years, the need for centers of excellence (COEs), for patients to receive the most innovative diagnostic work-up and best medical care, has become increasingly urgent. Simultaneously, health professionals also strive to work in COEs to increase the quality of their work as well as their professional satisfaction and academic prestige. However, health administrators worldwide debate the optimization of patient organization and the roles of clinicians to create the most cost-effective and suitable structures and increase the scientific contributions of their departments by publishing their most recent findings.

[a] Institute of Endocrinology, Università Vita-Salute San Raffaele, Via Olgettina Milano, 58, Milano, Milan 20132, Italy; [b] Division of Endocrinology, Complejo Hospitalario Universitario de Santiago (USC/SERGAS), Instituto de Investigacion Sanitaria de Santiago (IDIS), Rúa da Choupana, S/N, Santiago de Compostela, A Coruña 15706, Spain; [c] CIBER Fisiopatología de la Obesidad y la Nutrición (CIBERobn), Instituto de Salud Carlos III, Madrid, Spain
[1] Both authors contributed equally to this manuscript
* Corresponding author. Division of Endocrinology, Santiago de Compostela University, Choupana Street sn, Santiago de Compostela 15706, Spain.
E-mail address: felipe.casanueva@usc.es

Endocrinol Metab Clin N Am 49 (2020) 553–564
https://doi.org/10.1016/j.ecl.2020.05.010
0889-8529/20/© 2020 Elsevier Inc. All rights reserved.

endo.theclinics.com

COEs represent the gold standard in many clinical specialties (**Fig. 1**), such as breast cancer and bariatric surgery, particularly when surgical teams are involved in treatment. Recent experiences have shown outstanding improvements in the health care received by patients treated in COEs.[1] It is commonly thought that experts provide the best standard of care to patients and that COEs are particularly valuable when multidisciplinary teams, often including experts in both surgical techniques and medical treatments, are involved.[1–3] However, issues have arisen regarding the methods adopted to recognize COEs because there is currently no clear worldwide consensus on the definition of a COE. In this context, some centers might be driven by internal or external factors to nominate themselves as COEs without external or independent evaluation or accreditation processes, whereas, in other cases, the local, regional, or national accreditation procedures are not based on validated criteria.

COEs should be considered patient-centric organizations, because patient health is the core mission (**Fig. 2**). In real life, patient networks, engagement activities, family impact, educational platforms, digital infrastructure to facilitate care across primary and secondary health units, and specialties are essential for properly accredited COEs.[4]

PITUITARY TUMORS CENTERS OF EXCELLENCE

Increasing prevalence and incidence of pituitary tumors and hypopituitarism have been reported in recent decades,[5,6] particularly with the improvement of ultrasensitive biochemical assays,[7–10] advances in imaging procedures (particularly MRI),[11,12] and the availability of more efficacious drugs.[13,14]

However, despite this progress, diagnostic work-up and clinical management remain challenges for physicians. In many centers, endocrinologists and surgeons are connected but not integrated and the patients circulate between the different specialists. Pituitary tumors COEs (PTCOEs) require an integrated multidisciplinary group in a single location (**Fig. 3**). The best care for patients affected by pituitary disorders is provided by dedicated endocrinologists and experienced pituitary surgeons who work

> *A center of excellence is a program within a healthcare institution which is assembled to supply an exceptionally high concentration of expertise and related resources centered on a particular area of medicine, delivering associated care in a comprehensive, interdisciplinary fashion to afford the best patient outcomes possible*
>
> Elrod JK & Fortenberry JL 2017
>
> ***Mostly implemented when surgery is involved***

Fig. 1. The main characteristics of a COE. (*Data from* Elrod JK, Fortenberry JL Jr. Centers of excellence in healthcare institutions: what they are and how to assemble them. BMC Heath Serv Res. 2017; 17(Suppl 1):425.)

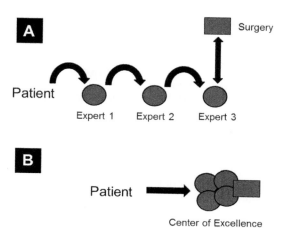

Fig. 2. (*A*) The usual process by which the patient passes from one expert to another, which is replaced by (*B*) the PTCOE as an integrated interdisciplinary center.

together as the leaders of interdisciplinary teams.[15,16] In the first phases, the endocrinologist should accompany the patient through the diagnostic work-up based on the most recent guideline recommendations and ensure the optimal clinical, psychological, and social conditions before handing the patient over to the neurosurgeon. Later, the same endocrinologist must follow the patient and should manage persistent or recurrent disease-related events and related comorbidities. The endocrinologist plays a key role in providing an individualized program of care that includes medical therapy, surgery, and, eventually, radiotherapy or radiosurgery, in addition to long-term follow-up. The ultimate goal is the elimination or reduction of excess morbidities and mortality associated with the tumor mass and hormonal hypersecretion while also addressing any complementary pituitary deficiencies.[15–17] The surgeon should be a well-trained, experienced, and dedicated neurosurgeon.

PTCOEs require support from a collaborative environment of other well-trained specialists, including neuroradiologists, neuropathologists, radiotherapists, neuro-

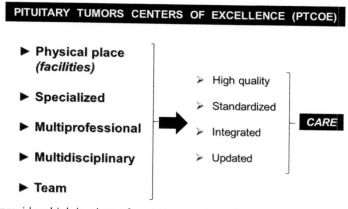

Fig. 3. To provide a high-level care for pituitary patients is the main target of a PTCOE. To reach that target, the organization of the PTCOE needs a physical place but also a multidisciplinary team organized to provide high-quality and standardized care

ophthalmologists, otorhinolaryngologists, bone experts, and cardiologists, in addition to trained nursing staff and psychologists to tackle both medical and psychological issues.[16,18]

The goals of these multidisciplinary teams include[4]:

1. Early tumor detection and diagnosis
2. Determination of the most suitable treatment based on a patient-centered approach to choose the most appropriate treatment at any time
3. Control of hormonal hypersecretion and its effects
4. Removal of the pituitary mass (and, possibly, hormonal hypersecretion) and preservation of the normal pituitary and nearby structures
5. Prevention of tumor recurrence
6. Recognition and care of both acute and delayed complications of the disease, including hypopituitarism

Research that indicates the need for PTCOEs either has mostly focused on the outcomes of surgical procedures or is based on health or administrative issues with the main goal of cost reduction. In several countries, pituitary units already feature effective high-level interdisciplinary workgroups; however, most of these groups are self-appointed structures without any formal acknowledgment.[16] Because explicit and practical definitions for a degree of excellence have not yet been defined, the measurement of patient outcomes remains unplanned and the fulfillment of the previously outlined goals remains undetermined.[19,20]

Notwithstanding the clinical activities, another purpose of PTCOEs is to enhance pituitary sciences through adequate participation in international meetings and publication of scientific reports. Several issues may arise in this regard because units formed by a single endocrinologist or neurosurgeon will not be very active in publishing original articles or actively participating in meetings and administrative organizations. In contrast, groups that are more successful are productive in terms of literature reports on the best outcomes, which seldom reflect the contributions of less experienced and less productive groups, leading to a communication bias. To reduce the impact of communication bias, the widespread use of disease-specific registries and files may be particularly effective, as shown by the different Scandinavian and European national health registries.[21,22]

NEUROSURGERY

Although the medical treatments for pituitary lesions have improved, PTCOEs could not exist without a pituitary-dedicated surgical group capable of performing both transsphenoidal endonasal (TNS) and transcranial approaches.[19,23] Despite the development of modern imaging techniques and neuronavigation, 1 or more experienced neurosurgeons are mandatory for safe and effective pituitary surgery.[24]

According to recent guideline recommendations, pituitary surgery remains a cornerstone for the treatment of pituitary adenoma and the most effective procedure for acromegaly, Cushing disease, thyroid-stimulating hormone (TSH)–secreting adenomas, resistant prolactinomas, and nonfunctioning pituitary adenomas causing mass symptoms, pituitary apoplexy, and rare cases of pituitary carcinomas.[25–27]

Although the end points for pituitary surgery include tumor removal with preservation of the normal pituitary and adjacent structures, the definition of excellence for individual pituitary surgeons is much more complex.[19,20]

Neurosurgeons devoted to pituitary tumors must have a deep knowledge of sellar anatomy and physiology and the principles of endocrine evaluation; from an education and training perspective, a residency program in neurosurgery with continuous exchanges with neuroendocrinologists is mandatory. After residency, depending on the training opportunities available, either completion of a formal postgraduate fellowship in pituitary surgery or skull-base/neuro-oncologic surgery or a postgraduate subspecialty training at a high-volume pituitary center have been suggested.[4,28] A fellowship at a high-quality center performing large numbers of TNS interventions each year is also routinely required to improve technical skills.[29–31]

However, a perfect residency and postspecialization training are not enough. A peculiarity of pituitary surgery is that neurosurgeons require continuous practice based on a high workload to maintain high levels of performance and capability. Several reports have shown that experienced surgeons have better outcomes and lower rates of complications than surgeons with lower workloads.[1,32–36]

For the fixed number of inhabitants covered by a PTCOE, a reduced number of pituitary surgeons must be enough to cover the clinical needs of that hospital because the outcomes are directly correlated with intense workloads. Thus, centers with few neurosurgeons have better outcomes than centers with several pituitary surgeons with low workloads.[32,33,35,37–39]

Nevertheless, a single neurosurgeon may face many bureaucratic and administrative challenges, including patient management during the neurosurgeon's absence, training of new fellows, or participation in clinical trials or research activities. Furthermore, the population served may be too small to permit an intense workload and artificially increasing the number of patients is not suitable or ethically acceptable.

One proposal to address these challenges is to concentrate up to 4 neurosurgeons at a given PTCOE to cover the neurosurgery requirements of a region ideally containing 2.5 million to 5 million inhabitants,[4] receiving patients living nearby as well as those who are referred from endocrine units in other regional hospitals.[40] These so-called regional PTCOEs should perform at least 100 interventions annually, receiving patients with already-confirmed diagnoses from different endocrinology units and sending the patients back for follow-up at the original hospitals after surgery.[4] Because pituitary diseases are not frequent, this organizational strategy could be effective and provide cost benefits for health administrators.

ENDOCRINOLOGY

A PTCOE requires that the neurosurgery group work closely with an endocrine unit devoted to pituitary disorders. Because pituitary disorders include not only tumors but also other pituitary pathologies, endocrinologists must be able to manage pituitary problems such as hormonal hypersecretion and deficiencies, disease-related complications, effects of tumor treatment, and mass symptoms.[14,25,41,42] Thus, in this clinical setting, endocrinologists play both a lifelong prominent role as well as a holistic role in managing all of the patients' problems. Although several studies have characterized the conditions required for surgeons to be considered experts pituitary surgeon, none has defined an expert pituitary endocrinologist.

Because of this deficiency in criteria, it is customary to rely on an endocrinologist's scientific activity instead, such as publications and participation in scientific meetings or randomized clinical trials. Although this solution is currently acceptable, concrete criteria such as workload and outcomes should in the future be adopted.

Although the established criteria for endocrinologist excellence may be more theoretic, in some ways it is easier to define than for a neurosurgeon because a high workload is, at present, not crucial. Similar to what was discussed earlier for neurosurgeons, basic training in internal medicine and endocrinology through residency, followed by postgraduate training with international experts in pituitary disorders, is mandatory for endocrinologists aiming to work in a PTCOE.

Because diagnosis is based on the accuracy of measurement of biochemical parameters and considering that high variability may affect the results of routine hormonal assays,[7–9] expert endocrinologists must have a thorough knowledge of the laboratory procedures for hormone analysis in basal conditions or during stimulatory/inhibitory tests as well as the reagents, calibrators, degree of standardization, and preanalytical and analytical variability. Deep knowledge of how hormonal assays work is currently a limitation in endocrinologist training. Interactions between clinicians and laboratory staff should be always recommended to maintain top-level international standards and implement the continuous updates in techniques. This approach is particularly helpful for the early detection of possible pitfalls during diagnostic work-up or long-term clinical management. Endocrinologists should be able to pass through national or regional protocols and guidelines that may differ between countries.[43]

Moreover, experts in pituitary diseases should have a rudimentary understanding of MRI and the clinical implications and limitations of anatomopathologic reports and tissue markers.

Another goal of the endocrinology unit in PTCOEs is to provide scientific advances in pituitary sciences, including consistent publication of original articles and reviews in peer-reviewed journals as well as chapters in monographs and participation in scientific congresses, consensus meetings, and multicenter trials. This goal should be included in the strategic planning for PTCOEs.

With evidence-based approaches, consensus recommendations address important clinical issues regarding multidisciplinary management of cardiovascular, endocrine, metabolic, and oncologic comorbidities; sleep apnea; and bone and joint disorders and their sequelae, as well as their effects on patient quality of life and mortality.[42,43] With the assistance of the different supporting units, endocrinologists are routinely charged with the management of these complications.

Secondary diabetes, dyslipidemia, and arterial hypertension are prevalent in many patients with growth hormone derangements, either in excess (ie, acromegaly)[44] or deficiency (growth hormone deficiency [GHD])[45] as well as those with cortisol hypersecretion.[46] Endocrinologists should be able to diagnose and manage these complications early, performing appropriate screening and prescribing innovative drugs to reduce the high cardiovascular risk associated with these conditions. At the same time, hypopituitarism may occur because of the pituitary lesion itself (eg, giant macroadenomas) or because of iatrogenic intervention neurosurgery, radiotherapy, and/or radiosurgery. Endocrinologists must manage all these conditions through the administration of replacement therapies and by monitoring both the advantages and possible side effects related to overtreatment and lack of sensitive and specific biochemical parameters.[47]

SUPPORTING UNITS

The close relationship between expert pituitary surgeons and pituitary endocrinologists requires additional support by several specialties to provide a high standard of care. These 2 core specialists coordinate the supporting units to guarantee the best standard of care in a patient-centered approach.

Imaging scans and analysis remain the cornerstones of diagnostic work-up, particularly in cases in which microadenoma is not easily identified. Therefore, the neuroradiology unit should perform not only high-field MRI with at least 1.5-T field strength and high-resolution depiction of the sellar region but also thin-collimation computed tomography for patients in whom MRI is contraindicated. To support radiological clinical trials and ensure reliable follow-up scans, neuroradiologists should be involved in the standardization of section orientation and image labeling. PTCOE supporting units should also have access to digital subtraction angiography and dynamic contrast-enhanced MRI,[48] whereas interventional radiologists should be experts in selective bilateral venous sampling of the inferior petrosal sinus.

The role of nuclear medicine units in the management of pituitary adenomas is increasing and the modern technique of PET scan may be useful in highly difficult cases.

Cardiovascular events are highly prevalent in patients with pituitary disorders and represent the major cause of death in most of these conditions, including acromegaly, Cushing, and adrenocorticotropic hormone (ACTH) deficiency.[47–49] Between collaborating units, the cardiology unit has an essential role both in the first phases of the diagnostic process and during long-term follow-up. The anesthesiologist is responsible for addressing any cardiac or circulation issues that may represent a contraindication for tumor neurosurgery or that may occur during the intervention.

The neuropathology unit is particularly useful for reaching a definitive diagnosis and should comprise several experienced neuropathologists or endocrine pathologists who perform routine classic assessment of histology (ie, mitoses, pleomorphism, giant cells, inclusions, inflammatory changes, stroma, hemorrhage, vascular features, proliferative indices) and routine pituitary hormone stains (ACTH, prolactin, growth hormone, TSH, luteinizing hormone, follicle-stimulating hormone, and, in some cases, α-subunit, chromogranin, P53, hormone receptor stains, and transcription factor assessments).[50,51] The pathologist is responsible for the report indicating the diagnosis, based on current World Health Organization (WHO) and Pituitary Society guidelines.[52,53] This final report should be always discussed with the core members of the PTCOE (neurosurgeon and endocrinologist) regarding its clinical implications on subsequent follow-up.[54–56] In addition, a tumor specimen bank may be included for basic and translational scientific progress.

PTCOEs may require close surgical collaboration between neurosurgeons and otolaryngologists for the execution of endonasal and other skull-base approaches, whereas neuro-ophthalmologists are required for the diagnosis and, in some cases, for follow-up of visual complications in macroadenomas and giant adenomas.

Stereotactic radiotherapy or gamma-knife radiosurgery are required for the treatment of pituitary tumors resistant to medical treatment, in cases of recurrence, in patients who refuse or cannot undergo surgery, or in cases of aggressive pituitary adenomas or carcinomas. Assisted by the most innovative computer technologies and imaging software and working with neurosurgeons, expert radiotherapists should have a deep knowledge of the tolerances of the optic systems, cranial nerves of the cavernous sinus, temporal lobes, and the normal pituitary gland.[57–59] Moreover, they should also try to establish a time lapse between radiation treatment and the development of complications such as hypopituitarism. Considering the different organizations of the national health systems and the very small number of units with very intense workloads, radiotherapy units are often located outside the referred PTCOE hospital; however, these should be formally included as a main part of the PTCOE architecture.

Skeletal fragility and high risk of fracture are common, although often underdiagnosed, complications in patients with pituitary diseases characterized by hypopituitarism or hormonal hypersecretion.[60] Therefore, bone specialists should work with the PTCOE to evaluate bone health in patients at diagnosis and during follow-up. In particular, this specialist may help with the diagnostic study of bone metabolism by selecting the optimal tools among bone markers, bone mineral density (BMD) measurements with classic dual-energy x-ray absorptiometry (DXA) scans, and vertebral morphometry. Fragility fractures, particularly vertebral fractures, are related to impaired bone quality more than bone quantity; thus, fractures may occur even when BMD is not severely reduced. In addition, bone specialists should advise on specific measures to prevent or treat bone loss in pituitary patients.

The management of psychiatric comorbidities requires a multidisciplinary approach[61]; namely, a psychologist to provide a more complete picture of the patient's symptoms and, most importantly, to help patients to feel understood, encourage patients to ask questions, and allow patients to be more comfortable with their therapeutic decisions.[62] A well-trained nursing group is also essential for the management of patients with pituitary tumors. Psychotherapy and/or medication may be recommended to some patients. After disease control, patients should be routinely checked for psychiatric symptoms and their results monitored based on the administration of specific disease-related questionnaires (eg, AcroQoL or CushingQoL), with psychological and/or medical treatment considered when necessary.[62]

Patients may also benefit from families and clinician support, participating in support groups, and receiving education on their diseases and the possible comorbidities, as recommended by recent guidelines.[42]

To better highlight the disease-related psychosocial impacts and address socioeconomic issues, patient associations might play a direct and active role by encouraging and supporting patients' requests based on patient perspectives and spreading knowledge on specific pituitary disorders.

NETWORKING PROCESSES

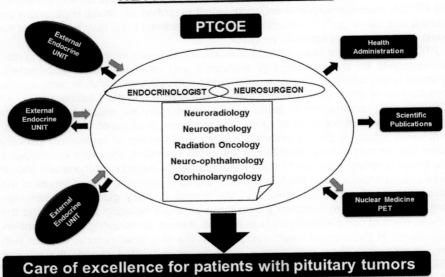

Fig. 4. Working procedure for a PTCOE. External endocrine units may send their patients to the PTCOE for treatment in addition to their own patients. After that, patients must return to their original centers for follow-up. In that way, PTCOEs and collaborating centers act as a network for effective patient care but also for research, clinical trials, and the development of pituitary science. Another task of a PTCOE is to assess health administrators and produce high-level publications while preserving its main target of providing excellent care to patients with pituitary tumors.

SUMMARY

In recent decades, a consistent body of evidence has supported the goal of providing the best possible care to patients with pituitary tumors. The PTCOEs represent this concept at the highest level and can be considered the future organizational gold standard for placing the patients at the center of decision-making processes. Modern PTCOEs devoted to these types of tumors include both expert neurosurgeons performing pituitary surgery as well as experienced neuroendocrinologists. Although these 2 specialties represent the core leadership, other specialties need to be included as supporting units to follow patients during the diagnostic work-up, the choice of different therapeutic options, and the management of any complications. PTCOEs at the regional level must also provide support to external high-level pituitary endocrine units. Patients should be able to move from those units to the PTCOE for final surgical treatment and outcome evaluation. After treatment, the patient should return to the center of origin (**Fig. 4**). Only patients going and returning makes the external units comfortable. Moreover, this system must be structured as a network not only for patient care but also for participation in meetings and publications, and performing clinical trials.

Performing these activities with a patient-centered approach by supporting units and coordinated by the endocrinology and neurosurgery units provides multiple benefits, including:

1. Providing the best standard of care with the most innovative techniques and the most effective drugs
2. Allowing scientific progress in neuroendocrinology and reducing possible bias
3. Creating a cost-effective organization, saving money for national health systems, and adding value to both physicians and administrative staff activities

DISCLOSURE

F.F. Casanueva is currently member of the Pituitary Society Executive Committee. The remaining authors have nothing to disclose.

REFERENCES

1. Pratt GM, McLees B, Pories WJ. The ASBS bariatric surgery Centers of Excellence program: a blueprint for quality improvement. Surg Obes Relat Dis 2006; 2:497–503.
2. Weisman CS, Squires GL. Women's health centers: are the National Centers of Excellence in Women's Health a new model? Womens Health Issues 2000;10: 248–55.
3. Champion JK, Pories WJ. Centers of excellence for bariatric surgery. Surg Obes Relat Dis 2005;148–51.
4. Casanueva FF, Barkan AL, Buchfelder M, et al. Criteria for the definition of Pituitary Tumor Centers of Excellence (PTCOE). Pituitary 2017;20:489–98.
5. Daly AF, Tichomirowa MA, Beckers A. The epidemiology and genetics of pituitary adenomas. Best Pract Res Clin Endocrinol Metab 2009;23:543–54.
6. Fernandez A, Karavitaki N, Wass JA. Prevalence of pituitary adenomas: a community-based, cross-sectional study in Banbury (Oxfordshire, UK). Clin Endocrinol 2010;72:377–82.
7. Schilbach K, Strasburger CJ, Bidlingmaier M. Biochemical investigations in diagnosis and follow up of acromegaly. Pituitary 2017;20:33–45.

8. Smith TP, Kavanagh L, Healy ML, et al. Technology insight: measuring prolactin in clinical samples. Nat Clin Pract Endocrinol Metab 2007;3:279–89.

9. Donegan DM, Algeciras-Schimnich A, Hamidi O, et al. Corticotropin hormone assay interference: A case series. Clin Biochem 2019;63:143–7.

10. Ceccato F, Boscaro M. Cushing's syndrome: screening and diagnosis. High Blood Press Cardiovasc Prev 2016;23:209–15.

11. Pressman BD. Pituitary imaging. Endocrinol Metab Clin North Am 2017;46:713–40.

12. Varrassi M, Cobianchi Bellisari F, Bruno F, et al. High-resolution magnetic resonance imaging at 3T of pituitary gland: advantages and pitfalls. Gland Surg 2019;8:S208–15.

13. Stormann S, Schopohl J. New and emerging drug therapies for Cushing's disease. Expert Opin Pharmacother 2018;19:1187–200.

14. Maffezzoni F, Formenti AM, Mazziotti G, et al. Current and future medical treatments for patients with acromegaly. Expert Opin Pharmacother 2016;17:1631–42.

15. Giustina A, Chanson P, Kleinberg D, et al. Expert consensus document: A consensus on the medical treatment of acromegaly. Nat Rev Endocrinol 2014;10:243–8.

16. Melmed S, Casanueva FF, Cavagnini F, et al. Guidelines for acromegaly management. J Clin Endocrinol Metab 2002;87:4054–8.

17. Barker FG, Klibanski A, Swearingen B. Transsphenoidal surgery for pituitary tumors in the United States, 1996-2000: mortality, morbidity, and the effects of hospital and surgeon volume. J Clin Endocrinol Metab 2003;88:4709–19.

18. Pertichetti M, Serioli S, Belotti F, et al. Pituitary adenomas and neuropsychological status: a systematic literature review. Neurosurg Rev 2019. https://doi.org/10.1007/s10143-019-01134-z.

19. Schwartz TH. A role for centers of excellence in transsphenoidal surgery. World Neurosurg 2013;80:270–1.

20. Faustini-Fustini M, Pasquini E, Zoli M, et al. Pituitary centers of excellence. Neurosurgery 2013;73:E557.

21. Esposito D, Ragnarsson O, Granfeldt D, et al. Decreasing mortality and changes in treatment patterns in patients with acromegaly from a nationwide study. Eur J Endocrinol 2018;178:459–69.

22. van Varsseveld NC, van Bunderen CC, Franken AA, et al. Fractures in pituitary adenoma patients from the Dutch National Registry of Growth Hormone Treatment in Adults. Pituitary 2016;19:381–90.

23. Swearingen B. Update on pituitary surgery. J Clin Endocrinol Metab 2012;97:1073–81.

24. Ammirati M, Wei L, Ciric I. Short-term outcome of endoscopic versus microscopic pituitary adenoma surgery: a systematic review and meta-analysis. J Neurol Neurosurg Psychiatry 2013;84:843–9.

25. Casanueva FF, Molitch ME, Schlechte JA, et al. Guidelines of the Pituitary Society for the diagnosis and management of prolactinomas. Clin Endocrinol 2006;65:265–73.

26. Katznelson L, Laws ER Jr, Melmed S, et al. Acromegaly: an endocrine society clinical practice guideline. J Clin Endocrinol Metab 2014;99:3933–51.

27. Mortini P, Barzaghi LR, Albano L, et al. Microsurgical therapy of pituitary adenomas. Endocrine 2018;59:72–81.

28. Mercado M, Gonzalez B, Vargas G, et al. Successful mortality reduction and control of comorbidities in patients with acromegaly followed at a highly specialized multidisciplinary clinic. J Clin Endocrinol Metab 2014;99:4438–46.

29. Knutzen R. Pituitary centers of excellence: for patients it is life or death. Neurosurgery 2014;74:E143.
30. Powell M, Grossman A. Quality indicators in pituitary surgery: a need for reliable and valid assessments. What should be measured? Clin Endocrinol 2016;84:485–8.
31. Snyderman C, Kassam A, Carrau R, et al. Acquisition of surgical skills for endonasal skull base surgery: a training program. Laryngoscope 2007;117:699–705.
32. Yamada S, Aiba T, Takada K, et al. Retrospective analysis of long-term surgical results in acromegaly: preoperative and postoperative factors predicting outcome. Clin Endocrinol 1996;45:291–8.
33. Gittoes NJ, Sheppard MC, Johnson AP, et al. Outcome of surgery for acromegaly the experience of a dedicated pituitary surgeon. An Int J Medicine 1999;92:741–5.
34. Erturk E, Tuncel E, Kiyici S, et al. Outcome of surgery for acromegaly performed by different surgeons: importance of surgical experience. Pituitary 2005;8:93–7.
35. Bates PR, Carson MN, Trainer PJ, et al. Wide variation in surgical outcomes for acromegaly in the UK. Clin Endocrinol 2008;68:136–42.
36. Koc K, Anik I, Ozdamar D, et al. The learning curve in endoscopic pituitary surgery and our experience. Neurosurg Rev 2006;29:298–305.
37. Ahmed S, Elsheikh M, Stratton IM, et al. Outcome of transphenoidal surgery for acromegaly and its relationship to surgical experience. Clin Endocrinol 1999;50:561–7.
38. Birkmeyer JD, Siewers AE, Finlayson EV, et al. Hospital volume and surgical mortality in the United States. N Engl J Med 2002;346:1128–37.
39. Barker FG, Curry WT, Carter BS. Surgery for primary supratentorial brain tumors in the United States, 1988 to 2000: the effect of provider caseload and centralization of care. Neuro Oncol 2005;7:49–63.
40. Luft HS, Bunker JP, Enthoven AC. Should operations be regionalized? The empirical relation between surgical volume and mortality. N Engl J Med 1979;301:1364–9.
41. Ascoli P, Cavagnini F. Hypopituitarism. Pituitary 2006;9:335–42.
42. Giustina A, Barkan A, Beckers A. A consensus on the diagnosis and treatment of acromegaly comorbidities: an update. J Clin Endocrinol Metab 2019. [Epub ahead of print].
43. Binder G, Reinehr T, Ibanez L, et al. GHD diagnostics in Europe and the US: an audit of national guidelines and practice. Horm Res Paediatr 2019;8:1–7.
44. Frara S, Maffezzoni F, Mazziotti G, et al. Current and emerging aspects of diabetes mellitus in acromegaly. Trends Endocrinol Metab 2016;27:470–83.
45. Hoybye C, Burman P, Feldt-Rasmussen U, et al. Change in baseline characteristics over 20 years of adults with growth hormone (GH) deficiency on GH replacement therapy. Eur J Endocrinol 2019;181(6):629–38.
46. Mazziotti G, Formenti AM, Frara S, et al. Diabetes in cushing disease. Curr Diab Rep 2017;17:32.
47. Mazziotti G, Formenti AM, Frara S, et al. Risk of overtreatment in patients with adrenal insufficiency: current and emerging aspects. Eur J Endocrinol 2017;177:R231–48.
48. Ragnarsson O, Olsson DS, Papakokkinou E, et al. Overall and disease-specific mortality in patients with cushing disease: A Swedish Nationwide Study. J Clin Endocrinol Metab 2019;104:2375–84.

49. Gadelha MR, Kasuki L, Lim DST, et al. Systemic complications of acromegaly and the impact of the current treatment landscape: An Update. Endocr Rev 2019;40: 268–332.
50. Evans CO, Young AN, Brown MR, et al. Novel patterns of gene expression in pituitary adenomas identified by complementary deoxyribonucleic acid microarrays and quantitative reverse transcription-polymerase chain reaction. J Clin Endocrinol Metab 2001;86:3097–107.
51. Gejman R, Swearingen B, Hedley-Whyte ET. Role of Ki-67 proliferation index and p53 expression in predicting progression of pituitary adenomas. Hum Pathol 2008;39:758–66.
52. Lloyd RV, Osamura RY, Klöppel G, et al. WHO classification of tumours of endocrine organs. 4th edition. IARC; 2017.
53. Ho K, et al. A tale of pituitary adenomas: to net or not to net a Pituitary Society position statement. Pituitary 2019;22:569–73.
54. Galland F, Lacroix L, Saulnier P, et al. Differential gene expression profiles of invasive and non-invasive non-functioning pituitary adenomas based on microarray analysis. Endocr Relat Cancer 2010;17:361–71.
55. Sheehan JM, Vance ML, Sheehan JP, et al. Radiosurgery for Cushing's disease after failed transsphenoidal surgery. J Neurosurg 2000;93:738–42.
56. Jane JA, Vance ML, Woodburn CJ, et al. Stereotactic radiosurgery for hypersecreting pituitary tumors: part of a multimodality approach. Neurosurg Focus 2003;14:e12.
57. Behbehani RS, McElveen T, Sergott RC, et al. Fractionated stereotactic radiotherapy for parasellar meningiomas: a preliminary report of visual outcomes. Br J Ophthalmol 2005;89:130–3.
58. Loeffler JS, Shih HA. Radiation therapy in the management of pituitary adenomas. J Clin Endocrinol Metab 2011;96:1992–2003.
59. Mortini P, Losa M, Barzaghi R, et al. Results of transsphenoidal surgery in a large series of patients with pituitary adenoma. Neurosurgery 2005;56:1222–33.
60. Mazziotti G, Frara S, Giustina A. Pituitary diseases and bone. Endocr Rev 2018; 39:440–88.
61. Santos A, Resmini E, Pascual JC, et al. Psychiatric symptoms in patients with cushing's syndrome: prevalence, diagnosis and management. Drugs 2017;77: 829–42.
62. Crespo I, Santos A, Resmini E, et al. Improving quality of life in patients with pituitary tumours. Eur Endocrinol 2013;9:32–6.

Moving?

Make sure your subscription moves with you!

To notify us of your new address, find your **Clinics Account Number** (located on your mailing label above your name), and contact customer service at:

Email: **journalscustomerservice-usa@elsevier.com**

800-654-2452 (subscribers in the U.S. & Canada)
314-447-8871 (subscribers outside of the U.S. & Canada)

Fax number: 314-447-8029

Elsevier Health Sciences Division
Subscription Customer Service
3251 Riverport Lane
Maryland Heights, MO 63043

*To ensure uninterrupted delivery of your subscription, please notify us at least 4 weeks in advance of move.

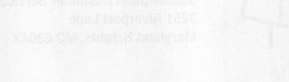

Printed and bound by CPI Group (UK) Ltd, Croydon, CR0 4YY

08/05/2025

01864692-0002